ADVANCES IN

Family Practice Nursing

Editor-in-Chief
Linda J. Keilman, DNP, MSN, GNP-BC, FAANP

Associate Editors
Melodee Harris, PhD, RN, FAAN

Sharon L. Holley, DNP, CNM, FACNM

Ann Sheehan, DNP, CPNP, FAANP

PHILADELPHIA   LONDON   TORONTO   MONTREAL   SYDNEY   TOKYO

Editor: Kerry Holland
Developmental Editor: Hannah Almira Lopez

Reprints: For copies of 100 or more of articles in this publication, please contact the Commercial Reprints Department, Elsevier Inc., 360 Park Avenue South, New York, NY 10010-1710. Tel: (212) 633-3812; Fax: (212) 462-1935; E-mail: reprints@elsevier.com.

Editorial Office:
Elsevier
1600 John F. Kennedy Blvd,
Suite 1800
Philadelphia, PA 19103-2899

International Standard Serial Number: 2589-420X
International Standard Book Number: 978-0-443-13159-2

ADVANCES IN
Family Practice Nursing

Editor-in-Chief

LINDA J. KEILMAN, DNP, MSN, GNP-BC, FAANP, Associate Professor, Gerontology Population Content Expert, Michigan State University, College of Nursing, East Lansing, Michigan

Associate Editors

MELODEE HARRIS, PHD, RN, FAAN, Associate Professor, University of Arkansas for Medical Sciences, College of Nursing, Little Rock, Arkansas

SHARON L. HOLLEY, DNP, CNM, FACNM, FAAN, Associate Professor of Nursing, Director of Nurse-Midwifery Pathway, University of Alabama at Birmingham School of Nursing, Birmingham, Alabama

ANN SHEEHAN, DNP, CPNP, FAANP, Assistant Dean for Practice and Associate Professor Health Professions, Michigan State University College of Nursing, East Lansing, Michigan

ADVANCES IN
Family Practice Nursing

CONTRIBUTORS

TAMATHA (TAMMY) ARMS, PhD, DNP, PMHNP-BC, NP-C, Associate Professor, University of North Carolina Wilmington, School of Nursing - College of Health and Human Sciences, Wilmington, North Carolina

NANCY BANASIAK, DNP, PPCNP-BC, APRN, Professor, Pediatric Nurse Practitioner, Yale University School of Nursing, Orange, Connecticut, USA

KELLIE BISHOP, DNP, APRN, CPNP-PC, PMHS, Clinical Instructor, College of Nursing, University of Arkansas for Medical Sciences, Little Rock, Arkansas

MARGARET T. BOWERS, DNP, FNP-BC, CHSE, AACC, FAANP, FAAN, Nurse Practitioner, Division of Cardiology at Duke Health, Professor, Duke University School of Nursing, Durham, North Carolina

KIM BRANNAGAN, PhD, RN, MSN, MBA, BS Ed, Associate Professor, Loyola University New Orleans, New Orleans, Louisiana

JUNE BRYANT, DNP, APRN, CPNP-PC, Assistant Professor, Department of Nursing, University of Tampa, Tampa, Florida

KRISTIN CASTINE, DNP, ANP-BC, Assistant Professor, Health Programs, Michigan State University College of Nursing, East Lansing, Michigan

EMILY DAVIS, MNSc, APRN, CPNP-AC, Clinical Instructor, University of Arkansas for Medical Sciences, College of Nursing, Little Rock, Arkansas

PALLAV DEKA, MS, PhD, AGACNP-BC, Assistant Professor, Michigan State University College of Nursing, East Lansing, Michigan

KIMBERLY J. ERLICH, MSN, RN, MPH, CPNP-PC, PMHS, CIMHP, Nurse Practitioner, The Healthy Teen Project, Los Altos, California; Lifestance Health, Burlingame, California

AMANDA C. FILIPPELLI, MPH, MSN, APRN, PPCNP-BC, AE-C, Pediatric Nurse Practitioner, Pulmonary Specialty Clinic, Connecticut Children's Medical Center, Hartford, Connecticut, USA

KATHY GRAY, DNP, Family Nurse Practitioners (FNP)-BC, CRNP, FAANP, Associate Professor, Thomas Jefferson University, Jefferson College of Nursing, Philadelphia, Pennsylvania

DEANNA GRAY-MICELI, PhD, GNP, FAAN, FGSA, FNAP, FAANP, Professor, Thomas Jefferson University, Jefferson College of Nursing, Philadelphia, Pennsylvania

MELODEE HARRIS, PhD, RN, FAAN, Associate Professor, University of Arkansas for Medical Sciences College of Nursing, Little Rock, Arkansas

LAURA HAYS, PhD, APRN, CPNP-PC, FAHA, Assistant Professor, College of Nursing, University of Arkansas for Medical Sciences, Little Rock, Arkansas

BARBARA J. HOLTZCLAW, PhD, RN, FGSA, FAAN, Professor, Fran and Earl Ziegler College of Nursing, University of Oklahoma Health Sciences Center, Oklahoma City, Oklahoma

KARMIE JOHNSON, DNP, CRNP, PMHNP-BC, CNE, Assistant Professor of Nursing, Department of Family, Community, and Health Systems, UAB, The University of Alabama at Birmingham School of Nursing, Birmingham, Alabama

SARAH ANN KEIL HEINONEN, DNP, APRN, CPNP-AC/PC, Pediatric Nurse Practitioner III, Division of Pediatric Pulmonology & Sleep Medicine, Children's Hospital Los Angeles, Los Angeles, California

LINDA J. KEILMAN, DNP, RN, GNP-BC, FAANP, Associate Professor, Gerontological Nurse Practitioner, Michigan State University, College of Nursing, East Lansing, Michigan

DEBORAH A. KERNOHAN, MSN, RN, NP-C, Nurse Practitioner, MedStar Health, Olney, Maryland

PAMELA J. LABORDE, DNP, APRN, CCNS, TTS, University of Arkansas for Medical Sciences, College of Nursing, Little Rock, Arkansas

MELISSA LEBRUN, DNP, MPH, APRN, FNP-C, FNP Program Director, Assistant Professor, Loyola University New Orleans, New Orleans, Los Angeles

VALERIE C. MARTINEZ, DNP, APRN, CPNP-PC, PMHS, Clinical Assistant Professor, Department of Nursing Practice, College of Nursing, University of Central Florida, Orlando, Florida

LAUREN MAYS, DNP, CRNP, FNP-BC, Assistant Professor, Family Nurse Practitioner Specialty Track Coordinator, Department of Family, Community, and Health Systems, UAB, The University of Alabama at Birmingham School of Nursing, Birmingham, Alabama

STEPHANIE MITCHELL, DNP, CNM, CPM, Birth Sanctuary Gainesville, Gainesville, Alabama

ELIZABETH MUÑOZ, DNP, CNM, FACNM, Assistant Professor of Nursing, Nurse-Midwifery Pathway, The University of Alabama at Birmingham, Birmingham, Alabama

ERIN O'CONNOR PRANGE, MSN, CPNP-PC, President Elect DelVal NAPAP, Pediatric Nurse Practitioner, Division of Neurology, Children's Hospital of Philadelphia, Philadelphia, Pennsylvania

LISA S. PAIR, DNP, CRNP, WHNP-BC, FAUNA, Assistant Professor, Department of Acute, Chronic, Continuing Care, The University of Alabama at Birmingham School of Nursing, Birmingham, Alabama

JYRISSA ROBINSON DNP, APRN, AGNP-C, Central Arkansas Veterans Healthcare System, Little Rock, Arkansas

LAQUADRIA S. ROBINSON, MSN, CRNP, PMHNP-BC, Instructor, Psychiatric Health Nurse Undergraduate Programs, Department of Family, Community, and Health Systems, UAB, The University of Alabama at Birmingham School of Nursing, Birmingham, Alabama

JANET ROOKER, MNSc, RNP, Clinical Associate Professor, University of Arkansas for Medical Sciences College of Nursing, Little Rock, Arkansas

KARA ELENA SCHRADER, DNP, FNP-C, Assistant Professor, Nurse Practitioner Program Director, Michigan State University College of Nursing, East Lansing, Michigan, USA

ANN SHEEHAN, DNP, CPNP, FAANP, Assistant Dean for Practice and Associate Professor Health Programs, Michigan State University, College of Nursing, East Lansing, Michigan

ELIZABETH R. SILVERS, MSN, RN, CPNP-PC, PMHS, Nurse Practitioner, UCSF Benioff Children's Hospital, San Francisco, California

ANTIQUA N. SMART, DNP, APRN, FNP-BC, PHNA-BC, COI, Assistant Professor, Loyola University New Orleans, New Orleans, Los Angeles

ELLEN SOLIS, DNP, CNM, FACNM, Teaching Associate and Track Lead, Nurse-Midwifery, University of Washington School of Nursing Health Sciences, Seattle, Washington; Quilted Health, Renton, Washington

WILLIAM E. SOMERALL Jr, MD, MAEd, Associate Professor, Acute, Chronic, and Continuing Care, The University of Alabama at Birmingham School of Nursing, Birmingham, Alabama

MATTHEW R. SORENSON, PhD, APRN, ANP-C, FAAN, Professor, Texas A&M University, College of Nursing, Bryan, Texas

PATRICIA M. SPECK, DNSc, CRNP, FNP-BC, AFN-C, DF-IAFN, FAAFS, DF-AFN, FAAN, Professor, Coordinator Advanced Forensic Nursing, Department of Family, Community, and Health Systems, UAB, The University of Alabama at Birmingham School of Nursing, Birmingham, Alabama

TERESA WHITED, DNP, APRN, CPNP-PC, Associate Dean for Academic Programs, Clinical Associate Professor, University of Arkansas for Medical Sciences, College of Nursing, Little Rock, Arkansas

VALLON WILLIAMS, DNP, APRN, AGNP-C, University of Arkansas for Medical Sciences, Translational Research Institute, Little Rock, Arkansas

CHRISTINA M. WILSON, PhD, CRNP, WHNP-BC, Assistant Professor, School of Nursing, Division of Gynecologic Oncology, Department of Obstetrics and Gynecology, The University of Alabama at Birmingham, and Heersink School of Medicine, Birmingham, Alabama

THANCHANOK WONGVIBUL, PhD Candidate, MSN, RN, College of Nursing, The Ohio State University, Columbus, Columbus, Ohio

ADVANCES IN
Family Practice Nursing

CONTENTS VOLUME 5 • 2023

Adult/Gerontology

Recognizing, Diagnosing, and Treating Posttraumatic Stress Disorder in Older Adults
Deborah A. Kernohan, Linda J. Keilman, and
Tamatha (Tammy) Arms

> Posttraumatic stress disorder (PTSD) is a mental health condition that is triggered by a disaster or traumatic event the individual has experienced or witnessed. Symptoms may include depression, anxiety, insomnia, nightmares, regularly reliving or thinking about the distressing memories or event, and severe emotional distress. These symptoms and others can affect daily life, work–life balance, relationships, and quality of life. Older adults are at higher risk for PTSD and have gone undiagnosed for months or years. Knowing how to recognize and screen for PTSD is important for primary care providers such as advanced practice registered nurses.

The Impact of Food Insecurity on Chronic Disease Management in Older Adults
Vallon Williams, Pamela J. LaBorde, and Jyrissa Robinson

Food insecurity among the older adult population not only centers on finances to purchase food. Food insecurity is impacted by the functional status of the individual to access food, to afford medical care in addition to food, and to have the needed social support to assist with access to food and decrease social isolation often caused by the lack of social support. Food insecurity in the aging population seriously impacts health conditions associated with increased disease burden.

Immunosenescence and Infectious Disease Risk Among Aging Adults: Management Strategies for FNPs to Identify Those at Greatest Risk
Deanna Gray-Miceli, Kathy Gray, Matthew R. Sorenson, and Barbara J. Holtzclaw

Age-related immune changes increase the risk for viral infections such as coronavirus disease-2019, its mutant variants, and common influenza outbreaks in long-term care settings. Utilization of evidenced-based nursing interventions such as cohorting practices and implications for testing and screening aims to reduce risk of infection and improve quality of life. Incorporating an infection control manager will add leadership in maintaining currency of information and case tracking.

Mild Cognitive Impairment in Older Adults
Melodee Harris, Janet Rooker, and Linda J. Keilman

Mild cognitive impairment (MCI) is more prevalent than dementia. The global population of older adults is growing and therefore the prevalence of MCI will continue to grow. MCI is *not* dementia. Cognition in persons diagnosed with MCI may progress to dementia, stay the same, or revert to normal cognition. More research is needed to prevent the progression of MCI to dementia.

Heart Failure in Older Adults
Margaret T. Bowers

There is an increasing prevalence of heart failure in older adults. Early recognition and intervention are important to enhance the quality of life and moderate heart failure symptoms. Universal definitions of heart failure provide a framework to tailor therapies that include new medications. Addressing goals of care should guide therapeutic treatments that may include pharmacologic agents, devices, referral for advanced therapies as well as lifestyle changes.

A Life Course Approach to Understanding Urinary Incontinence in Later Life
Thanchanok Wongvibul

Urinary incontinence (UI) is a highly prevalent condition that affects individuals at any stage of life, especially in older adults. The presence of UI can seriously affect the overall quality of life, leading to feelings of shame, embarrassment, as well as stigmatization. To prevent or delay the progression of this condition, it is very important to understand the risk factors that contribute to the development of UI across the life span. A better understanding of UI will help indicate the development of interventions to reduce UI.

The Three-Generation Pedigree: Elucidating Family Disease Patterns to Guide Genetic Screening, Testing, and Referral
Laura Hays

A family history pedigree, a three-generation pedigree of a person's biological relatives with attached pertinent health information, is a standard tool used to more readily recognize patients who may benefit from genetics services. The depiction of both relationships and disorder traits advantage the pedigree over a simple genealogy for identifying patterns of disease expression and risk of disease inheritance.

Peripheral Arterial Disease in Primary Care
Kara Elena Schrader, Kristin Castine, and Pallav Deka

Peripheral artery disease is the stenosis of the peripheral arteries due to atherosclerosis that reduces perfusion to the extremities. The risk is increased in older adults aged 65 and older. Complications include claudication, nonhealing ulcers, gangrene, critical limb ischemia, and amputation. PAD is underrecognized, with diagnosis occurring late in the condition. Patients have an elevated risk for atherosclerotic cardiovascular disease and require evidence-based management strategies to reduce risk. Strategies include the management of associated conditions such as smoking, diabetes, hypertension, and hyperlipemia. It is essential for nurse practitioners to identify risk factors and symptoms to institute early guideline-directed medical treatment.

Women's Health

Assessment and Management of Pelvic Organ Prolapse for the Rural Primary Care Provider

Lisa S. Pair and William E. Somerall

Pelvic organ prolapse is a common condition occurring in more than 50% of female patients. Patients may be asymptomatic or have complaints of pelvic pressure, pelvic fullness, or bulging around the vaginal opening. They may also have urinary, bowel, or sexual function complaints including urinary incontinence or voiding or bowel dysfunction. Educating rural primary care providers in the assessment, diagnosis, and nonsurgical management of pelvic organ prolapse including lifestyle modifications, pelvic floor muscle training, and the use of a vaginal support device can provide access to care for rural patients and increase their quality of life.

Care for Women with Past Trauma Using Trauma-Informed Care

Patricia M. Speck, LaQuadria S. Robinson, Karmie Johnson, and Lauren Mays

Violence against women is prevalent in all societies. Healthcare providers have the opportunity to care compassionately by implementing person-centered trauma-informed care practices, furthering safety and trustworthiness by using methods that encourage transparency, mutuality, and collaboration during all aspects of healthcare. The article promotes interventions for recognition of the person with traumatic experiences, assisting healthcare providers in the delivery of trauma-informed care, suggesting interventions to address person-centered cultural, historical, and gender issues. Using trauma-informed person-centered approaches, authors propose intervention tools to assist the healthcare provider in recognition and intervention, promoting self-efficacy and confidence in persons overcoming their complex personal traumas.

Care for Women with past Trauma: The Physiology of Stress and Trauma

Patricia M. Speck, LaQuadria S. Robinson, Karmie Johnson, and Lauren Mays

When traumas are continuous or toxic, the body increases the hormonal response, and the sensory perception is that environments are unsafe and unpredictable. In these situations, increasing anxiety and fear are the overarching demonstrative emotions. The initial trauma responses release hormones to preserve life. The sensory memory is activated and the next time the senses detect a similar stimulus, the hormones release again. When the environment is toxic, there is continuous release of hormones that manifest in early organ system failure and muted memories. This article discusses the physiologic response to trauma, explaining formative causes of disease and inheritance.

Cannabis Use in Pregnancy and Postpartum: Understanding the Complicated History and Current Recommendations to Facilitate Client-Centered Discussions

Elizabeth Muñoz, Ellen Solis, and Stephanie Mitchell

Cannabis use in pregnancy can lead to poor pregnancy outcomes and negatively affect the health of the pregnant person and fetus. Its use is also highly stigmatized and can even lead to legal ramifications for the pregnant person in some states. Health care professionals need to be ready to answer questions from clients regarding cannabis use in pregnancy and be able to do so in a bias-informed and evidence-based manner using client-centered language. This article examines the history of cannabis use and explores care considerations if a client is using the substance in pregnancy.

Gaps in Social Determinants of Health History Taking, Clinical Documentation, and Billing/Coding Errors During Women's Health Patient Encounters

Melissa LeBrun, Kim Brannagan, and Antiqua N. Smart

Defining social determinants of health (SDOH) and identifying key areas in which they influence health is pertinent in health care and health-care education. The objectives of this article are to define SDOH and identify key areas in which they affect health, discuss SDOH as they relate to issues faced primarily by women, common screening tools used to assess SDOH, clinical documentation pearls for health assessment, including areas specific to preventative care for women, and SDOH Z-codes used for billing purposes. Common SDOH documentation errors are also addressed along with solutions to reduce them.

Sexual Dysfunction in Biologic Females for Family Practice Providers: Assessment, Diagnosis, and Treatment
Christina M. Wilson

Sexual health is an important part of many individuals' lives, and when there are problems with sexual function, it can disrupt or have a significant impact in their life. Sexual dysfunction typically occurs in one of the areas of the sexual response cycle (desire, arousal, orgasm) or is related to a lack of lubrication and/or pain. Sexual dysfunction affects a substantial proportion of both premenopausal and postmenopausal women. Both nonpharmacologic and pharmacologic options are available to help treat sexual dysfunction but are commonly used in conjunction with one another depending on the diagnosis.

Pediatrics

The Importance of Sleep for Normal Growth and Development
Ann Sheehan

Sleep is a period of intense brain growth and restoration. Quality sleep is an important part of physiologic, emotional, and cognitive development. Individual variability in sleep need is influenced by behavioral, medical, environmental, and cultural factors. This article provided an overview of the development of the sleep-wake cycle, how achievement of developmental milestones can affect the sleep-wake cycle, and the elements for creating a bedtime routine that support quality and quantity of sleep throughout childhood and adolescence. The consequences of poor sleep results in chronic health conditions, mood dysregulation, school failure, obesity, and an increase in risk taking behaviors.

Fever of Unknown Origin in Pediatrics

Emily Davis and Teresa Whited

Fever of unknown origin (FUO) is defined as fever lasting at least 3 weeks without an apparent source after 1 week of investigation. The cause of FUO includes infectious, autoimmune, malignancy, neurologic, genetic, pharmacologic, and iatrogenic. Workup for FUO includes a comprehensive history from the patient, a thorough physical examination, and discontinuance of any nonessential medications. Initial laboratory and radiology workup include a complete blood count with differential, blood culture, C-reactive protein, erythrosedimentation rate, procalcitonin, liver enzymes, renal function tests, lactate dehydrogenase, urinalysis, urine culture, and chest radiograph.

Pediatric Asthma for the Primary Care Provider
Sarah Ann Keil Heinonen, Amanda C. Filippelli, and
Nancy Banasiak

Asthma, one of the most common pediatric chronic
diseases, disproportionately affects children living in low-
income households. Characterized by airway
hyperresponsiveness, inflammation, and obstruction,
asthma causes symptoms including wheezing, coughing,
chest tightness, and shortness of breath. Asthma control
remains a primary goal through guidelines, education,
appropriate medication, specialist referrals, asthma action
plans, and access to health care providers. Poorly
controlled asthma remains the leading cause of
absenteeism from school and work and an economic
burden despite medical advances. This review article
provides an overview of pediatric asthma, diagnosis, and
the most current guideline-based management for the
primary care provider.

The Weight of Body Image
Elizabeth R. Silvers and Kimberly J. Erlich

Prevalence of eating disorders (EDs) in the adolescent and
young adult (AYA) population has increased since the
start of the COVID-19 pandemic, which correlates with
increased engagement with social media and negative
body image in AYAs. In addition, increased severity of
EDs at presentation is evidenced by higher rates of
hospitalization since the start of the pandemic,

underscoring the need for health-care providers to obtain further training in managing EDs and appropriately referring to higher levels of care when indicated.

Emerging Mental Health Issues in Children and Adolescents Secondary to the Coronavirus Disease-2019 Pandemic
Kellie Bishop and Teresa Whited

This article examines and compares the incidence and prevalence of mental health issues, including depression, anxiety, and suicide, among adolescents before and during the coronavirus disease-2019 pandemic. It discusses contributing factors, clinical presentation, screening tools, treatment options, and implications for advance practice nurses. This article prepares the advance practice nurse to promote mental wellness and identify, screen for, and appropriately manage emerging mental health issues in this vulnerable population.

Attention-Deficit/Hyperactivity Disorder Update 2022: New Medications Are Here!
Erin O'Connor Prange

Over the last 5 years, there has been an explosion of new attention-deficit/hyperactivity disorder (ADHD) medications US Food and Drug Administration approved and available for clinical use on the market. Trying to discern what is the same, different, and best for a specific patient can prove challenging. To ease this burden, this article will review the pharmacokinetics of stimulants and non-stimulants and highlight the benefits of these newly available medications. In addition, the article will discuss the most common side effects and describe options to manage these potential concerns. It is not the intention of this article to review the diagnostic criteria for an ADHD diagnosis.

Primary Care Management of Autonomic Dysfunction
June Bryant

Autonomic dysfunction (AD) in the primary care setting can often be masked by other conditions or met with provider bias due to subjectivity of symptoms. Without specific diagnostic test markers, underdiagnosis or misdiagnosis is common in those conditions that fall under the umbrella of dysautonomia. This article gives a broad overview of the common types of AD presenting in the primary care setting, how advanced practice nurses should recognize, diagnose, and manage these types of AD, as well as when and what patients should be referred to a specialist.

When It Is Not Just Attention-Deficit Hyperactivity Disorder: Coexisting Depression and Anxiety in Pediatric Primary Care
Valerie C. Martinez

Attention-deficit hyperactivity disorder (ADHD) often exists along with other psychiatric disorders, such as depression and anxiety, but these conditions may be misdiagnosed or undertreated due to often overlapping symptomatology. Because of significant systemic and structural barriers to accessing specialized mental health care, pediatric primary care providers (PCPs) must possess a comprehensive understanding of ADHD and coexisting depression and/or anxiety to effectively diagnose and treat their patient's symptoms. The purpose of this article is to review the prevalence of ADHD with coexisting depression and anxiety and outline assessment, diagnostic, and management considerations for PCPs when it is not just ADHD that requires clinical decision-making.

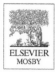

ELSEVIER
MOSBY

ADVANCES IN FAMILY PRACTICE NURSING

PREFACE

Applying Words and Concepts to Transform Nursing Practice

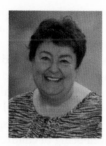

Linda J. Keilman, DNP, MSN, GNP-BC, FAANP
Editor-in-Chief

As I was writing the Preface in January 2023, the US Department of Health and Human Services extended, for the twelfth time since January 2020, the COVID-19 public health emergency for 90 days. The evidence for this decision was based on the increasing cases of the Omicron subvariant XBB.1.5. In January, Omicron XBB.1.5 was considered the most contagious subvariant that was continuing to mutate and was becoming better at evading antibodies.[1] What will things be like with COVID-19 at the time of this fifth issue printing and publication? Will the world still be in the pandemic? Will there continue to be emergence of new mutant subvariants impacting public health and the world population? How will advanced practice nursing be different, if at all? It is important for health care professionals to stay current in understanding the pandemic. The American Nurses Association has a robust COVID-19 Resource Center that is regularly updated. You can find information at the following link[2]: https://www.nursingworld.org/practice-policy/work-environment/health-safety/disaster-preparedness/coronavirus/what-you-need-to-know/covid-19-vaccines/.

Whether we are still in the middle of a pandemic or not, there will always be emerging and transformative health information to read about and apply to quality patient care and the innovation of visionary and equitable health care systems. We are constantly learning and understanding that health and health

https://doi.org/10.1016/j.yfpn.2023.01.004
2589-420X/23/© 2023 Published by Elsevier Inc.

care in the United States need to drastically change, especially related to systemic/institutional bias and racism, health disparities, and skyrocketing costs. COVID-19 has unearthed many of the issues that we may have suspected in the past but did not quite internalize the depth and detriment of the impact on both people and health systems. Many of us have been inspired "to move from hopeful intention to skilful action."[3] As the editor-in-chief of this journal, I hope we are meeting this action through the selection of varied topics we bring to our issues—and you, our readers.

We cover some of the most relevant health care topics that are important for advanced practice registered nurses (APRNs) in this issue. Topics are across three relevant populations: adult/gerontology, women's health, and pediatrics. Some of the topics include information that has been magnified during the pandemic. Posttraumatic stress disorder, trauma-informed care, human trafficking, food insecurity, genetics, marijuana use by women of childbearing age, attention-deficit/hyperactivity disorder, body image, and mental health issues across the lifespan. We investigate how COVID-19 has specifically impacted older adults and the mental health and well-being of children and adolescents. Some authors share new insight and suggestions for diagnosing and managing chronic conditions, such as mild cognitive impairment, heart failure, urinary incontinence, uterine and bladder prolapse, peripheral artery disease, and female sexual dysfunction. In pediatrics, we learn more about how sleep impacts growth and development, how to assess for the source of fever, how to teach parents and children to manage childhood asthma, and autonomic dysfunction. Many words with many meanings!

I hope you will learn from reading and engaging in the information presented here for you. We know that reading, learning, and then applying evidence lead to improved quality of life for our patients and improved health care outcomes. We also know that education is a lifelong journey that we bring to the care of our patients on a regular basis. As APRNs, we are advocating for our patients, ourselves, and the betterment of health care systems. I hope you will learn and grow in your knowledge and care for all human beings.

> For he who has health has hope; and he who has hope, has everything.
>
> —Arabian Proverb

Linda J. Keilman, DNP, MSN, GNP-BC, FAANP
Gerontological Nurse Practitioner
Michigan State University
College of Nursing
1355 Bogue Street, A126 Life Science Building
East Lansing, MI 48824, USA

E-mail address: keilman@msu.edu

References

[1] Zimmer C., Health experts warily eye XBB.1.5, the latest Omicron subvariant, *The New York Times*. Matters Column. 2023. Available at: https://www.nytimes.com/2023/01/07/science/covid-omicron-variants-xbb.html. Accessed February 02, 2023.

[2] American Nurses Association Enterprise. COVID-19 vaccines. COVID-19 Resource Center. Published January 12, 2023. Available at: https://www.nursingworld.org/practice-policy/work-environment/health-safety/disaster-preparedness/coronavirus/what-you-need-to-know/covid-19-vaccines/. Accessed January 14, 2023.

[3] Jana T, Mejias AD. Erasing institutional bias: how to create systemic change for organizational inclusion. Oakland, CA: Berrett-Koehler Publishers, Inc; 2018.

INTRODUCTION

A Celebration of Words

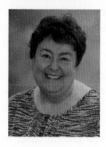

Linda J. Keilman, DNP, MSN, GNP-BC, FAANP
Editor-in-Chief

D id you realize you are part of a celebration? According to an online website, the definition of a celebration is "a special enjoyable event that people organize because something pleasant has happened."[1] What pleasant event has occurred? The publication of our fifth issue of *Advances in Family Practice Nursing*–that is what we are celebrating! It is very exciting for all of us, and we could not have accomplished this without you–our loyal *readers.* We thank you for reading the words that are an accumulation of thoughts and ideas that eventually emerge into finished articles of interest to you.

Thank you to our *authors* who volunteer to share their wisdom, expertise, and time on topics related to adult/gerontology, women's health, and pediatrics. If not for the expert authors, we could not put our journal to print.

That brings me to the incredible professional *Elsevier management and production staff*, who organize, edit, manage, and produce this great journal. We celebrate your multifactorial roles and expertise. A special shout-out to our fearless leaders at Elsevier, *Kerry K. Holland*, who is Senior Editor at Elsevier/Global Content Partners, and *Hannah Lopez*, who is the Developmental Editor for Elsevier/Global Content Partners. Both are integral in keeping us on track, on time, and motivated to birth another issue of exciting words that we can apply to our ever-increasing nursing knowledge. I don't know the names of all the people behind the scenes who do all the publishing work. But names or not–we celebrate YOU! Thanks for putting the words together to achieve

https://doi.org/10.1016/j.yfpn.2023.01.001
2589-420X/23/© 2023 Published by Elsevier Inc.

quality scholarly work in the form of a hardbound journal. We applaud you and appreciate you!

As editor-in-chief, I am blessed to work with three amazing *associate section editors* (Doctors Harris, Holley, and Sheehan), who search for authors for each of their sections. It takes a lot of time trying to secure authors to commit to delivery of a timely and quality article. I admire your work and persistence while carrying out your full-time academic teaching and clinical practice roles. You are a top-notch team; I am grateful for the opportunity to work with each of you!

This fifth issue is full of wonderful, meaningful words–many of which are medical terminology. We all know words matter. Their accurate and appropriate use is imperative in health care literature. Trying to define and explain some of the words is important for the reader–they need to know to grow! Professional and personal growth leads to improved patient care, which leads to better outcomes, better quality of life, and decreased health care costs. A WIN-WIN for everyone!

I hope you will celebrate our fifth issue with us! If you have ideas or would like to be considered as a future author, please reach out to me at keilman@msu.edu. We have our 2024 sixth issue already planned; we are working on ideas for 2025! Share your words and wisdom with us and our nursing readers. All of us associated with the *Advances in Family Practice Nursing* journal want *our* journal to have meaning for *you*–our readers. Looking forward to another five celebratory years!

Linda J. Keilman, DNP, MSN, GNP-BC, FAANP
Gerontological Nurse Practitioner
Michigan State University
College of Nursing
1355 Bogue Street, A126 Life Science Building
East Lansing, MI 48824, USA

E-mail address: keilman@msu.edu

Reference

[1] Collins Dictionary. Definition of celebration. Available at: https://www.collinsdictionary.com/us/dictionary/english/celebration. Accessed January 9, 2023.

Adult/Gerontology

Advances in Family Practice Nursing 5 (2023) 1–13

ADVANCES IN FAMILY PRACTICE NURSING

Recognizing, Diagnosing, and Treating Posttraumatic Stress Disorder in Older Adults

Deborah A. Kernohan, MSN, RN, NP-C[a],
Linda J. Keilman, DNP, GNP-BC, FAANP[b],*,
Tamatha (Tammy) Arms, PhD, DNP, PMHNP-BC, NP-C[c]

[a]MedStar Health, Olney, MD, USA; [b]Michigan State University, College of Nursing, 1355 Bogue Street, A 126 Life Sciences Building, East Lansing, MI 48824, USA; [c]University of North Carolina Wilmington, School of Nursing - College of Health and Human Sciences, 601 South College Road, McNeill 2034A, Wilmington, NC 28403, USA

Keywords
• Posttraumatic stress disorder • PTSD • Older adults • Veterans

Key points

- The symptoms of posttraumatic stress disorder (PTSD) go back to ancient times when traumatic events, such as wars and disasters, occurred. During World War I, military personnel reported a variety of symptoms that were called shell shock or combat fatigue.

- It was not until 1980 when the American Psychiatric Association published the third edition of the Diagnostic and Statistical Manual of Mental Disorders when the term PTSD was coined.

- When compared with the younger population, adults aged 65 years and older are at higher risk for developing PTSD. This includes veterans who were on active duty and experienced combat.

- Risk factors along with signs and symptoms of PTSD should be important aspects of all patient encounters in primary care. Knowing the patient's story from birth helps the advanced practice registered nurse (APRN) to consider experienced traumas that may be contributing to current mental health issues.

- Treatment of PTSD consists of specific medications combined with therapy. The APRN needs to know what therapies are available in their practice community so they can make appropriate referrals for patient recovery from PTSD.

*Corresponding author. E-mail address: keilman@msu.edu

https://doi.org/10.1016/j.yfpn.2023.01.002
2589-420X/23/

One of our cultural myths has been that only weaklings break down psycholog-
ically [and that] strong men with the will to do so can keep going indefinitely [1]

A HISTORICAL PERSPECTIVE

The origin of the symptoms now referred to as posttraumatic stress disorder
(PTSD) are embedded in world military history going back to ancient times.
It was not until World War I (WWI) that the military lived experience of
active duty highlighted the combat activities that exposed personnel, and civil-
ians in war-zones, with an assortment of events they most likely had never
personally experienced before WWI. Many of the veterans involved in
WWI experienced both physical and mental health issues. Veterans reported
symptoms of anxiety, nightmares, impaired sight and hearing, tremors, and
grief/loss [2]. Physical conditions were more easily treated; mental wounds
were more difficult and labeled with terms such as *shell shock, combat fatigue,
war neurosis*, and *soldier's heart* [2]. Whether living with physical or mental health
wounds, many veterans of WWI were permanently disabled related to their
injuries [3].

During World War II (WWII), traumatic responses were reported by active-
duty personnel in both the United States (US) and Great Britain [2]. Military
personnel were deployed for long periods in battlefields and were on constant
alert for altercations and engagements. Some soldiers were sent home and then
discharged for their inability to perform their duties based on combat exhaustion and fatigue [4]. These symptoms were similar to those reported by WWI
veterans but were labeled *battle fatigue, combat fatigue*, and *combat stress reaction* [2].
During WWII, it was understood that with constant stress, everyone has a
breaking point [4]. The American Psychiatric Association coined the term *Guadalcanal Disorder* in 1943 [4]. Symptoms reported by US soldiers stationed in the
Solomons included panic attacks, tremors, sensitivity to noise, forgetfulness,
tense muscles, and inability to control their hands when trying to perform basic
activities [4]. Soldiers also reported more severe symptoms (Box 1) and with
these, especially bowel/bladder incontinence, also came feelings of humiliation,
embarrassment, and shame [4].

Numerous factors contributed to the symptoms experienced by veterans that
participated in the world wars. Since the Civil War, battle fatigue has been

---

Box 1: Guadalcanal Disorder Symptoms
- Frantic heart rate
- Uncontrollable trembling
- Sweating
- Periods of weakness
- Sleep deprivation [1]
- Vomiting
- Involuntary urination and defecation [4]

recognized by military physicians [5]. A definitive and accurate diagnosis and appropriate treatment and management of these symptoms took many decades to come to fruition. With the increased understanding of evidence-based (EB) research related to trauma and its sequalae [6], more research was conducted trying to discern a more appropriate diagnosis and effective treatment of the symptoms experienced by veterans.

In the first edition (1952) of the American Psychiatric Association Diagnostic and Statistical Manual (DSM-I), the stress-related symptoms previously discussed were coined *gross stress reaction* and categorized as stressful environmental events such as war or natural disasters [6]. In the 1968 second edition of the DSM (II), gross stress reaction became *transient situational disturbance* [6] with the etiology focused on the event versus the individual [7]. The philosophy assumed that "if the patient has good adaptive capacity his symptoms usually recede as the stress diminishes" [7]. Relative to experiences of military personnel during the Vietnam War, the third edition of the DSM (III; 1980) introduced the term *PTSD* associated with symptoms related to exposures to a significant stressor or situation [6]. Classification of PTSD in DSM-IV (1994) was found under the anxiety disorders category and in the DSM-5 edition (2013), PTSD is currently categorized within trauma and stressor-related disorders [6]. All the conditions in this category require exposure to a traumatic or stressful event [8].

Generations of veterans with symptoms of PTSD were stigmatized, discriminated against, considered cowardly and weak, and did not receive adequate or appropriate treatment or disability benefits for their symptoms. When it became apparent that symptoms of PTSD were caused from a mixture of life events and could happen to anyone, more focus was directed into an appropriate diagnosis and treatment. PTSD is long-term and generally influences quality of life (QoL) and the ability to engage in activities of daily living (ADL) and instrumental activities of daily living (IADL). Approximately 12 million Americans have been, or are, diagnosed with PTSD; 11% of the US population will be diagnosed with PTSD in their lifetime [8]. Women are at greater risk for experiencing trauma than men, when considering sexual and physical/mental abuse. Approximately 8 out of 100 women, compared with 4 out of 100 men, will experience trauma in their lives [8], leading to a diagnosis of PTSD.

OLDER ADULTS AND POSTTRAUMATIC STRESS DISORDER
When compared with the general population, it is theorized that older adults (OAs) are at higher risk of developing PTSD [8]. Aging, ageism, bias, role changes, accumulated grief and loss, past traumatic events (military service, social determinants of health [SDOH], abuse, the depression, conflict during the Civil Rights Movement, discrimination, the Holocaust, gun violence, substance use disorders, 9/11, and so forth), dealing with physical and mental changes that accompany aging, retirement, and functional and cognitive decline just scratch the surface of the accumulation of life challenges that can be traumatic.

In OAs, greater lifetime trauma exposure was related to poorer self-rated health, more chronic health problems, and more functional difficulties [9].

One in 5 OAs in the US have experienced a mental health disorder such as depression, anxiety, or substance use disorder [10]. In the US in 2020, approximately 53 million adults aged older than 18 years had *Any Mental Illness*, which is defined as an emotional, mental, or behavioral disorder, ranging from mild-to-severe impairment [10]. Increasing rates of social isolation, lack of personal engagement, and loneliness that were perpetuated by the coronavirus disease 2019 (COVID-19) pandemic have also highlighted gaps in care for mental health concerns. The increased risk of suicide, as well as a 220% increase in the number of adults aged 55 and older seeking emergency department care for opioid misuse, all point to why all health-care professionals (HCPs), and advanced practice registered nurses (APRNs) specifically, must address the mental health needs of older Americans [11].

The aim of this article is to provide the reader with understanding how SDOH, past military service, and past life experiences of OAs need to be part of the collected health record data, so the individual's life story is clearly documented. Just because an OA has never been diagnosed with PTSD, does not mean they have not experienced the symptoms during their lifetime. Moreover, an accurate assessment of their cognitive and functional status will help to determine whether a diagnosis of PTSD may be of value.

RECOGNIZING POSTTRAUMATIC STRESS DISORDER

The diagnostic criterion for PTSD implies specific cause [7]. A variety of theories exist as to why some individuals experiencing similar traumas can live through the experience without treatment and move on in their life without issues, whereas others are diagnosed with PTSD. Some current thoughts have moved away from the traumatic event itself and are based on PTSD research that postulates variance can be accounted for by.

- Peritraumatic processes,
- Previous trauma,
- Psychological history, and
- Posttrauma factors [7].

PTSD is an extremely common diagnosis after military service [12]. However, not every individual diagnosed with PTSD has experienced a dangerous event or served in the military [13]. It is important to know the individual's story including any adverse childhood experiences, SDOH, personal or family history of mental illness or substance use, sexual trauma, death, loss, and risk factors that increase the possibility of developing PTSD with aging. Additional identified risk factors are found in Box 2.

PTSD is a mental health disorder that occurs when an individual experiences, observes, or hears about a traumatic event that has such a powerful impact on them that intrusive thoughts, persistent avoidant behaviors, and negative alterations in cognition and mood last more than 1 month [14]. To

Box 2: Posttraumatic Stress Disorder Risk Factors
- Dangerous event
- Getting injured or seeing other people injured or killed
- Feeling horror, helplessness, hopelessness, or extreme fear
- Having little or no social support after the event
- Illness, death, or loss of a loved one
- Loss of a job, home, possessions, and faith [13].

be diagnosed with PTSD, adults need to exhibit the following for a minimum of 1 month.

- At least 1 reexperiencing symptom: including flashbacks, bad dreams, and frightening thoughts that affect ADLs and IADLs
- At least 1 avoidance symptom: not attending events, going out to places, or handling objects that are reminders of the traumatic experience
- At least 2 arousal and reactivity symptoms: easily startled, feeling tense or edgy, difficulty sleeping, and angry outbursts
- At least 2 cognition and mood symptoms: difficulty remembering the sequala of the event, pessimistic and negative thoughts about the world or oneself, feelings such as guilt or blame, and loss of interest in previously enjoyable activities [13].

Understanding where an OA is in their life course helps the APRN to guide their assessment along the individual's current life and what they may be experiencing. Symptoms of PTSD may not appear for several months or years after the experience has occurred. Approximately 66% of OAs are not receiving the care they need for PTSD, despite the current availability of effective treatments [15]. Persons presenting with a variety of physical, emotional, and/or behavioral health symptoms may be candidates for PTSD screening. PTSD can be underrecognized and undertreated because presenting symptoms resemble a variety of common conditions for which persons seek health care. HCP awareness of PTSD as part of their differential diagnosis may identify candidates for PTSD screening. Screening and identification allow for timely appropriate treatment and the journey toward recovery [16].

A common issue in aging is the risk of falls, which can increase the risk of developing PTSD. In 2014, it was reported that 27 out of 100 OAs aged 65 years or older were hospitalized after a fall and had PTSD symptoms [17]. Because the OA population is growing and living older globally, assessing for fall risk and history of falls is imperative. It is also imperative to assess what the OA coping strategies have been during their life. With aging, some coping strategies become less available (working long hours, going out for drinks with work colleagues, inability to drive, and so forth), forcing the OAs to deal with trauma in a different way for the first time. Knowing the signs/symptoms of PTSD is very important. Knowing additional symptoms that an OA may experience is imperative (Boxes 3 and 4).

Box 3: Signs/Symptoms of Posttraumatic Stress Disorder in Older Adults

- Aggression (increased)
- Anxiety disorders
- Apathy
- Difficulty concentrating
- Disengagement
- Emotional numbness
- Falls (frequent)
- Fear
- Insomnia
- Increased or new substance use/abuse
- Lower psychosocial functioning [9]
- Mood disorders (including depression)
- Purposeful isolation
- Reckless or aggressive behavior
- Reliving the trauma through recollections of the event including during sleep
- Report less depression, hostility, and guilt than younger adults [17]
- Somatic complaints regarding appetite, sleep, pain, or memory issues increase [17].

Being diagnosed with PTSD is a risk factor in developing dementia [9]. Now, let us put some of the information you have read about to this case study.

CASE STUDY

Mr Jones is a 75-year-old man, pleasant, social, retired accountant, living alone in his own home. He does not drive. His family provides support with errands, and they provide him transportation to church twice a week. He also receives home health aide services twice weekly.

Mr Jones receives regular routine health care with a consistent provider. His medical history includes hypertension, osteoarthritis, colon cancer with resection, generalized anxiety (GAD), subjective mild cognitive impairment,

Box 4: PTSD Acronym

"The PTSD patient Remembers Atrocious Nuclear Attacks"

    R–Reexperiencing the trauma via intrusive memories, flashbacks, or nightmares

    A–Avoidance of stimuli associated with trauma

    N–Negative alterations in cognitions and mood

    A–Arousal increase, such as insomnia, irritability, hypervigilance gastroesophageal reflux disease, obesity, and peripheral vascular disease. His colon resection resulted in the complete removal of lesions without evidence of metastatic disease. He did not need a colostomy and did not receive any additional radiation or chemotherapy treatment. Cancer surveillance consisted of bloodwork and computed tomography scan of the abdomen every 6 months and a yearly colonoscopy. During the course of 3 years, there was no evidence of new or recurrent lesions. Surveillance monitoring was extended to yearly, without further need for colonoscopies unless indicated by abnormal diagnostics.

Mr Jones frequently presented to the clinic with multiple repetitive concerns: abdominal pain, back pain, blurred vision, insomnia, and headaches. Laboratory and diagnostic workups were consistently within the patient's baseline, without changes or newly identified issues. His symptoms resolved with conservative nonpharmacologic interventions and no new medications. EB tools were used, and Mr Jones scored as follows.

- Mini mental status Examination: 30/30
- Geriatric depression scale: 2/15
- Functional assessment staging test: stage 2/7
- Palliative performance scale: 80%–90%

Home health aides reported Mr Jones frequently had episodes of irritability, anger, anxiousness, argumentativeness, and uncooperative behavior, which was outside of his normal interactions. Additional investigative medical workup yielded no identifiable underlying cause.

Because the physical and diagnostic workup were within the patient's baseline, using motivational interviewing techniques during his clinic visit revealed new information about Mr Jones.

Mr Jones was involved as a passenger in a motor vehicle accident as a teenager; his father was driving, and his sibling was killed. Mr Jones was seriously injured with a skull fracture and other serious multiple fractures that required an 8-month hospital and then acute rehabilitation stay. Mr Jones parents would not talk to him about the accident or the death of his sibling. He was unable to attend funeral services due to his injuries and hospitalization. When he was discharged home, all evidence of his sibling had been removed. His parents forbid him to ever speak of the accident or his sibling's death.

As the clinic visit progressed, Mr Jones shared episodes of flash backs, increased anxiety regarding his mortality, lack of closure and processing of his sibling's death, increased anger, difficulty sleeping, and increased muscle tension. Perhaps, you have already guessed that Mr Jones had an undiagnosed condition—which was PTSD. He was taking Sertraline for GAD. He was referred to a mental health provider for medication management and therapy. Mr Jones also worked with physical therapy (PT) to help reduce his anxiety symptoms and improve his mood. He was able to decrease his physical symptoms with the PT interventions and realize his potential in the recovery journey.

RESILIENCE FACTORS

When caring for individuals such as Mr Jones, it is important to understand how they can overcome stressors and challenges—or how resilient they are. In health care, resilience has been described as the psychological mindset in the face of chronic disease and major life stressors [18]. Resilience has also been referred to as the phenomenon that maintains positive adjustment under challenging conditions such that the (*individual*) emerges from those conditions strengthened and more resourceful [19]. The authors have swapped out the word organization for individual in the above definition because this outlook can apply to human beings with PTSD.

Resilience factors that may reduce the likelihood of developing PTSD include the following:

- Seeking out support from friends, family, or support groups
- Learning to feel okay with one's actions in response to a traumatic event
- Having a coping strategy for getting through and learning from a traumatic event
- Being prepared and able to respond to upsetting events as they occur, despite feeling fear [10].

In the case study, as a child Mr Jones was not allowed by his parents to discuss his traumatic event or even mourn the loss of his deceased sibling. From the resilience factors above, it can be assumed that he was never able to explore his feelings and his catastrophic injuries with his family, which most likely led to many, if not all, of his chronic comorbid conditions. Having a mindful APRN who listened to the patient and asked the appropriate questions made all the difference in the life of Mr Jones. Resilience is also a characteristic APRN should assess in all OA patients, including during the current pandemic.

IMPACT OF CORONAVIRUS DISEASE 2019 ON THE DEVELOPMENT OF POSTTRAUMATIC STRESS DISORDER

There has been a recognized link between COVID-19 experiences and the development of PTSD [20]. Early data suggest approximately 26% of the general population have PTSD symptoms precipitated by fear of the illness, social isolation, feelings of guilt, economic impact, and an individual's health status. The increase in persons developing and experiencing progressive PTSD symptoms is expected to grow due to continued uncertainty surrounding the impact of COVID-19 [12,20]. Those diagnosed with PTSD often experience increased physical symptoms related to being diagnosed with COVID-19 and may include increased anxiety related to safety of public areas, feeling more guarded and isolated, experience more triggers of past trauma, increased negative thoughts, difficulty with sleep, and decreased ability to engage in activity deemed safe during the pandemic [12,20]. Similar to the impact of personal and historic events contributing to current PTSD diagnoses, COVID-19 will have a long-lasting effect on the public health of the global population. Awareness and early identification of PTSD by HCP allow opportunity for early, and appropriate interventions [12,20].

COMORBIDITY POSTTRAUMATIC STRESS DISORDER AND DEMENTIA

Recent studies have demonstrated that PTSD can be a risk factor for all-cause dementia and persons diagnosed with PTSD have a higher risk of dementia diagnosis over time than those without PTSD [21,22]. Recurrent stress exposure in PTSD may activate changes in neurobiological pathways negatively affecting social and cognitive response to stressors and thereby, increasing the risk of dementia [21,22]. Brain imaging changes, smaller hippocampi, and hippocampal atrophy are seen with both PTSD and dementia [21]. Recent studies of 3 Veteran populations identified that comorbid rates of PTSD and dementia were between 4.7% and 7.8% [21,22]. Also identified was the general population with PTSD had twice the risk of being diagnosed with dementia, whereas veterans had one and one-half times higher risk [21,22]. The assumption of the lower risk in veterans could be attributed to increased access to mental health care and actively receiving services for PTSD, which could modify the dementia risk. There are many opportunities for increased research into the relationship of PTSD as a modifiable risk factor for dementia. Research has demonstrated persons with PTSD experience symptoms and behaviors that contribute to decreased cognitive function: social isolation, heightened anxiety, fear, triggers, and substance abuse being the most common.

ADVANCED PRACTICE REGISTERED NURSE ROLE

APRNs practice and serve in multiple types of diverse community healthcare settings. In the APRN role, they function as clinicians, educators, prescribers, counsellors, change agents, collaborators, consultants, and many additional types of roles. The APRN is in a unique position to incorporate behavioral health services and techniques into their patient interactions regardless of the reason for the encounter. Self-awareness of the impact APRNs have during patient encounters can assist in identifying mental health symptoms and conditions presenting as an array of conditions not typically recognized as a mental health conditions. Establishing a routine of including mental health symptoms and diagnoses in the differential to common complaints will ensure early identification and intervention for mental health disorders.

One of the many roles of the APRN is interviewing. Simply asking, "What has changed recently" can get the interview started. The APRN should keep in mind during patient interaction the acronym for PTSD [22].

Using EB tools is also important when working with an OA who may present with a variety of symptoms that could indicate a variety of conditions as well as PTSD. The OA patient may report difficulty sleeping but the APRN needs to know if the issue is difficulty getting to sleep (an indication of anxiety) or difficulty staying asleep (an indication of depression). There are several tools a provider can use to screen for PTSD. Two that have higher than 80% sensitivity and specificity are the Primary Care-PTSD-5 and the PTSD checklist civilian version [23,24]. The APRN should consider screening for PTSD in persons with signs and/or symptoms of depression, social isolation, substance abuse, use of avoidant techniques such as working excessively, increased aggression, anxiety, fear, and/or insomnia.

TREATMENT

There are only 2 medications approved by the United States Food and Drug Administration to treat PTSD–Sertraline and Paroxetine. However, many other serotonin reuptake inhibitors and serotonin and norepinephrine reuptake inhibitors are commonly used off-label to treat PTSD. Prazosin is commonly prescribed to treat the nightmares associated with PTSD and propranolol can be used to treat the social anxiety that accompanies the disorder [24]. If the older adult seems to have significant amounts of anxiety, the APRN may want to consider buspirone. However, be cautious of serotonin syndrome when prescribing 2 medications that increase serotonin levels. The overall goal of treatment is always symptom remission but should also include improved QoL through better sleep, decreased hypervigilance, decreased intrusive thoughts, and improved relationships and functional status.

Thinking back to the case study–because Mr Jones was already on sertraline, the APRN should ensure the dose is being maximized. The APRN could also add a low dose of prazosin to treat nightmares during sleep.

The OAs with PTSD may have suffered only one or multiple traumatic events throughout their lifetime. Evidenced-based practice has shown that persons engaged in therapy do better than those only taking medications. A referral for therapy is essential. Types of therapies that have proven beneficial for treating PTSD are as follows:

- Cognitive behavioral therapy: talk therapy focused on modifying negative thoughts, behaviors, and emotional responses associated with psychological distress
- Trauma-focused cognitive behavioral therapy: addresses safety and stabilization, formal gradual exposure, and consolidation/integration
- Eye movement desensitization reprocessing (EMDR): reduces the stress of traumatic events through eye movements
- Exposure therapy: helps patients safely face both situations and memories that are painful or frightening so the individual can learn coping strategies to deal with the thoughts and feelings [25].

For Mr Jones, the APRN needs to ask direct questions about suicidal ideation and intent and collaborate with his therapist on the most beneficial treatment regimen.

IMPLICATIONS FOR PRACTICE

OAs seek primary care services for an array of mental health disorders but generally concentrate on physical complaints. Recognition of signs and symptoms of PTSD expedites accurate diagnosis and interventions. Personal biases or knowledge deficits may contribute to limited screening for PTSD. As an APRN, commit to understanding personal and professional challenges related to mental health care and ensure that all patients receive timely, appropriate care. If APRNs are to practice holistically, they need to consider the mind/ body/spirit in all encounters and remember the head (emotions, feelings, thoughts, ideas) *is* attached to the body (physical concerns). Interacting with all patients as a whole, versus segmenting out mental health from physical health, will increase positive patient outcomes because they face seeking wellness and an improved QoL! PTSD is treatable; APRNs just need to step up to the plate and ask the questions to get to the diagnosis.

CLINICS CARE POINTS

- PTSD is currently categorized in the trauma and stressor-related disorders in the DSM-5.
- Women are at higher risk than men for developing PTSD, but all human beings should be questioned, and if appropriate, screened to determine an accurate diagnosis.
- Determining the cognitive and functional status of OA is extremely important. Utilizing evidence-based tools for both is essential. The APRN should consider using any of the following EB tools in practice:
  - Clock Drawing Test (CDT) https://www.cgakit.com/m-1-clock-test
  - The Short Portable Mental Status Questionnaire (SPMSQ) https://geriatrics.stanford.edu/wp-content/uploads/downloads/culturemed/overview/assessment/downloads/spmsq_tool.pdf
  - Mini-Cog© https://mini-cog.com/download-the-mini-cog-instrument/
  - Montreal Cognitive Assessment (MoCA) https://mocacognition.com/
  - St. Louis University Mental Status Examination (SLUMS) https://www.slu.edu/medicine/internal-medicine/geriatric-medicine/aging-successfully/pdfs/slums_form.pdf
  - Katz Index of Independence in Activities of Daily Living (ADL) https://www.alz.org/careplanning/downloads/katz-adl.pdf
  - Lawton/Brody Instrumental Activities of Daily Living (IADL) https://www.alz.org/careplanning/downloads/lawton-iadl.pdf
- If PTSD is suspected, becoming familiar with, and utilizing one of the EB tools specifically for PTSD is prudent.
  - Primary Care PTSD Screen for DSM-5 (PC-PTSD-5 – military version) https://www.ptsd.va.gov/professional/assessment/documents/pc-ptsd5-screen.pdf
  - PTSD CheckList – Civilian Version (PCL-C) https://www.mirecc.va.gov/docs/visn6/3_ptsd_checklist_and_scoring.pdf

- Keeping in mind that OA have been shown to have increased depression, anxiety, social isolation, and loneliness since the onset of the COVID-19 pandemic. Asking questions or utilizing EB tools to quantify patient feelings may help with alleviating the situation and improving the OAs outlook.

DISCLOSURE

The authors have nothing to disclose.

References

[1] Helmus TC, Glenn RW. The lessons of war: the causations of battle fatigue. Steeling the mind: combat stress reactions and their implications for urban warfare. Santa Monica, CA: Rand Corporation; 2005. p. 23–38.

[2] History.com. PTSD and shell shock. History. 2017. Available at: https://www.history.com/topics/inventions/history-of-ptsd-and-shell-shock#:~:text=Post%2Dtraumatic%20stress%20disorder%20was,the%20%E2%80%9CGreat%20War%E2%80%9D%20began Updated August 21, 2018. Accessed January 08,2023.

[3] Reft R. World War I: injured veterans and the disability rights movement. Library of Congress blog. 2017. Available at: https://blogs.loc.gov/loc/2017/12/world-war-i-injured-veterans-and-the-disability-rights-movement/. Accessed January 08, 2023.

[4] Schultz D. Combat fatigue: how stress in battle was felt (and treated) in WWII. Warfare History Network. 2021. Available at: https://warfarehistorynetwork.com/combat-fatigue-how-stress-in-battle-was-felt-and-treated-in-wwii/. Accessed January 08, 2023.

[5] Chermol BH. Wounds without scars: treatment of battle fatigue in the U.S. armed forces in the second world war. Military Affairs 1985;49(1):9–12.

[6] Finch J. The history of the diagnosis of PTSD. Centre for Clinical Psychology; 2017. Available at: https://psychpd.com.au/history-diagnosis-ptsd/. Accessed January 08, 2023.

[7] Schubert S, Lee CW. Adult PTSD and its treatment with EMDR: a review of controversies, evidence, and theoretical knowledge. Journal of EMDR Practice and Research 2009;3(3):117–32.

[8] U. S. Department of Veterans Affairs. PTSD: National Center for PTSD. PTSD and DSM-5. 2022. Available at: https://www.ptsd.va.gov/professional/treat/essentials/dsm5_ptsd.asp. Accessed January 08, 2023.

[9] Kaiser AP, Schuster Wachen J, Potter C, et al. with the Stress, Health, and Aging Research Program. Posttraumatic Stress Symptoms among Older Adults: A Review. U.S. Department of Veterans Affairs. 2022. Available at: https://www.ptsd.va.gov/professional/treat/specific/symptoms_older_adults.asp#:~:text=Prevalence%20and%20symptoms&text=Older%20Veterans%20report%20more%20somatic,Veterans%20(18%2C%2019). Accessed January 08, 2023.

[10] National Institute of Mental Health. Mental Illness. 2022. Available at: https://www.nimh.nih.gov/health/statistics/mental-illness. Accessed January 08, 2023.

[11] Mason M, Soliman R, Kim HS, et al. Disparities by sex and race and ethnicity in death rates due to opioid overdose among adults 55 years or older, 1999 to 2019. JAMA Netw Open 2022;5(1):e2142982.

[12] Veterans and PTSD: understanding causes, signs, symptoms, and treatment. Wounded Warrior Project. 2022. Available at: https://www.woundedwarriorproject.org/programs/mental-wellness/veteran-ptsd-treatment-support-resources. Accessed January 08, 2023.

[13] National Institute of Mental Health. Post-traumatic stress disorder. 2022. Available at: https://www.nimh.nih.gov/health/topics/post-traumatic-stress-disorder-ptsd. Accessed January 08, 2023.

[14] Magruder KM, McLaughlin KA, Elmore Borbon et al. Trauma is a public health issue. Eur J Psychotraumato 2017;8(1):1375338.

[15] National Council on Aging. Center for Healthy Aging for Professionals. Get the Facts on Health Agine. 2022. Available at: https://www.ncoa.org/article/get-the-facts-on-healthy-aging. Accessed January 08, 2023.

[16] Miao XR, Chen QB, Wei K, et al. Posttraumatic stress disorder: from diagnosis to prevention. Military Medical Research 2018;5(1):32.

[17] Jayasinghe N, Sparks M, Kato K, et al. Posttraumatic stress symptoms in older adults hospitalized for fall injury. Gen Hosp Psychiatry 2014;36(6):669–73.

[18] Martin CM. Resilience and health (care): a dynamic adaptive perspective. J Eval Clin Pract 2018;24:1319–22.

[19] Martin CM. What matters in "multimorbidity"? arguably resilience and personal health experience are central to quality of life and optimizing survival. J Eval Clin Pract 2018;24(6):1282–4.

[20] Hong S, Kim H, Park MK. Impact of COVID-19 on post-traumatic symptoms in the general population: an integrative review. Int J Ment Health Nurs 2021;30(4):834–46. Available at: https://pubmed.ncbi.nlm.nih.gov/33884723/. Accessed January 08, 2023.

[21] Sobczak S, Olff M, Rutten B, et al. Comorbidity rates of posttraumatic stress disorder in dementia: a systematic literature review. Eur J Psychotraumatol 2021;12(1):1883923. Available at: https://doi.org/10.1080/20008198.2021.1883923. Accessed January 08, 2023.

[22] Gunak M, Billings J, Carratu E, et al. Post-traumatic stress disorder as a risk factor for dementia: systematic review and meta-analysis. Br J Psychiatry 2020;217:600–8.

[23] Spottswood M, Davydow DS, Huang H. The prevalence of posttraumatic stress disorder in primary care: a systematic review. Harv Rev Psychiatry 2017;25(4):159–69.

[24] Stahl SM. Prescribers Guide: Stahl's Essential Psychopharmacology. (6th edition). Cambridge, England: Cambridge University Press; 2017.

[25] U.S. Department of Veterans Affairs. PTSD Treatment. 2022. Available at: https://www.va.gov/health-care/health-needs-conditions/mental-health/ptsd/. Accessed January 08, 2023.

Advances in Family Practice Nursing 5 (2023) 15–25

ADVANCES IN FAMILY PRACTICE NURSING

The Impact of Food Insecurity on Chronic Disease Management in Older Adults

Vallon Williams, DNP, APRN, AGNP-C[a],*,
Pamela J. LaBorde, DNP, APRN, CCNS, TTS[b],
Jyrissa Robinson, DNP, APRN, AGNP-C[c]

[a]University of Arkansas for Medical Sciences, Translational Research Institute, 4301 West Markham Street, Slot 577, Little Rock, AR 72205, USA; [b]University of Arkansas for Medical Sciences, College of Nursing, 4301 West Markham Street, Slot 529, Little Rock, AR 72205-7199, USA; [c]Central Arkansas Veterans Health care System, 4300 West 7th Street, Little Rock, AR 72205, USA

Keywords

- Food insecurity - Food security - Chronic diseases - Mental health - Depression
- Cardiovascular - Diabetes - Older adults

Key points

- Food insecurity increases the susceptibility of chronic diseases and impacts health status.
- Combating food insecurity could potentially improve health outcomes, hospital readmissions, and financial burdens.
- Nurse practitioners should be knowledgeable of local and national resources to provide interventions for food insecurity in their patient population.
- It is helpful to have a holistic approach to the management of food insecurity in older adults as it is a multifaceted health issue.
- Health disparities continue to wedge health care outcomes; therefore, health care providers must understand risk factors, cultural awareness, literacy, history, systems, and their relationship to food insecurity.

CASE PRESENTATION

Sandra Polite is a 66-year-old African American woman with a past medical history of pulmonary sarcoidosis, hypertension, depression, prediabetes, obesity, and chronic vitamin D deficiency. She is seeing the advanced practice

*Corresponding author. E-mail address: vwilliams@uams.edu

https://doi.org/10.1016/j.yfpn.2022.12.001
2589-420X/23/© 2022 Elsevier Inc. All rights reserved.

registered nurse (APRN) at the internal medicine clinic for a 6-month checkup. Ms Polite's blood pressure is 145/91 and her hemoglobin A1C is 6.2%. Current medications include atenolol, nifedipine, prednisone, vitamin D, calcium, ipratropium–albuterol nebulizer, budesonide–formoterol inhaler, and albuterol inhaler as needed. She resides in an income-based housing apartment in rural Arkansas. Ms Polite receives $930 in Social Security disability benefits and $65 in Supplemental Nutrition Assistance Program (SNAP) payments monthly. She has two adult children who live 45 miles away. Ms Polite has limited access to fresh food as the closest grocery store is 15 miles from her home and she does not own a vehicle. A family friend takes her to the grocery store at the beginning of the month. However, because fresh food is likely to spoil before her next visit to the grocery store, Ms Polite makes limited fresh food selections. She has a hard time preparing meals as she becomes dyspneic easily, so she purchases packaged or frozen food that is easier to prepare. Ms Polite's response to the Hunger Vital Sign screening tool indicates that she is at risk for food insecurity (FI). Her responses prompted the APRN to administer the US Adult Food Security Survey Module, which revealed that Ms Polite is experiencing low food security. The APRN contacted the local Area Agency on Aging to initiate an application for the Meals on Wheels program.

INTRODUCTION

Erin Brockovich once said, "most of our citizenry believes that hunger only affects people who are lazy or people who are just looking for a handout, people who don't want to work, but, sadly, that is not true. Hungry people are members of households that simply cannot provide enough food or proper nutrition. And to think of the older adult suffering from malnutrition is just too hard for most of us." [1]. FI attributes to this suffering and is a topic of concern in the Healthy People 2030 Social Determinants of Health [2]. Food security is described as "access by all people at all times to enough food for an active, healthy life." [3] The US Department of Agriculture (USDA) provides the following definitions for the types of food security:

Food security
- High food security (old label = Food security): no reported indications of food-access problems or limitations.
- Marginal food security (old label = Food security): one or two reported indications—typically of anxiety over food sufficiency or shortage of food in the house: little or no indication of changes in diets or food intake.

Food insecurity
- Low food security (old label = Food insecurity without hunger): reports of reduced quality, variety, or desirability of diet: little or no indication of reduced food intake.
- Very low food security (old label = Food insecurity with hunger): reports of multiple indications of disrupted eating patterns and reduced food intake [4].

The USDA states that many households are subjected to FI which can be sporadic throughout the year due to limited money and access to resources, or more severe, characterized by a reduction or disruption in the person's normal eating patterns [5]. "In 2020, 89.5% of US households were food secure throughout the year. The remaining 10.5% of households were food insecure at least sometime during the year, including 3.9% (5.1 million households) that had very low food security." [5] According to the *State of Senior Hunger in 2020*, 5.2 million seniors aged 60 years and older (one in 15) experienced FI [6]. Shockingly compared with the 2007 Great Recession, this statistical notes a higher percentage of older adults experiencing FI.

ASSOCIATED FACTORS

As one ages, more challenges may be experienced related to overall health, economic struggles, and nutritional intake. Such challenges can exacerbate FI among older adults. Demographic and socioeconomic categories that contribute to FI in this population include disabilities, types of housing (renting vs homeowner), financial income, household makeup (especially multigenerational households), and race and ethnicity [7]. Older adults who experience FI have a noted decrease in consuming key nutrients such as protein and iron. In addition, FI contributes to chronic health conditions such as depression, asthma, diabetes, heart failure, obesity, decreased quality of life, and myocardial infarctions [7]. Before delving into some of these chronic conditions, a discussion regarding the associated factors contributing to FI among older adults is warranted to help shine a light on this public health issue.

Mobility-related conditions and disabilities

Functional limitations and mobility-related disabilities have been linked to FI. These conditions can create transportation issues that limit the older adult's ability to work, thus decreasing resources to access and purchase food. In addition, some mobility-related conditions and disabilities restrict independence for meal preparation and feeding oneself, resulting in FI and malnutrition. These types of disabilities may be more prevalent among older adults, especially if they live alone and have no one to rely on to help them in obtaining food, prepare meals, and assist with feeding [8]. Functional limitations may also contribute to diminished participation in social interactions centered on food and eating outside the home, which are other accesses to food and social support among older adults.

Economic factors

Older adults often live on a limited or fixed income resulting in choosing between eating healthy foods or paying for medical services and medications. Out-of-pocket medical-related costs can take precedence over healthy food choices. FI affects adherence to treatment plans or medical conditions, such as diabetes, heart disease, or obesity [7]. Seligman and colleagues [9] found that food-insecure households purchase less expensive foods with poor nutritional value and higher caloric content, which is associated with adverse health consequences. In a study by Bengle and colleagues,[10] food-insecure individuals had a threefold increase in medication cost nonadherence than those not experiencing FI. Bhargava and colleagues [11] reported that food-insecure individuals are likely to describe their health as poor and more likely to have more chronic diseases. Making difficult choices between paying for medical expenditures or food places the older adult in a predicament of not investing in their health and negative outcomes. Over time, poor choices can lead to public health concerns that need to be addressed by understanding FIs health-related factors, in food-insecure older adults.

Food assistance programs are aimed at relieving economic burdens. These programs provide the recommended macronutrients by national dietary guidelines. However, participation in such programs is linked to increased depression and emotional distress among some participants. This linkage is centered around the stigma of relying on government assistance or assistance of any kind. This stigma may have social and cultural implications such as laziness or failure to obtain food independently [12].

Government programs also help to relieve comorbidities. In one longitudinal study [12], older adults who receive the SNAP may prevent the development of some chronic diseases. However, they found that participation in SNAP was a risk factor for depressive symptoms, possibly associated with the stigma of being on welfare, leading to lower self-esteem. More research is needed to investigate food assistance programs and the emotional stress of food assistance recipients [12].

FOOD INSECURITY AND CHRONIC DISEASE

FI in the aging population has detrimental effects on chronic disease management, and they are more likely to have multiple chronic conditions compared with their food-secure counterparts [13]. This article examines the impact of FI on managing cardiovascular disease (CVD), diabetes, and mental health disorders in older adults.

Food insecurities and cardiovascular disease

CVD is the number one leading cause of death in the United States [14]. It encompasses a range of heart-related morbidities including hypertension, heart failure, myocardial infarction, angina pectoris, stroke, and atherosclerosis [14]. Despite a rate decrease in the general US population, heart disease mortality in adults 65 years and older has increased in recent years [15]. Contributing factors to this growth include a rapidly increasing aging population combined with climbing rates of diabetes and obesity [15]. Inadequate access to food resources is associated with poor CVD outcomes [16,17]. The association between increased atherosclerotic CVD (ASCVD) risks in persons with FI is compounded by nutrition, psychological, and access to care pathways [18]. Factors related to FI lead to increased ASCVD risks such as consuming less expensive calorie-dense foods, increased psychological stressors, and deferred medical treatment [18]. One systematic review found FI has a two to four times greater likelihood of CVD [16]. Another systematic review showed a direct relationship between FI and cardiometabolic risk factors, including excess weight, hypertension, dyslipidemia, and stress [17]. One cross-sectional data analysis [19] showed that older adults at the marginal, low, and very low levels of FI have a higher risk of peripheral artery disease potentially due to inflammation caused by the inability to maintain a nutrient-dense diet. Further, heart failure mortality is linked to limited access to food [20].

Food insecurity and diabetes
Diabetes is a major chronic disease in the United States. Compared with 13% of the general adult population, 26.8% of persons 65 years and older have diagnosed and undiagnosed diabetes [21]. Potential diabetes-related morbidities in older adults include macrovascular (hypertension, hyperlipidemia, congestive heart failure, and atherosclerosis) and microvascular (retinopathy, neuropathy, and chronic kidney disease) complications [22]. Older adults with diabetes who face FI are more likely to have emergency department visits, hospitalizations, and elevated A1C levels [23].

Walker and colleagues [24] studied the association between FI and diabetes-related health outcomes. The investigators found that FI has a direct relationship to glycaemic control and an indirect relationship with self-care via perceived stress in persons with type II diabetes (DM) [24]. A cross-sectional study of food pantry clients revealed a dose–response association between the increased levels of FI and more difficulties with DM self-management [25]. Related factors to higher rates of FI and persons with DM are likely associated with impaired nutrition quality and consumption, reduced access to healthier dietary options, and competing needs such as medication and housing costs [26,27]. Diabetes-related morbidity, particularly kidney complications, is a mediator for depressive symptoms in older adults [28].

Food insecurities and depression
Depression is another significant health condition experienced by older adults and affects 7% of this population [29]. FI among aging persons has been associated with increased depressive symptoms [30–33]. There is a bidirectional association between mental health and FI [27]. Prior research revealed that adults 65 years and older with depression had a sixfold increased chance of experiencing very low food security versus those reporting high food security [31]. The ability to purchase and prepare food is positively related to depressive symptoms in older adults [30]. One study listed anxiety, sleep problems, depression, and cognition as associated factors to fall-related injury in aging persons with severe FI. FI almost doubled the odds of fall-related injuries in older adults, with mental health complications as the primary mediating factor [34]. Further, food deprivation has been linked to suicidal thoughts and suicide attempts in older adults [35]. FI affects those who care for older adults, especially when the caregiving duration exceeded 6 months [36].

Table 1
Food insecurity screening tools

Survey model	Web site
https://www.ers.usda.gov/topics/food-nutrition-assistance/food-security-in-the-u-s/survey-tools/	1. US Household Food Security 2. 10-Item Adult Food Security 3. Spanish: US Household Food Security 4. Chinese: US Household Food Security 5. Six-Item Short Form of the Food Security
https://www.census.gov/data/experimental-data-products/household-pulse-survey.html	1. Household Pulse Survey for COVID 2. Household Pulse Survey for COVID-Spanish

HEALTH CARE ASSESSMENTS

Chronic diseases, psychological symptoms, nutritional disorders, and social economics disparities are associated with increased susceptibility to FI in the older adult population. Therefore, health care screenings are implemented to wedge this gap. The 2-Item Food Insecurity, also known as the Hunger Vital Sign, has a 94.5% of specificity in adults greater than 60 year old [37]. This tool identifies households at risk by asking the following questions. "Within the past 12 months, we worried whether our food would run out before we got money to buy more." [38] Within the past 12 months, the food we bought just didn't last and we didn't have money to get more." [38] FI is identified if the answers are often true or sometimes true [38]. Although this option is a quick and efficient tool to use, it will not determine the level of FI, nor will it address contributing factors compared with the USDA full eighteen-item screening tool [39].

The USDA screening tool (U.S. Household Food Security Survey Module) is used nationally to determine the FI category and central variables across various ethnicities and geographic locations [40]. The 10-item Adult Food Security Survey Module is a shorter version that focuses on the targeted population and excludes children from the equation. Per Economic Research Services [40], the items include:

- Worried food will run out before one got money to buy more
- Food bought didn't last and no money for more
- Couldn't afford a balanced meal
- Cut the size of meal or skipped it
- Ate less than one should
- Cute size or skipped meal in 3 months or more
- Hungry but no money to purchase food
- Weight loss
- No food for 1 day
- Did not eat for 1 day in 3 months or more

The responses, "yes, often, almost every month, and some months but not every month," are scored as 1, resulting in their FI status [40]. The statuses are as follows: High security (0), Marginal security (1–2), Low security (3–5), and

Very low security (6–10) [40]. Once the category is established, appropriate interventions are implemented. However, alternative survey tools identify FI and its contributing factors.

In 2022, the Household Pulse Survey (HPS) was created to measure how the Coronavirus impacts food security, mental health, physical ability, vaccination status, and other economic variables [41]. The HPS is a 20-minute self-administered assessment taken online to provide near real-time data [41]. The HPS questions one's household income and its effect on food security, utilities, transportation, and health maintenance. In addition, screening tools such as the patient health questionnaire (PHQ-2) for depression and general anxiety

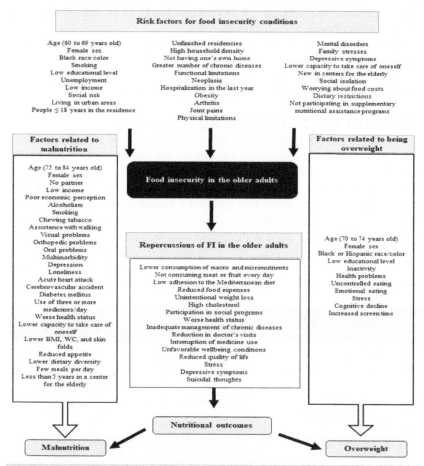

Fig. 1. Model detailing food insecurity in older adults and associated nutritional outcomes. (Reproduced with permission from Oxford University Press. Pereira MHQ, Pereira MLAS, Campos GC, Molina MCB. Food insecurity and nutritional status among older adults: a systematic review. Nutrition Reviews. 2022;80(4):631–644. https://doi.org/10.1093/nutrit/nuab044.)

disorder (GAD-2) for anxiety are included. Hence, the survey has multiple questions outside our targeted population. However, the focused data help frame the picture so the provider can fill in the missing pieces to the puzzle.

Screenings vary in detail, depth, and time just like patients vary in language, ethnicity, and culture. However, most of the instruments listed in Table 1 are validated, with the 10-Item Adult Security Survey being the most reliable [42]. Even though there is not enough research to support the validity of the HPS, it is an efficient tool for data collection [41].

INTERVENTIONS

Interventions for FI are a health imperative for older adults. Initially, providers must understand and identify the risk factors for FI to prevent chronic and mental health disease exacerbation (Fig. 1).

Once core variables are identified, clinicians connect patients with national and substantial community resources that will promote reliable public health solutions. In addition to national programs, churches, food pantries, and community gardens are local programs considered (Table 2).

ADVANCED PRACTICE REGISTERED NURSE ROLE

Recognizing FI in conjunction with its associated factors is a challenge. Interventions should be implemented to address the contributing variables. In 2011, the Patient Protection and Affordable Care Act initiated annual wellness visits to address preventive health needs and chronic concerns in Medicare Part B recipients [45]. This yearly visit includes a Health Risk Assessment and a personalized preventative plan that specifically identifies and addresses internal and external links to FI along with chronic disease, mental illness, and disabilities. Also, it allows the nurse to build a rapport with patients and organizations in the community. Clinicians begin to collaborate with dietitians, social workers, physical and occupational therapists, psychologists, and nursing

Table 2
Community and national resources [39,43,44]

Community	National
• Churches • Food banks • Community gardens • Anti-hunger advocacy groups • Senior centers • Public health department	• National Hunger Hotline: will assist with locating local food resources, call 1-(866)-3-HUNGRY, 1-(877)-8-HAMBRE, or text 1-(914)-342-7744 • SNAP: provides eligible participants funds to purchase food • Commodity Supplemental Food Program: offers nutritious eats and supporting education • Senior Farmers' Market Nutrition Program: provides fresh fruit and vegetables from local establishments • Emergency Food Assistance Program: provides food based on income and employment status • Meals on Wheels Program: brings meals to people's homes with limited mobility

facilities to optimize healthy aging and reduce the prevalence of FI. Last, nurses can advocate FI concerns at the local, state, and national levels [43]. Ensuring that policies provide additional funding to community organizations, importing healthier food, and streamlining applications to national programs would simultaneously decrease FI and chronic conditions while promoting a better quality of life.

SUMMARY

FI is a socioeconomic issue that has multiple implications for controlling chronic diseases such as diabetes, CVD, and depression in older adults. The inability to obtain adequate food resources can hinder the proper management of chronic illnesses due to products of FI such as a reduced nutrient-dense diet and prioritizing other life necessities above healthier foods. Further, poor mental health status as a result of FI leads to worsening health outcomes such as increased falls. Resourceful tools including the adult FI 10-item survey can be administered in the clinical setting to identify FI in aging Americans. Health care providers such as APRNs can positively impact this multifactorial issue with early screening, appropriate interventions, and political advocacy.

CLINICS CARE POINTS

- Food insecurity is related to poor quality of life, adverse outcomes, and increased susceptibility to chronic diseases.
- Food insecurity variables are multidimensional.
- Food security screening decreases comorbidities, reduces hospital admissions, and increases health outcomes.

DISCLOSURE

The authors have nothing to disclose.

References
[1] Erin B. The Emily Fund for a Better World. Available at: https://doonething.org/heroes/-pages-b/brockovich-quotes.htm. Accessed February 28, 2022.
[2] Office of Disease Prevention and Health Promotion. Food insecurity. 2022. Available at: https://health.gov/healthypeople/priority-areas/social-determinants-health/literature-summaries/food-insecurity. Accessed October 01, 2022.
[3] United States Department of Agriculture. Definitions of food security. Updated September 07, 2022. Accessed October 01, 2022. Coleman-Jensen A, Rabbitt MP, Gregory CA, Singh A. Household Food Security in the United States in 2021. Economic Research Service, United States Department of Agriculture; September 2022. ERR-309. Accessed October 01, 2022.
[4] Economic Research Service. US Department of Agriculture. Definitions of Food Security. 2022. Available at: https://www.ers.usda.gov/topics/food-nutrition-assistance/food-security-in-the-u-s/definitions-of-food-security. Accessed September 30, 2022.

[5] Economic Research Service. US Department of Agriculture. Food insecurity and nutrition assistance. 2022. Available at: https://www.ers.usda.gov/data-products/ag-and-food-statistics-charting-the-essentials/food-security-and-nutrition-assistance. Accessed February 28, 2022.

[6] Zilliak JP, Gundersen C. The state of senior hunger in 2020. Feeding America. 2022. Available at: https://www.feedingamerica.org/research/senior-hunger-research/senior. Accessed February 28, 2022.

[7] Fernandes SG, Rorigues AM, Nunes C, et al. Food insecurity in older adults: results from the epidemiology of chronic diseases cohort study 3. Front Med (Lausanne) 2018;5:203.

[8] Heflin CM, Altman E, Rodriquez LL. Food insecurity and disability in the United States. Disabil Health J 2019;12(2):220–6.

[9] Seligman HK, Bindman AB, Vittinghoff E, et al. Food insecurity is associated with diabetes mellitus: results from the National Health Examination and Nutrition Examination Survey (NHANES) 1999-2002. J Gen Intern Med 2007;22(7):1018–23.

[10] Bengle R, Sinnett S, Johnson T, et al. Food insecurity is associated with cost-related medication non-adherence in community dwelling, low-income older adults in Georgia. J Nutr For Elder 2010;29(2):170–91.

[11] Bhargava V, Lee JS, Jain R, et al. Food insecurity is negatively associated with home health and out-of-pocket expenditures in older adults. J Nutr 2012;142(10):1888–95.

[12] Pak TY, Kim G. Food stamps, food insecurity, and health outcomes among elderly Americans. Prev Med 2020;130:105871.

[13] Leung CW, Kullgren JT, Malani PN, et al. Food insecurity is associated with multiple chronic conditions and physical health status among older US adults. Prev Med Rep 2020;20: 101211.

[14] Benjamin EJ, Muntner P, Alonso A, et al. Heart disease and stroke statistics-2019 update: a report from the American Heart Association. Circulation 2019;139(10):e56–528.

[15] Sidney S, Go AS, Jaffe MG, et al. Association between aging of the us population and heart disease mortality from 2011 to 2017. JAMA Cardiol 2019;4(12):1280–6.

[16] Parekh T, Xue H, Cheskin LJ, et al. Food insecurity and housing instability as determinants of cardiovascular health outcomes: a systematic review. Nutr Metab Cardiovasc Dis 2022;32(7):1590–608.

[17] da Silva Miguel E, Lopes SO, Araújo SP, et al. Association between food insecurity and cardiometabolic risk in adults and the elderly: a systematic review. J Glob Health 2020;10(2): 1–7.

[18] Palakshappa D, Ip EH, Berkowitz SA, et al. Pathways by which food insecurity is associated with atherosclerotic cardiovascular disease risk. J Am Heart Assoc 2021;10(22):e021901.

[19] Redmond M, Dong F, Jacobson L, et al. Food insecurity and peripheral arterial disease in older adult populations. J Nutr Health Aging 2016;20(10):989–95.

[20] Gondi K, Sifuentes A, Hummel SL. Food insecurity is independently associated with heart failure mortality in The United States. J Card Fail 2022;28(5 suppl 015):S7.

[21] Centers for Disease Control and Prevention. National Diabetes Statistics Report. 2020. Available at: https://www.cdc.gov/diabetes/pdfs/data/statistics/national-diabetes-statistics-report.pdf. Accessed July 6, 2022.

[22] LeRoith D, Biessels GJ, Braithwaite SS, et al. Treatment of diabetes in older adults: an endocrine society* clinical practice guideline. J Clin Endocrinol Metab 2019;104(5):1520–74.

[23] Schroeder EB, Zeng C, Sterrett AT, et al. The longitudinal relationship between food insecurity in older adults with diabetes and emergency department visits, hospitalizations, hemoglobin A1c, and medication adherence. J Diabetes its Complications 2019;33(4):289–95.

[24] Walker RJ, Joni SW, Egede LE. Pathways between food insecurity and glycaemic control in individuals with type 2 diabetes. Public Health Nutr 2018;21(17):3237–44.

[25] Ippolito MM, Lyles CR, Prendergast K, et al. Food insecurity and diabetes self-management among food pantry clients. Public Health Nutr 2017;20(1):183–9.

[26] Gucciardi E, Vahabi M, Norris N, et al. The intersection between food insecurity and diabetes: a review. Curr Nutr Rep 2014;3(4):324–32.

[27] Flint KL, Davis GM, Umpierrez GE. Emerging trends and the clinical impact of food insecurity in patients with diabetes. J Diabetes 2020;12(3):187–96.

[28] Bergmans RS, Zivin K, Mezuk B. Depression, food insecurity and diabetic morbidity: evidence from the Health and Retirement study. J Psychosom Res 2019;117:22–9.

[29] World Health Organization. Mental health of older adults. 2017. Available at: https://www.who.int/news-room/fact-sheets/detail/mental-health-of-older-adults. Accessed July 06, 2022.

[30] Jung SE, Kim S, Bishop A, et al. Poor nutritional status among low-income older adults: examining the interconnection between self-care capacity, food insecurity, and depression. J Acad Nutr Diet 2019;119(10):1687–94.

[31] Brostow DP, Gunzburger E, Abbate LM, et al. Mental illness, not obesity status, is associated with food insecurity among the elderly in the Health and Retirement study. J Nutr Gerontol Geriatr 2019;38(2):149–72.

[32] Jih J, Nguyen TT, Jin C, et al. food insecurity is associated with behavioral health diagnosis among older primary care patients with multiple chronic conditions. JGIM: J Gen Intern Med 2020;35(12):3726–9.

[33] Bergmans RS, Wegryn-Jones R. Examining associations of food insecurity with major depression among older adults in the wake of the Great Recession. Soc Sci Med 2020;258; https://doi.org/10.1016/j.socscimed.2020.113033.

[34] Smith L, Shin JI, López-Sánchez GF, et al. Association between food insecurity and fall-related injury among adults aged ≥65 years in low- and middle-income countries: the role of mental health conditions. Arch Gerontol Geriatr 2021;96:104438.

[35] Cabello M, Miret M, Ayuso-Mateos JL, et al. Cross-national prevalence and factors associated with suicide ideation and attempts in older and young-and-middle age people. Aging Ment Health 2020;24(9):1533–42.

[36] Goswami S, Korgaonkar S, Bhattacharya K, et al. Food Insecurity in a Sample of Informal Caregivers in 4 Southern US States. Preventing Chronic Dis 2022;19:1–10.

[37] Gundersen C, Engelhard EE, Crumbaugh AS, et al. Brief assessment of food insecurity accurately identifies high-risk US adults. Public Health Nutr 2017;20(8):1367–71.

[38] Hager ER, Quigg AM, Black MM, et al. Development and validity of a 2-item screen to identify families at risk for food insecurity. Pediatrics 2010;126(1):e26–32.

[39] Saffel-Shrier S, Johnson MA, Francis SL. Position of the Academy of Nutrition and Dietetics and the Society for Nutrition Education and Behavior: food and nutrition programs for community-residing older adults. J Acad Nutr Diet 2019;119(7):1188–204.

[40] Economic Research Service. US Department of Agriculture. Survey tools. 2022. Available at: https://www.ers.usda.gov/topics/food-nutrition-assistance/food-security-in-the-u-s/survey-tools/. Accessed August 11, 2022.

[41] United States Census Bureau. Measuring household experience during the coronavirus pandemic. 2022. Available at: https://www.census.gov/data/experimental-data-products/household-pulse-survey.html. Accessed August 11, 2022.

[42] Bickel G, Nord M, Price C, et al. Guide to measuring household food security. United States Department of Agriculture. 2000. Available at: https://www.fns.usda.gov/guide-measuring-household-food-security-revised-2000. Accessed August 11, 2022.

[43] Reid A. Older adults with chronic disease and food insecurity in the United States. J Gerontol Nurs 2021;47(12):7–11.

[44] Food and Nutrition Service. US Department of Agriculture. National Hunger Hotline. 2019. Available at: https://www.fns.usda.gov/partnerships/national-hunger-clearinghouse. Accessed September 26, 2022.

[45] Cuenca AE. Making Medicare annual wellness visits work in practice. Fam Pract Management 2012;19(5):11–6. Accessed August 11, 2022.

Advances in Family Practice Nursing 5 (2023) 27–40

ADVANCES IN FAMILY PRACTICE NURSING

Immunosenescence and Infectious Disease Risk Among Aging Adults

Management Strategies for FNPs to Identify Those at Greatest Risk

Deanna Gray-Miceli, PhD, GNP-BC, FAAN[a],*,
Kathy Gray, DNP, FNP-BC, CRNP, FAANP[a],
Matthew R. Sorenson, PhD, APRN, ANP-C, FAAN[b],
Barbara J. Holtzclaw, PhD, RN, FAAN[c]

[a]Thomas Jefferson University, Jefferson College of Nursing, 130 South Ninth Street, Edison Building, Suite 864, Philadelphia, PA 19107, USA; [b]Texas A&M University, College of Nursing, Clinical Building 1, 8441 Riverside Parkway, Bryan, TX 77807, USA; [c]Fran and Earl Ziegler College of Nursing, University of Oklahoma Health Sciences Center, 1100 North Stonewall, Oklahoma City, OK 73117, USA

Keywords
• COVID-19 • Immunosenescence • Leadership • Nursing • Pandemic

Key points

- Immunosenescence is a progressive contributing risk for the development of viral infection.
- Cohorting can be an effective means of reducing overall population risk.
- Immunosenescence is a progressive contributing risk factor for the development of viral infection and infectious disease among the older adult population, especilly for those residing in nursing homes.
- The use of interventions such as cohorting by nurse leaders in nursing homes can be an effective strategy for reducing overall population risk among older adult residents.

*Corresponding author. Professor of Nursing, Thomas Jefferson University, Jefferson College of Nursing, 901 Walnut Street, Suite 707, Philadelphia, PA 19107. *E-mail address:* Deanna.Gray-Miceli@jefferson.edu

https://doi.org/10.1016/j.yfpn.2022.11.004

INTRODUCTION

Nurses at the point of care face several challenges and concerns related to protecting older adult patients over 65 years who are at the highest risk for coronavirus disease-2019 (COVID-19)-related infections. These age-associated immunologic changes that occur among this age-group are referred to as *immunosenescence*. Progressive decline in immune processes over each passing decade reduces the ability to trigger effective antibodies and cellular responses to infectious diseases and vaccines [1]. It is necessary to understand the risks posed by immunosenescence to plan protective adjuvants and interventions. This article is designed to provide the reader basic information on immunosenescence and its predictable effects on immunocompetence. Implications for decision-making on the part of nursing leadership to protect the vulnerable and control outbreaks are guided by a recommendation framework developed by the *Coronavirus Commission for Safety and Quality in Nursing Homes* [2]. Such strategies include appointing an infection control manager, cohorting, and establishment of consistent testing and monitoring. These concepts are reviewed and followed by a case exemplar to facilitate application to practice.

PATHOPHYSIOLOGY

Innate and adaptive immune systems

The innate immune system: Immunosenescence emerges from changes to both the innate and adaptive immune systems [3]. The *innate immune system* includes physical barriers and select immune cell classes that are activated without the presence of an antigen. The main cells of the innate immune system and its soluble mediators include cytokines, hormones, and free radicals that remain well preserved throughout aging, but lose their ability to effect protective responses in advanced age. Examples of these age-related changes include decreases in phagocytic capability of neutrophils and diminished functional ability of natural killer cells (refer to Box 1). Blunted febrile responses are seen in response to pyrogenic cytokines [4].

The adaptive immune system: Although innate immune changes place the older adult at increased risk for developing infection, changes in the adaptive arm of the immune system are of greater concern for vaccine responsiveness and defense against viral infection.

The *adaptive immune system*, also known as the acquired immune system, includes elements of two intimately linked aspects: *humoral* and *cell-mediated* immunity. Humoral immunity includes a combination of peptides, complement proteins, and antibodies produced by B cells. Cell-mediated immunity affects T-cell responses, which progressively lose their potency with aging. As a result, advancing age is associated with an increase in the number of B cells, to compensate for the progressive decrease in their functional ability. The effectiveness of the antibody released from immunosenescent B cells is diminished and is produced in lower amounts. There are also fewer naïve T cells and a large accumulation of memory T cells. The lower number of naïve T cells reflects a decline in responsiveness to new antigens. Together, reduced responsiveness to new

Box 1: Main features of immunosenescence

Cell population	Aging-associated change
B cells	Number of cells increases while the functional ability of these cells decreases. Antibody is produced in lower amounts and generally is of lower quality.
Macrophages	The number of macrophages remains consistent, but phagocytic ability is decreased.
Natural killer	Increased number of cells, with concomitant decrease in functional ability.
Neutrophils	No significant change in the number of cells produced but decrease in functional capacity and a shorter life span.
T cells	• Decrease in number of naïve T cells, resulting in diminished response to new antigens. • Increased number of memory cells lineage committed to specific antigen. In other words, large number of cells programmed to respond to other viruses.

Adapted from Sorenson, M. (2010). Immunosenescence: An Unappreciated Risk. MedSurg Matters, 1, 6-8; with permission.

antigen and increased numbers of memory T cells indicates consequences of the older adult's lifelong exposure to viral infections. Common viral etiologies targeting the respiratory system in older adults are provided in Box 2.

Increases in memory T cells, reduced naïve T cells, and lower B cell functional ability, results in less ability to produce an effective response to vaccination. In studies of influenza vaccines, even adding adjuvant immune response enhancers fails to produce the desired antibody responses in older adults [5]. Similar findings are being seen in emerging trials of select COVID-19 vaccine with antibody levels manifesting lower in adults over age 70 [6]. Such findings show the need for nursing leadership to implement protections beyond using vaccination programs.

Immunosenescence presents a dilemma faced in previous pandemics: Immunization is required to achieve immunity, whereas at the same time aging is associated with a reduction in vaccination responsiveness. Responsibly, we

Box 2: Common respiratory viral etiologies in older adult populations

Adenovirus

Coronaviruses

Human metapneumovirus

Influenza A and B

Parainfluenza

Respiratory syncytial virus

must decrease the older resident's exposure to the virus even as the influx of new infections increase. To best address an action plan that informs safer, healthier, resilient nursing homes, in the existing context of immunosenescence, the conceptual framework for this article is aligned with recommendations from the *Coronavirus Commission for Safety and Quality in Nursing Homes* [2].

Conceptual framework

The task of nursing leadership in any setting to prepare for a pandemic response requires specific considerations and steps. Many of these same steps are necessary to manage care of an individual at risk for immunosenescence. The conceptual model developed by the *Coronavirus Commission for Safety and Quality in Nursing Homes* [2] was developed to reduce risk of exposure to COVID-19, but can also inform the care to reduce any viral infection that may be encountered by a population facing immunosenescence (refer to Fig. 1). Regardless of viral etiology, protective measures implemented in response to the latest coronavirus-associated pandemic apply. The model presented here deals not only with nursing leadership but also it shows the importance of collaboration, delegation, and shared responsibility to carry out protective recommendations. These can be readily applied by nursing in facing infectious outbreaks in long-term care situations.

In the model, systemic challenges place older adults at increased risk. Although there are institutional variables that influence implementation of protective actions, select interventions can be readily implemented by nursing leadership to reduce risk and enhance protection of uninfected older adults.

HISTORY

Severe acute respiratory syndrome coronavirus-2 (SARS-CoV-2), the pathogen responsible for COVID-19, was first identified in in Wuhan, China in

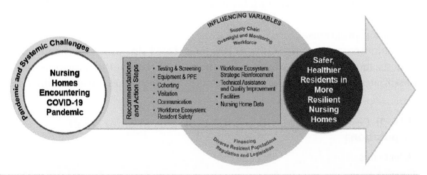

Fig. 1. Commission recommendation framework. Recommendations and action steps are designed to improve the ability of long-term care settings to respond to the challenges raised by COVID-19. Implementation of recommendations would result in enhanced resident safety. (© 2020 The MITRE Corporation. All Rights Reserved. Reprinted with permission of The MITRE Corporation.)

December of 2019 and by March of 2020 was declared a pandemic. Older adults, especially in nursing home settings, were affected by the virus by virtue of the proximity of residents and the fact that the transmission of the virus occurs by respiratory droplets. This mode of transmission made it impossible for long-term care residents to avoid contracting the virus especially as mask wearing was not the norm initially.

COVID-19 presents with a wide range of symptomatology, from mild-to-severe life-threatening. Age remains the strongest risk factor for severe COVID-19 outcomes accounting for 81% of US COVID-19-related deaths in people over the age of 65 years. Residents of long-term care facilities accounted for more than 35% of all COVID-19 deaths [7] even though only 1% of the US population lives in long-term care facilities.

The older adult population, many of whom suffer from multiple chronic disease states affecting the cardiovascular, pulmonary, endocrine, and renal systems, are at a higher risk for the development of severe illness from COVID-19. Symptomatology of COVID-19 includes the following: fever or chills, cough, shortness of breath, fatigue, muscle or body aches, headache, new loss of taste or smell, sore throat, congestion, nausea or vomiting and diarrhea [8]. Fatigue and cognitive impairment are the most common debilitating symptoms of post-COVID-19 syndrome (refer to Box 3) [9].

Family and adult nurse practitioners

Family and adult primary care nurse practitioners are the key primary care providers working in long-term care facilities. As key providers they need to be vigilant in the management of this resident population by recognizing symptoms early and initiating screening and up to date treatment protocols. Screening for the virus using the reverse transcription polymerase chain reaction (RT-PCR) method has been shown to be the gold standard for making an accurate diagnosis of COVID-19 [10]. Early diagnosis is important as treatment options such as monoclonal antibodies and antivirals need to be started

---

Box 3: Nonspecific signs and symptoms of viral infection in older adults

Increasing weakness

Delirium, confusion, and restlessness

Nausea, vomiting, or anorexia

Partial or total anosmia

Tremor and ataxia

Increased urinary incontinence

Sore throat

Nasal congestion or drainage

Diarrhea

early in the disease state and have been shown to reduce the risk of hospitalization and death. It is also important to ensure that all residents have been vaccinated and adequately boosted according to the CDC 2022 guidelines.

The older adult resident is subject to multiple comorbidities and nurse practitioners practicing in long-term care and outpatient care are experts in the management of chronic disease, a predisposition to developing severe COVID-19 symptoms. The treatment goal is to keep residents stable and improving the quality of life among older adults through the practice of primary, secondary, and tertiary prevention.

Assessment: testing and screening

Vigilance and steady surveillance are essential elements for weathering the "perfect storm" describing this pandemic and nursing homes [11]. The congregate nature of living, underlying comorbidities and immunosenescence of residents, low numbers of registered nurse (RN) staff and minimal preparation of other caregivers combined with staffing shortages due to the pandemic, all converge in a society aching to break confinement and return to normal.

Concern for the rapid spread of the virus affects both nursing home residents and the staff that attends them. Nearly all nursing home personnel are intimately connected to risk; made clear with Centers for Mediciare and Medicaid (CMS's) estimate of 1632 COVID-19-related nursing home staff deaths at the end of March 2021. Although the country reeled from the waves of rising incidence and deaths, the needs of long-term care facilities for material resources gave way to the priorities of overcrowded acute care settings needing more beds, isolation space, respiratory care, and protective gear. Refer to Box 4 for viral screening tests.

Although some of the current viral pandemic situation may have reached a lull and appeared to subside, the threat persists, and variants of the originating virus have emerged. Older adults will need reimmunization when guidelines are developed. Immunosenescence plays an important part in this equation for the following reasons:

- The length of time (durability) of immunity from current vaccines is still not fully known.
- *Moderna* vaccines show protective antibodies up to 6 months after the second dose in younger and middle-age adults, but these are diminished in older adults.
- Decline in antibody activity, from sensitive "live virus neutralization tests were geometrically lower as adults reached ages 56 and above [6].

Clinical management: maintaining a screening and testing plan: staffing

The importance of a manager. The centers for disease control (CDC) recommends [2] a full-time role of COVID-19 infection prevention and control (IPC) Manager of at least one person in care facilities with 100 residents, or in residences that also maintain their own ventilator or hemodialysis services. Specific CDC recommendations for the role are available from the online CDC site. There should also be no ambiguity as to who has been assigned to coordinate and monitor IPC practices in each facility. This can be a new addition to the staff, or a qualified individual already serving the facility. Assigning a central manager with the authority to act, implement immediate changes and relocate the resident, if the situation arises, can avoid issues that arise from segmented roles with differing priorities.

Vaccine protection for older adults
Ideally, in response to viral outbreak, all residents and staff of nursing homes should be immunized against the threatening virus. Especially as immunization is expected to be less effective in older immunosenescent residents. However, in the early months of the COVID-19 outbreak in the United States, neither the vaccine nor its availability existed. Now, there are still regions in the country that have insufficient vaccine to inoculate their population. Even with the growing availability of vaccines, there are shifting waves of demand for vaccinations by some and anti-vax disinclination by others, along with confusing evidence about the length or durability of the initial vaccination series. There are indications from recent evidence that by the time the majority of the population could be immunized, a booster immunization will be required, particularly for the older adult [6]. These changing scenarios make it essential for the facility's IPC Manager to keep abreast of weekly notices from CDC, CMS, and the state and local infection reports for the nursing home setting. Weekly meetings with all staff are recommended to keep everyone aware of the numbers of active

Box 4: Viral screening tests

Description	Concerns	Implications
Antibody serology test Detects antibodies present in the blood soon after infection or vaccination.	• Cannot distinguish between current coronavirus infection or vaccination [7]. • Negative result can emerge if resident is tested during window of antibody development	• While of value, such testing cannot be completely relied upon due to variability in individual's ability to generate antibody [4,12]. • Those with negative results should still be subject to protective measures.
Viral COVID test Detects presence of virus through use of real-time reverse-transcriptase polymerase chain reaction.	• Will likely require a laboratory outside the facility.	• Nasal swabbing may be uncomfortable for residents. • Rather than a specific viral test, may be more beneficial to consider use of a screening panel to assess for other causative agents.

cases, suspected cases, isolations, and relocations of the facility. Transparency will help avoid rumors or feelings of distrust.

Screening and testing of older adults
Why are we so concerned? Navigating symptoms, symptom severity and progression related to COVID versus age-related changes (change in function)––it is reasonable to suspect.

Screening and testing methods are an important part of maintaining vigilance against infection, but each approach has its values and limitations. Continuous screening is necessary throughout a resident's stay during a pandemic situation. It should consist of a regular checklist of assessments, and determinations for testing. Some signs and symptoms are tried and true warnings of infection in younger adults and children but provide confusing information in the case of older adults. The following screening steps are examples.

Hazards of over-reliance on fever in assessment
Fever for example, is widely being used as a screen for COVID-19 infection in the general population. In some cases, screening temperatures with a hand-held or wall device is used to allow admission to facilities if no temperature elevation is detected. This screening approach, while useful in younger or middle-aged persons, is less reliable as a person ages. Clinical studies, done two decades ago, showed that older adult body temperatures run a lower baseline and age incrementally produces a lower febrile response for each decade of life [12]. The older adult is therefore less likely to mount a temperature elevation, even if infected. The exact mechanisms for this decline have been speculated more recently to implicate immunosenescence as the source of this blunted febrile response [4]. To use body temperature as a screen for elevation in an older adult requires a record of an individualized "norm" for that older resident. Keeping track of their non-febrile or "well" baseline temperatures, with any detectable increase, will be more meaningful when combined with the more reliable surrounding signs and symptoms of any suspected illness. Other important signs of infection in older adults besides temperature elevation are generalized malaise, loss of appetite, acute cognitive changes and/or increase in respiratory rate (tachypnea) at rest.

Non-specific signs of infection do not designate the presence of infection, nor can they specify COVID-19 or coronavirus infection specifically. However, they can signal a need for action, which may include observation, specific testing, relocation, isolation, or even evaluation for a different infection source. Some of these signs of infection are shown by older adults, without an infection, and with possibility of blunted febrile response, can challenge assessment. However, the key to recognition is greater severity and often the confluence of several signs at once.

Testing for coronavirus disease-2019 in nursing homes
As with all guidelines for testing, screening, immunizing and treatment of COVID-19, the prudent IPC Manager will follow evolving CDC, CMS, and

State guidelines that are often reported as "Interim" recommendations. New testing measures and devices are under research and development by government, academic, and commercial groups, but the two most prevalent in use today are the antibody serology test and the viral COVID-19 test of respiratory secretions (see Box 3 [6,13,14]).

Communicating the differences in test capabilities to residents, visitors, and personnel can help them understand why many quarantine decisions are necessary:

Testing of older adults in nursing homes
- The IPC Manager will ideally align CDC recommendations [13,14] with state and federal requirements to clarify process for testing residents.
  - Triggers for testing (eg, routine admission to facility, symptoms consistent with COVID-19, new resident with active infection in facility).
  - Identify available access to tests capable of viral tests and arrangements with laboratories to process or carry out and process point-of-care tests on-site.
  - Establish the process and capacity to perform testing for all residents and staff.
  - Train health care staff to collect and process specimens correctly and safely using personal protective equipment.
  - Prepare health care staff to deal with situations where residents decline or refuse to be tested.
  - Prepare a plan for responding to test results before initial testing.
- The IPC Manager will periodically explore additional information about testing residents by State and local health departments and other nursing homes.

Management: isolation and cohorting

Isolation is seldom a possibility when residents or new admissions rapidly multiply. Cohorting refers to the grouping of individuals with the same condition in the same location (eg room, wing, or building). Concerning this article, the term cohorting refers to keeping residents who are COVID-19 positive or are suspected to have COVID-19 in the same space (wing, floor, etc.), that is separate from those who are COVID-19 negative or do not have exposure to COVID-19. Cohorting was a universal prevention and control approach from the World Health Organization (WHO) early in the COVID-19 pandemic [15]. It continued as part of a national disaster mitigation strategy recommended by the Centers for Medicare and Medicaid Services (CMS), the American Health Care Association (AHCA), and the National Center for Assisted Living, to deal with the US outbreak in skilled nursing facilities and long-term settings [6,15]. Cohorting was also a strategy recommended by the CMS in their *COVID-19 Long Term Care Facility Guidance alert* with actions needed to prevent the virus transmission [2]. This announcement included unprecedented flexibility with blanket waivers allowing facilities to transfer residents within the facility, to another facility, or to other non-certified locations to cohort older adults based on their COVID-19 status [2].

Cohorting patients is not a new approach; it has long been used in hospitals to locate patients, with the same or similar conditions, in the same space for efficiency, specialization of staff, and proximity to condition-specific equipment. In pandemics, however, the primary reason for cohorting in nursing homes is to reduce or prevent interaction between infected and uninfected residents. Rates of morbidity and disease severity are particularly high for older adults during outbreaks of infectious diseases because of their age, comorbidities, and associated immunosenescence.

A collaborative model. The declaration of COVID-19 as a US national emergency was followed by a collective outbreak of new cases in Michigan nursing homes, where cases rose from 1 case to 1,035 cases in two weeks [16,17]. Three nursing homes in southeast Michigan took rapid action to cohabit that provides a model of collaboration, cooperation, and communication with positive containment of spread. It involved moving together residents from across facilities into categories of positive infection, need for isolation, and freedom from infection. Moving, isolation, and separation from familiarity provided some downsides for residents and staff, and these are issues that also bear consideration in one-facility cohorting [13,14]. The report credits the preexistence of the collaborations of local hospitals and public health officials, infectious disease experts, and an academic health system, for their impressive outcomes to lower mortality and reduce hospitalization. These affiliations were reasons for choosing cohorting as a reasonable way to mitigate transmission. But recognition of the power of collaboration offers lessons about the need for heightened readiness to meet possible resurgence or new mutant strains of existing infectious diseases. The key in this case was proactive collaboration across local skilled nursing facilities, hospitals, laboratory services, parent corporations and health care providers. Laboratory testing for the SARS-CoV-2 positive residents by the local the hospital is also credited for early identification, testing at points of prevalence, and cohorting of infected patients. Environmental cleaning and protected traffic patterns for staff and provided separate entry and exits to the facility.

Isolation and cohorting of residents within the facility
Given the lack of preexisting facility collaborations, most nursing homes are faced with decisions of how to manage isolation and cohorting in their own facility. CMS offers some guidance in recommending a period of assessment for all new admissions or transfers. If space allows, a separate area, or if this is not possible, waivers in the codes are recommended that would allow them to be observed in a separate facility [12]. The availability of rapid diagnosis is difficult for nursing homes without close or affiliated laboratories. But as unit-based tests for COVID-19 become more reliable and available, they will become essential to streamline the process of triage and identification of infected residents. In the meantime, one hospital has developed a triage tool that uses physical signs (temperature, cough, shortness of breath, myalgia, sore throat), computed tomography (CT) of chest (pneumonia), low lymphopenia, neutrophilia, and existing comorbid conditions, to categorize patients into four groups: (1) high risk of poor outcome/low risk of infection, (2) low risk of

poor outcome/high risk of infection, (3) low risk of poor outcome/low risk of infection, and (4) low risk of poor outcome/high risk of infection. This kind of categorization, administered in the emergency department with a nursing home resident becomes ill, may be a useful way of early assessment that necessitates hospital admission for those at highest risk while identifying those needing cohort accommodation in the nursing home.

Resident perspectives of cohorting. Two action points designated by the CMS Coronavirus Commission for Safety and Quality in Nursing Homes [1] address the tensions existing between rigorous infection control measures and quality of life issues that exist in cohorting and visitation policies. Their recommendations and action steps reflect the intent to update cohorting guidance to balance resident and staff psychological safety with IPC. Action steps are to prioritizes resident social and emotional health and minimize disruption of resident daily routines. They point out the need to be transparent with the needs of isolation or cohorting, and any possibilities of moving to different facilities [1]. The Michigan example also emphasizes the anticipatory *Collaboration* as key to their project's success, and addresses the value in partnering with local agencies, care facilities, and care providers in a way not addressed by the CMS Commission [2]. Communication methods included in this report were emphasized between residents, health care personnel, and families, informing all of the planned response. Residents received updates of their testing results or exposure to infected roommates. Additional daily communication with other skilled nursing facilities not only kept them informed, it allowed these allied groups to plan a collaborative response that included allocation of personal protection equipment (PPE), distribution of staffing (nurses, nurse assistants, occupational and physical therapists, and equipment technicians) across facilities. Universal testing of residents allowed mapping of prevalence at specific points. Separate break rooms, eating areas, and free meals and beverages were provided to dedicated COVID unit staff, with incentive pay for dedicated nursing staff. These attributes were only possible by cooperation and shared responsibility with preexisting partnerships that are a model for possible preparation for an uncertain future in infectious disease.

SUMMARY

The impact of viral infections to the older adult residing within the long-term care setting poses a significant threat not only to their physical health, but to their emotional well-being. Although beneficial for containing viruses, primary care providers' use of isolation or other cohorting measures described in this article can cause emotional damage. These measures must be instituted along with practice measures to ensure regular human contact [18]. Many of the frail older adults residing in long-term care are particularly vulnerable to social isolation and feelings of loneliness because of their limited mobility, reduced stamina or fatigue. The presence of cognitive impairment compounds limitations in mobility and significantly increases risk of loneliness or isolation—especially if they are placed in isolation. All residents placed in isolation will be susceptive to social isolation. Research evidence has shown frail older adults who are lonely or socially isolated experience higher rates of mortality [16]. In response to the National Workforce Recommendations made by the Coronavirus Commission For Safety And Quality In Nursing Homes, the panel of Nurse Experts in Aging of the American Academy of Nursing developed a must-read of important guidelines for practitioners working with older residents in long-term care settings [18]. These guidelines detail nursing interventions such as frequent communication and reassurance, walking rounds, daily contact with trusted significant others and altering the plan of care to focus on bedside nursing care. These nursing interventions are protective measures which caregivers may use to keep the resident engaged with staff, family caregivers and significant others. The family nurse practitioner working as primary provider in the long-term care setting must use the public health framework of primary, secondary and tertiary levels of prevention to contain the virus, screen at-risk residents for social isolation and enact protective measures.

CLINICS CARE POINTS: IMMUNOSENESCENCE
Nursing leadership needs to maintain an awareness of the risks posed by immunosenescence, not only in terms of increased risk for acquisition of coronavirus disease-2019 (COVID-19) but infection in general. Key points for leadership to remain focused upon:

1. Progressive immunosenescence raises the vulnerability of the older adult resident, regardless of vaccination status.
2. Blunted febrile responses makes fever a less reliable indicator of infection in older adults.
3. Older adults should be regularly screened for other indicators of infection besides a febrile response, such as loss of appetite, cognitive changes and/or tachypnea at rest.
4. Immunosenescence poses a unique risk for the development of viral infection.
5. Vaccination of the older adult provides some seroprotection but may require a repeat immunization 6 to 7 months later.
6. Mutations in viruses (COVID-19 and influenza) require boosters and repeat vaccination when available.
7. Antibody tests are unable to distinguish COVID-19 from other coronavirus infection.
8. An aging staff force is also at risk for viral infection along with residents.

CLINICS CARE POINTS: IMPLICATIONS FOR LEADERSHIP
1. Nursing leadership needs to maintain an effective tracking system for not only routine immunization but for tracking of pandemic-associated vaccination and monitor for symptom development.
2. Awareness is needed related to concerns tied to testing, and effective testing plan needs to be established for each setting.
3. An infection prevention and control (IPC) Manager is a key person to stay abreast of local, state, and national information to guide care.

4. The IPC Manager is necessary to coordinate, consult, and communicate with personnel, residents, and families in an informative, transparent manner.
5. Some residents will not be able to understand or tolerate masking. Seeing others masked may be confusing or frightening to cognitively impaired residents. Alternative considerations require leadership investigation.
6. Maintaining an isolated location is the safest way to protect the older adult but can deeply affect the quality of life for the resident and the family, and lead to social isolation, depression, and worsening mobility.
7. Keeping a reliable cohort of infection-free personnel to attend uninfected and infected cohorts of residents is desirable.

DISCLOSURE

The authors have no financial or commercial conflicts associated with the information presented in this article.

References

[1] Aiello A, Farzaneh F, Candore G, et al. Immunosenescence and its hallmarks: how to oppose aging strategically? A review of potential options for therapeutic intervention. Front Immunol 2019;10:2247.
[2] Coronavirus Commission for Safety and Quality in Nursing Homes Commission Final Report 2020 Available at: https://sites.mitre.org/nhcovidcomm/. Accessed January 11, 2023.
[3] Oh SJ, Lee JK, Shin OS. Aging and the immune system: the impact of immunosenescence on viral infection, immunity and vaccine immunogenicity. Immune Netw 2019;19(6):e37.
[4] Martín S, Pérez A, Aldecoa C. Sepsis and immunosenescence in the elderly patient: a review. Front Med 2017;4:20.
[5] Joshi SR, Shaw AC, Quagliarello VJ. Pandemic influenza H1N1 2009, innate immunity, and the impact of immunosenescence on influenza vaccine. Yale J Biol Med 2009;82(4): 143–51.
[6] Doria-Rose N, Suthar MS, Makowski M, et al. Antibody Persistence through 6 Months after the Second Dose of mRNA-1273 Vaccine for Covid-19. N Engl J Med 2021; https://doi.org/10.1056/NEJMc2103916.
[7] (CDC, 2019). Re: COVID-19 Risks and Vaccine Information for Older Adults Available at: https://www.cdc.gov/aging/covid19/covid19-older-adults.html. Accessed January 11, 2023.
[8] (CDC, 2019). Re: Symptoms of Covid-19 Available at: https://www.cdc.gov/coronavirus/2019-ncov/symptoms-testing/symptoms.html. Accessed January 11, 2023.
[9] Ceban F, Ling S, Lui LMW, et al. Fatigue and cognitive impairment in Post-COVID-19 Syndrome: A systematic review and meta-analysis. Brain Behav Immun 2022;101:93–135.
[10] Böger B, Fachi MM, Vilhena RO, et al. Systematic review with meta-analysis of the accuracy of diagnostic tests for COVID-19. Am J Infect Control 2021;49(1):21–9.
[11] Ouslander JG, Grabowski DC. COVID-19 in Nursing Homes: Calming the Perfect Storm. J Am Geriatr Soc 2020;68(10):2153–62.
[12] Roghmann MC, Warner J, Mackowiak PA. The relationship between age and fever magnitude. Am J Med Sci 2001;322(2):68–70.
[13] Interim Guidance for Managing Healthcare Personnel with SARS-CoV-2 Infection or Exposure to SARS-CoV-2. Available on the Internet at: https://www.cdc.gov/coronavirus/2019-ncov/hcp/guidance-risk-assesment-hcp.html#. Accessed January 11, 2023.
[14] Centers for Disease Control and Prevention. Testing guidelines for nursing homes : interim SARS-CoV-2 testing guidelines for nursing home residents and health care personnel (2020). Available at: https://www.cdc.gov/coronavirus/2019-ncov/hcp/infection-control-recommendations. Accessed January 11, 2023.

[15] Centers for Disease Control and Prevention. CDC 24/7: Saving Lives PP. Updated Health care Infection Prevention and Control Recommendations in Response to COVID-19 Vaccination. Centers for Disease Control and Prevention. Updated April 22, 2021. Available at: Centers for Disease Control and Prevention (cdc.gov). Accessed January 11, 2023.

[16] Hoogendijk EO, Smit AP, van Dam C, et al. Frailty Combined with Loneliness or Social Isolation: An Elevated Risk for Mortality in Later Life. J Am Geriatr Soc 2020;68(11):2587–93.

[17] Gray-Miceli D, Bouchaud M, Mitchell AB, et al. Caught off guard by covid-19: Now what? Geriatr Nurs 2020;41(6):1020–4.

[18] Bakerjian D, Boltz M, Bowers B, et al. Expert nurse response to workforce recommendations made by The Coronavirus Commission For Safety And Quality In Nursing Homes. Nurs Outlook 2021;69(5):735–43.

Advances in Family Practice Nursing 5 (2023) 41–53

ADVANCES IN FAMILY PRACTICE NURSING

Mild Cognitive Impairment in Older Adults

Melodee Harris, PhD, RN[a,*], Janet Rooker, MNSc, RNP[a],
Linda J. Keilman, DNP, RN, GNP-BC[b]

[a]University of Arkansas for Medical Sciences College of Nursing, 4301 West Markham Street Slot #529, Little Rock, AR 72205, USA; [b]Michigan State University, College of Nursing, 1355 Bogue Street, A126 Life Sciences, East Lansing, MI 48824, USA

Keywords

- Mild cognitive impairment • Dementia • Mild neurocognitive disorder
- Major neurocognitive disorder • Subjective cognitive decline • Normal cognition

Key points

- Mild cognitive impairment (MCI) is not dementia.
- MCI is often unrecognized, undiagnosed, and untreated.
- Dementia is a generalized term whereas Alzheimer's disease is a specific brain disease.
- There are no evidence-based interventions to prevent MCI.
- More research is needed to prevent the progression of MCI to dementia.

INTRODUCTION

Compared with Alzheimer's disease, mild cognitive impairment (MCI) is not well understood [1]. To begin, dementia is a general or umbrella term whereas Alzheimer's disease is a specific brain disease. MCI is an enigma to many health care providers (HCPs), patients, and the public who must distinguish between normal aging, dementia, and what lies in between. MCI is often unrecognized, undiagnosed, and untreated.

One in 100 people age successfully without developing cognitive impairment [2]. The prevalence of MCI is 6.7% to 25.2% in adults older than 60 years of age [3]. It is estimated that adults 65 years and older are twice as likely to have MCI rather than dementia [4]. It is estimated that 5 million Americans are living with a diagnosis of MCI attributed to Alzheimer's disease [5].

*Corresponding author. E-mail address: harrismelodee@uams.edu

https://doi.org/10.1016/j.yfpn.2023.01.003
2589-420X/23/

According to surveys conducted by the Alzheimer's Association across racial and ethnic populations, less than 20% of Americans (one in five) are aware of MCI, 43% have never heard of MCI and 55% perceive MCI as normal aging [5]. A diagnosis of MCI due to Alzheimer's disease is described as worrisome for 42% of Americans [5]. Survey data show that minority populations worry more about a diagnosis of MCI attributed to Alzheimer's dementia (50% Asian, 49% Hispanic, 47% Black and 41% American Indian) than white populatins (39%) [5]. Overall, even though Americans may not understand the diagnosis, over half of those who have MCI (54%) want to know if they have Alzheimer's disease compared with 15% of Americans who have a diagnosis of late-stage Alzheimer's disease [5].

MCI is not dementia and is not a specific disease state. MCI is a syndrome [6]. A syndrome is a group of signs and symptoms that do not have a determined underlying cause. Not all persons living with MCI will convert to a dementia. Each year, there are 10% to 15% of persons living with MCI that converts to dementia [5]. Within 5 years from diagnosis, one-third of persons living with MCI progress to some type of dementia [5,7]. This article is a primer on the definition, early recognition, diagnosis, and treatment guidelines for MCI.

DEFINITION

MCI is a neuropsychological (cognition and behavior) syndrome [1]. Mild neurocognitive disorder (NCD) and MCI are two closely associated terms and are used interchangeably. According to the Diagnostic and Statistical Manual of Mental Disorders (DSM)-IV, mild NCD is based on a signal criterion or testing score [6,8]. The DSM-5 expands the meaning of mild NCD to include cognitive and related criteria [6,8]. The term MCI refers to the older adult population based on research that supports the concept [6]. Mild NCD refers to a cognitive state across the lifespan [6,8]. Mild NCD is interchangeable with MCI as used by the DSM-5 [1,8]. Although not agreed upon by all experts, the term MCI is more widely used [6].

There are two types of MCI: amnestic MCI and non-amnestic MCI [8,9]. Memory is impaired in amnestic MCI; there is no impairment in non-amnestic MCI [8,9]. MCI can coexist with mood disorders such as depression and anxiety that may be present early in the diagnosis [8]. Apathy, sleep disorders, and behavioral symptoms may also occur [8]. Fig. 1 is a schematic representation of the MCI subtypes.

RISK FACTORS

MCI is a risk factor for dementia [10]. Depression, anxiety, and apathy [10] are neuropsychiatric symptoms that are common in MCI and may lead to disease progression and dementia. Age is a strong risk factor for mild and major NCDs [6]. Genetic risk factors also play a role. Beta-amyloid is a potential biomarker for Alzheimer's disease and dementia [6,11]. In one study that collected genetic data, apolipoprotein E (APOE) was associated with the progression of MCI to dementia [12]. Other risk factors include mental and physical conditions

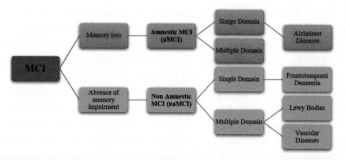

Fig. 1. MCI subtypes. (*From* Tomino C, Ilari S, Solfrizzi V, et al. Mild cognitive impairment and mild dementia: the role of ginkgo biloba (EGb 761®). Pharmaceuticals (Basel) 2021;14(4):305. Published 2021 Apr 1. https://doi.org/10.3390/ph14040305.)

including medications, social isolation, depression, sedentary lifestyle, diabetes, smoking, hypertension, and high cholesterol [5]. Fig. 2 depicts the risk factors for possible MCI development.

PREVALENCE

The prevalence of MCI increases with age [9,13]. Because MCI occurs long before dementia appears [14], the prevalence of MCI is greater in adults younger than 65 years old [5]. The prevalence of MCI is lower in persons with higher levels of education [13]. MCI is more common in men [9,15]. Amnestic MCI is the most common subtype of MCI [14].

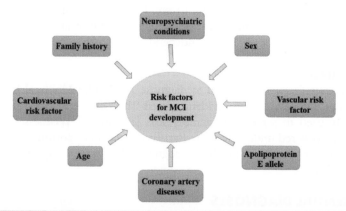

Fig. 2. Risk factors for MCI development. (*From* Tomino C, Ilari S, Solfrizzi V, et al. Mild cognitive impairment and mild dementia: the role of ginkgo biloba (EGb 761®). Pharmaceuticals (Basel) 2021;14(4):305. Published 2021 Apr 1. https://doi.org/10.3390/ph14040305.)

PATHOPHYSIOLOGY

The diagnosis of MCI was initially based on the clinical presentation without including any evidence for biomarkers [14]. The pathophysiology of MCI is multifactorial [14]. The hallmark of MCI is amyloid-beta plaques throughout the brain [14]. In early phases of disease pathology, amyloid is seen in the neocortex, then in the allocortices, and into the basal ganglia, thalamus, and hypothalamus [14]. In the fourth phase, amyloid is found in the midbrain and medulla oblongata; in the fifth stage, the pons and cerebellum [14]. It is unknown if amyloid is generated from dying neurons or precisely how amyloid plays a role in dementia [14]. Amyloid beta plaques occur long before the disease manifests in cognitive decline [14]. Genetic factors also play a role in the initiation of amyloid as a trigger for dementia [14]. Oxidative stress and inflammation is thought to play a role in MCI as well [9].

SYMPTOMS

In MCI, changes are subtle. Symptoms may not be detected by family, caregivers, or friends [8]. Persons living with MCI may describe daily tasks as becoming more difficult, taking longer to perform, and requiring accommodations to complete them [8]. Neuropsychiatric symptoms that sometimes occur with dementia are also present in MCI [10]. Anxiety, depression, and apathy are common neuropsychiatric symptoms that can simultaneously occur with MCI [10]. In fact, compared with normal cognition, persons living with MCI experience higher rates of depression [10]. Symptoms may be undetected by HCPs or attributed to a variety of medical or mental health conditions [8]. The focus must be on changes rather than lifelong characteristics [8]. The person may not seek help until later stages of the disease process. It is imperative for HCPs to monitor older adults regularly and closely for changes in cognitive function, physical function, and behavior to avoid the progression of the syndrome [9]. In contrast with Alzheimer's disease, symptoms are typically less severe, personality changes do not occur, and independent function is maintained [16].

SCREENING

Memory screening tests are used to diagnose MCI. The Montreal Cognitive Assessment (MoCA) is an evidence-based (EB) 30-item assessment tool commonly used to screen for memory loss [3]. Annual Wellness Examinations/Visits (covered under Medicare Part B) include an opportunity for assessing memory. For suspicion of MCI or cognitive deficits, it is important to refer to a specialist.

DIFFERENTIAL DIAGNOSES

There are several cognitive states in the differential diagnoses for MCI including normal and subjective cognitive impairment as well as dementia [3,17]. Depression, anxiety, and other mental health conditions are also a consideration. Persons with normal cognition and depression or apathy, experience higher rates of progression to MCI [10]. Delirium is also in the differential. Normal cognition is the product of successful/optimal aging and occurs when neuropsychiatric testing and performance of activities of daily living (ADLs) are intact [17]. Subjective cognitive decline is a self-report of a personal experience without any objective testing [18]. One in nine adults reports subjective cognitive decline [19].

DIAGNOSIS

It is important for HCPs to recognize MCI early and make a diagnosis of MCI subtypes as well as differentiating between normal cognition, subjective cognitive impairment, and dementia [1]. The following criteria meet the requirement for a diagnosis of MCI.

- Complaint of a defective memory
- Normal ADLs
- Normal general cognitive function
- Absence of dementia [20].

The DSM-5 defines MCI (also referred to as mild NCD) as the evidence of modest cognitive decline from a previous level of performance in one or more cognitive domains (complex attention, executive function, learning and memory, language, perceptual motor, or social cognition) based on.

1. Concern of the individual, a knowledgeable informant, or the HCP that there has been a mild decline in cognitive function.
2. A modest impairment in cognitive performance, preferably documented by standardized neuropsychological testing or, in its absence, another quantified clinical assessment.
3. Evidence of decline above what is expected for age without crossing over to the diagnostic dementia range.

   In addition, the following criteria must also be considered.

   - The cognitive deficits do not interfere with the capacity for independence in everyday activities (ie, complex instrumental activities of daily living [IADLs] such as paying bills or managing medications are preserved, but greater effort, compensatory strategies, or accommodation may be required)
   - The cognitive deficits do not occur exclusively in the context of a delirium
   - The cognitive deficits are not better explained by another mental disorder (eg, major depressive disorder, schizophrenia, etc.) [8].

The diagnosis of subtypes is based on cognitive, behavioral, and functional symptoms to differentiate etiologies for neurodegeneration such as Alzheimer's disease, Parkinson's disease, Lewy body dementia, frontotemporal lobar (frontal/temporal lobes) dementia (sometimes referred to as Pick's disease), and other dementias [8]. Amnestic and non-amnestic are two subtypes of MCI [1]. Persons living with amnestic MCI have the same underlying pathophysiology as dementia [1]. In amnestic MCI, memory is affected [5]. Non-amnestic MCI involves skills that do not involve memory such as visual perception, making decisions, or the ability to judge time [5].

Diagnostic guidelines for MCI include an abnormal cerebral spinal fluid (CSF) test for amyloid-beta protein or a positron emission tomography (PET) scan [5]. Amyloid-beta protein is a biomarker for Alzheimer's disease [5].

WORKUP

A thorough health/medical workup is critical in the careful consideration of MCI and cannot be overestimated. A data baseline should be established for comparison on follow-up visits. Neuropsychiatric testing early in the disease process is imperative [8]. Family, caregivers, and friends may provide important and useful observations and pertinent information–utilize their input [5]. Symptoms due to brain tumors can mimic neuropsychiatric symptoms of dementia. Magnetic resonance imaging (MRI–with and without contrast, as indicated) can rule out tumors, vascular conditions such as stroke, and detect cerebral atrophy associated with dementia. A flurodeoxyglucose (FDG)–-PET will show hypometabolism of glucose in areas of the brain associated with Alzheimer's disease [6]. Table 1 lists the components of an appropriate and thorough assessment/workup for MCI, which may not occur all in one visit. The primary goal of the workup is to differentiate MCI from normal aging or dementia and to identify possible reversible forms of MCI related to other conditions (infection, renal failure, vitamin/mineral deficiencies, and hypo/hyper calcium, glucose, magnesium, and thyroid) [8,21].

TREATMENT

Early diagnosis is critical for initiating treatment before the progression to dementia occurs [5]. International and national EB guidelines vary [1]. Historically, research has focused on risk reduction [1]. A multimodal approach is used for treatment to include appropriate nutrition and hydration, physical activity, brain health activities, mental stimulation, social engagement, and QOL [1]. HCPs *must individualize* treatment based on unique patient symptoms [1].

SUPPLEMENTS AND MEDICATIONS

There are no specific Food and Drug Administration (FDA)-approved medications to treat MCI [9]. Ginko Biloba leaf extract (EGb 761) has been studied extensively; more research is needed to support its use in MCI [9]. Diabetes is a risk factor for MCI [5]. One example of research on pharmacology and MCI is a randomized double-blind clinical trial ($n = 289$) on intranasal insulin with participants diagnosed with MCI and Alzheimer's disease, conducted at 27 clinical sites [28]. After 12 months of treatment with intranasal insulin, data analyzed on MRI and CSF biomarkers did not show any cognitive benefit [28]. Donepezil (aricept) was also studied. Because it is thought that cognitive deficits associated with MCI are not due to cholinergic dysfunction, anticholinesterase inhibitors are not effective in deterring MCI [4]. It is thought the hippocampus and cortical cholinergic projection system provides compensatory

Table 1
Workup Components for Possible Mild Cognitive Impairment

Assessment Components	
Health history: *comprehensive, detailed, in-depth, subjective and objective data, holistic, age-appropriate, formative, and person-centered*	Head-to-toe physical examination (PE): *comprehensive, individualized to the unique person*
• Reason for visit or presenting illness; the "persons story"	• Vital signs
• Past health and surgical history	• Height/weight/body mass index (BMI)
• Family health history	• Current level of comfort
• Social history	• Inspection ⎫
• Social determinants of health (SDOH)	• Palpation ⎬ *Appropriate to*
• Allergies with reactions/consequences	• Percussion ⎬ *body region and*
• Vaccinations	• Auscultation ⎭ *organ system*
• Medications	
• Nutrition intake including fluids	• Observation
• Physical activity	• Head, neck, eyes, ears, nose, oral cavity/ mouth, and throat
• History of falls, fear of falling (FOF)	• Lungs
• Sleep pattern	• Heart
• Socialization/engagement	• Abdomen
• Sexual orientation and gender identity (SO/GI)	• Skin
• Relationship status including sexual activity and pertinent sexual habits	• Genitalia
• Religion/faith/spirituality	• Musculoskeletal
• Safety/prevention interventions in place	○ Agility
• Occupation—past and current	○ Endurance
• Work/life balance	○ Flexibility
• Hobbies/areas of interest	○ Range of motion (ROM)
• Psychological well-being	○ Stamina
• Determine how the individual defines themself related to their health	○ Strength
• Life/health values and meaningful goals	• Neurological
• Advance care planning (ACP)	○ Cranial nerves
○ Advance directives	○ Gait (balance and coordination)
	○ Mental status:
	■ Folstein test
	■ MoCA
	○ Motor system
	○ Reflexes
	○ Sensory system
	○ Station
Functional assessment: *measures level of function and ability to consistently perform daily tasks; use of EB tools, patient or others reports; can be accomplished during history and PE*	Mental status examination: *structured; can help distinguish between mood disorders, thought disorders, and cognitive impairment* [22]
• Ability to perform ADLs and IADLs	• Abstract reasoning
• Continence	• Alertness
• Living environment (home, work, etc.)	• Appearance
• Mental status (cognition and affect)	• Attentiveness
	• Attitude and insight
	(continued on next page)

Table 1
(continued)

Assessment Components	
• Mobility • Nutrition • Social support • Socialization and engagement • Vision and hearing Some EB tools to consider: • Brody IADL scale • Functional activities questionnaire • Katz index of independence in ADLs	• Behavior (overall) • Constructional ability and praxis • Language • Level of consciousness (LOC) • Memory • Mood • Motor and speech activity • Thought and perception

Mood and affect: *affect is the outward expression of current emotions and feelings; mood is the sustained emotional makeup of one's overall personality and how they view the world*
• Anxiety: includes generalize anxiety disorder (GAD), phobias, posttraumatic stress disorder (PTSD), pain disorder, and obsessive–compulsive disorder (OCD) [24]
  ○ Davison Trauma Scale (DTS) [25]
  ○ GAD-7
  ○ Geriatric Anxiety Inventory (GAI)
  ○ PTSD Scale for DSM-5 (CAPS-5) [25]
• Depression [26]
  ○ Beck Depression Inventory (BDI)
  ○ Center for Epidemiologic Studies Depression Scale (CES-D)
  ○ Geriatric Depression Scale (GDS)
  ○ Patient Health Questionnaires (PHQ-2; PHQ-9)
	Laboratory testing: *individualized; completed to rule out potentially reversible forms of MCI* [21]
	• Complete blood count (CBC)
	• Electrolytes
	• Glucose
	• Calcium
	• Thyroid function
	• Vitamins D and B12
	• Others as indicated

Medication Review: *specific classes and combinations of medications contribute to cognitive impairment* [21]
• Current and past prescriptions
• Herbal and homeopathic use
• Home remedies
• Lotions, rubs, and ointments
• Over-the-counter
• Vitamin/mineral supplements
Brown bag medication review: asking patients to bring all their medications (as above) to their health care appointment and review everything in the "brown bag" with them [27]
	Biomarkers: *measurable indicators of what is going on in the body; when combined with other diagnostic tests may help determine whether an individual has risk factors for possibly developing some of the dementias* [23]
	• Blood
	  ○ Limited; guidelines available through the Food and Drug Administration (FDA); not routinely used
	• Body fluids
	  ○ Cerebrospinal fluid (CSF): looking for changes in levels of fluid; lumbar puncture (spinal tap)
	• Organs
	• Tissues

(continued on next page)

Table 1 (***continued***)
Assessment Components

Brain imaging [23]: *techniques that determine the interaction between brain tissue and forms of energy*
- *Computerized tomography* (CT): uses radiation to produce images of the brain and other body parts
- MRI: use of magnetic fields and radio waves produce detailed images of the brain including the size, shape, and brain regions
- *Positron emission tomography* (PET): radioactive substance (tracer) measures specific activity or molecule in different brain regions
  - *Amyloid PET scans*: measure abnormal deposits of beta-amyloid and presence of amyloid plaques (hallmark of Alzheimer's disease)
  - *Tau PET scans*: detect abnormal accumulation of tau protein—tangles within nerve cells
  - *FDG-PET scans*: measure energy use in the brain including amount of glucose present

mechanisms that delay the transition from MCI to dementia [4]. Guidelines address that research on pharmacological interventions, such as donepezil, does not show conclusive evidence of benefit for MCI [29].

However, pharmacological research is beginning to show more promise. Aducanumab (aduhelm) is the first FDA-approved infusion that is indicated for persons living with MCI or early-stage Alzheimer's disease [30]. Lecanemab (leqembi) is another study drug that reduces amyloid levels in persons with MCI and early Alzheimer's disease [30]. Amyloid-related imaging abnormalities, known as ARIA, are a side effect of aducanumab and lecanemab [30]. More research is needed to determine the safety and efficacy of these monoclonal antibody infusions [30].

NONPHARMACOLOGICAL INTERVENTIONS

Because there are no pharmacological treatments to prevent MCI from progressing to dementia, lifestyle changes are very important [31]. Although there is no research to support causality, physical activity shows a protective factor against converting from MCI to dementia [31]. Nonpharmacological interventions are important in the treatment of MCI. Physical activity is shown to lower the risk of Alzheimer's disease in persons living with MCI [31]. A Consensus Study Report appointed by the National Academies of Sciences, Engineering, and Medicine (formerly the Institute of Medicine) showed encouraging but inconclusive, evidence that blood pressure (BP) control, physical activity, appropriate nutrition, hydration, music therapy, brain health activities, and cognitive training may prevent MCI [32,33].

CORONAVIRUS DISEASE-2019

In one cross-sectional survey study of caregivers of loved ones living with MCI or dementia ($n = 204$), results showed an overall decline (78.8%) attributed to a lack of support resources (59.7%) [34]. Specific decline was noted in mood, communication, movement, and adherence to COVID-19 protocols [34]. The study also showed there was an increase in physical (64.7%) and psychological (80%) caregiver burden during this time [34].

TRANSITION TO DEMENTIA

There is no evidence from randomized controlled trials to support utilizing pharmacological or nonpharmacological interventions to prolong the transition from MCI to dementia [1]. Although evidence is inconclusive, research shows that BP control, physical activity, and cognitive training show promise for the prevention of dementia [32]. Although the cognitive function may stay the same or improve in persons with MCI, during 1 year it is estimated that 10%-20% of adults age 65 or older transition from MCI to dementia [35]. Owing to the lack of standardized screening, diagnostic testing, differences in population settings, and changes in guidelines, there are various rates of conversion from MCI to dementia [7]. Cognitive reserve takes education level into account and is an important factor in converting from MCI back to normal cognition [17]. Results from the Nun Study showed for those with higher education levels, a 30.3% transition from MCI to normal cognition occurred; 83.9% never developed dementia [17]. Approximately 21% of older adults with normal cognition progress to MCI, and when compared with normal cognition, those with MCI are 2.8 times more likely to progress to dementia [36]. Approximately half (47%) of those with MCI remain unchanged; 31% return to normal cognition [36]. Impaired cognition and language were predictors for transition to dementia [36]. One study ($n = 688$) of cognitively intact older adults who were taking anticholinergic medications, were at increased risk for progressing to MCI, especially those with CSF biomarkers and APOE genotypes; an important issue to acknowledge in support of deprescribing [37]. Medications and managing/treating conditions such as depression can reverse MCI [2]. However, MCI is a risk factor for dementia [10]. Neuropsychiatric symptoms such as depression, apathy, and anxiety can contribute to further cognitive decline and dementia [10].

SUMMARY

There is a need to operationalize MCI and standardize treatment globally. Mild NCD, as presented in the DSM-5, is more inclusive and may better reflect international common denominators [6]. More research is needed due to the growing population of older adults, the increasing prevalence of MCI, and the need to prevent the conversion of MCI to dementia. Treatment of MCI may serve the following goals.

1. Symptom improvement including cognitive function, and
2. Disease modification that would prevent or delay further cognitive decline and progression to a dementia diagnosis [1].

As HCPs, the responsibility to reach the above goals is within the advanced practice registered nurse (APRN) scope of practice. Therefore,

APRNs have an ethical obligation to make a difference in the lives of older adults facing cognitive decline that can potentially be prevented, controlled, or reversed. The use of EB guidelines, along with practicing holistic, compassionate, person-centered care, is the foundation for moving forward and making a difference in older adults' mental health, well-being, and QOL. APRNs CAN!

CLINICS CARE POINTS

- Early identification of MCI and referral to specialists is vital to an appropriate plan of care.
- Differentiate MCI from Major Neurocognitive Disorder.

DISCLOSURE

The authors have no financial or commercial conflicts associated with the information presented in this article.

References

[1] Kasper S, Bancher C, Eckert A, et al. Management of mild cognitive impairment (MCI): the need for national and international guidelines. World J Biol Psychiatry 2020;21(8): 579–94.

[2] Petersen RC. Mild cognitive impairment. N Engl J Med 2011;364:2227–34.

[3] Jongsiriyanyong S, Limpawattana P. Mild cognitive impairment in clinical practice: a review article. Am J Alzheimers Dis Other Demen 2018;33(8):500–7.

[4] Mufson EJ, Counts SE, Perez SE, et al. Cholinergic system during the progression of Alzheimer's disease: therapeutic implications. Expert Rev Neurother 2008;8(11): 1703–18.

[5] 2022 Alzheimer's disease facts and figures. Alzheimer's Dement. 2022;18(4):700–89.

[6] Stokin GB, Krell-Roesch J, Petersen RC, et al. Mild neurocognitive disorder: an old wine in a new bottle. Harv Rev Psychiatry 2015;23(5):368–76.

[7] Ward A, Tardiff S, Dye C, et al. Rate of conversion from prodromal Alzheimer's disease to Alzheimer's dementia: a systematic review of the literature. Dement Geriatr Cogn Dis Extra 2013;3(1):320–32.

[8] American Psychiatric Association. In: Neurocognitive disorders. Diagnostic and Statistical Manual of Mental Disorders: DSM 5. 5th edition. Arlington VA; 2013. p. 591–644.

[9] Tomino C, Ilari S, Solfrizzi V, et al. Mild cognitive impairment and mild dementia: the role of ginkgo biloba (EGb 761®). Pharmaceuticals 2021;14(4):305.

[10] Ma L. Depression, anxiety, and apathy in mild cognitive impairment: current perspectives. Front Aging Neurosci 2020;12:9.

[11] Jack CR Jr, Knopman DS, Jagust WJ, et al. Hypothetical model of dynamic biomarkers of the Alzheimer's pathological cascade. Lancet Neurol 2010;9(1):119–28.

[12] Angevaare MJ, Vonk JMJ, Bertola L, et al. Predictors of incident mild cognitive impairment and its course in a diverse community-based population. Neurology 2022;98(1):e15–26.

[13] Sachdev PS, Lipnicki DM, Kochan NA, et al. The prevalence of mild cognitive impairment in diverse geographical and ethnocultural regions: the COSMIC collaboration. PLoS One 2015;10(11):e0142388.

[14] Mufson EJ, Binder L, Counts SE, et al. Mild cognitive impairment: pathology and mechanisms. Acta Neuropathol 2012;123(1):13–30.

[15] Petersen RC, Roberts RO, Knopman DS, et al. Prevalence of mild cognitive impairment is higher in men. The Mayo Clinic Study of Aging. Neurology 2010;75(10):889–97.

[16] National Institute of Health. What is mild cognitive impairment 2021. Available at: https://www.nia.nih.gov/health/what-mild-cognitive-impairment. Accessed January 08, 2023.

[17] Iraniparast M, Shi Y, Wu Y, et al. Cognitive reserve and mild cognitive impairment: predictors and rates of reversion to intact cognition vs progression to dementia. Neurology 2022;98(11):e1114–23.

[18] Howard R. Subjective cognitive decline: what is it good for? Lancet Neurol 2020;19(3): 203–4.

[19] Centers for Disease Control and Prevention (CDC). Subjective cognitive decline. Available at: https://www.cdc.gov/aging/data/subjective-cognitive-decline-brief.html. Accessed January 08, 2023.

[20] Petersen RC, Smith GE, Waring SC, et al. Aging, memory, and mild cognitive impairment. Int Psychogeriatr 1997;9(S1):65–9.

[21] Langa KM, Levine DA. The diagnosis and management of mild cognitive impairment: a clinical review. JAMA 2014;312(23):2551-1561.

[22] Snyderman D, Rovner BW. Mental status examination in primary care: a review. Am Fam Physician 2009;80(8):809–14.

[23] National Institute of Aging. How biomarkers help diagnose dementia 2022. Available at: https://www.nia.nih.gov/health/how-biomarkers-help-diagnose-dementia. Accessed January 08, 2023.

[24] The Centre for Addiction and Mental Health. Anxiety in Older Adults. Available at: https://www.camh.ca/en/health-info/guides-and-publications/anxiety-in-older-adults. Accessed January 08, 2023.

[25] American Psychological Association. PTSD Assessment Instruments. Available at: https://www.apa.org/ptsd-guideline/assessment. Accessed January 08, 2023.

[26] American Psychological Association. Depression Assessment Instruments. Available at: https://www.apa.org/depression-guideline/assessment. Accessed January 08, 2023.

[27] Agency for Healthcare Research and Quality. Brown Bad Medication Review. Available at: https://health.gov/hcq/trainings/pathways/assets/pdfs/AHRQ-Tool8.pdf. Accessed January 08, 2023.

[28] Craft S, Raman R, Chow TW, et al. Safety, efficacy, and feasibility of intranasal insulin for the treatment of mild cognitive impairment and Alzheimer disease dementia: a randomized clinical trial. JAMA Neurol 2020;77(9):1099–109.

[29] Petersen RC, Lopez O, Armstrong MJ, et al. Practice guideline update summary: Mild cognitive impairment: report of the guideline development, dissemination, and implementation subcommittee of the american academy of neurology. Neurology 2018;90(3):126–35.

[30] van Dyck CH, Swanson CJ, Aisen P, et al. Lecanemab in Early Alzheimer's disease [published online ahead of print, 2022 Nov 29]. N Engl J Med 2022; https://doi.org/10.1056/NEJMoa2212948.

[31] Kim YJ, Han KD, Baek MS, et al. Association between physical activity and conversion from mild cognitive impairment to dementia. Alzheimer's Res Ther 2020;12(1):136.

[32] National Academies of Sciences, Engineering, and Medicine 2017. Preventing cognitive decline and dementia: a way forward. Washington, DC: The National Academies Press; 2017; https://doi.org/10.17226/24782. Accessed January 08, 2023.

[33] Yang J, Chen J, Lui Y, et al. Integrated nonpharmacological intervention for patients with MCI—a preliminary study in Shanghai, China. Int J Integr Care 2022;1(21):1–10.

[34] Tsapanou A, Papatriantafyllou JD, Yiannopoulou K, et al. The impact of COVID-19 pandemic on people with mild cognitive impairment/dementia and on their caregivers. Int J Geriatr Psychiatry 2021;36(4):583–7.

[35] National Institute of Aging. What is mild cognitive impairment?. Available at: https://www.alzheimers.gov/alzheimers-dementias/mild-cognitive-impairment. Accessed January 08, 2023.
[36] Manly JJ, Tang MX, Schupf N, et al. Frequency and course of mild cognitive impairment in a multiethnic community. Ann Neurol 2008;63(4):494–506.
[37] Weigand AJ, Bondi MW, Thomas KR, et al. Association of anticholinergic medications and AD biomarkers with incidence of MCI among cognitively normal older adults. Neurology 2020;95(16):e2295–304.

Advances in Family Practice Nursing 5 (2023) 55–65

ADVANCES IN FAMILY PRACTICE NURSING

Heart Failure in Older Adults

Margaret T. Bowers, DNP, FNP-BC, CHSE, AACC

Division of Cardiology at Duke Health, Duke University School of Nursing, 307 Trent Drive, Durham, NC 27710, USA

Keywords
- Heart failure • Heart failure with reduced ejection fraction
- Heart failure with preserved ejection fraction • Older adults • Universal definition

Key points
- Discuss new heart failure definitions and stages.
- Discuss therapeutic treatments for heart failure including newer medications.
- Describe considerations for treatment when caring for older adults with heart failure in the ambulatory setting.
- Apply a triage strategy to correlate signs and symptoms of heart failure to determine the appropriate treatment setting.

INTRODUCTION

Heart failure (HF) is a clinical syndrome that is associated with a shorter life-span and the prevalence increases in adults over the age of 60 and almost double in those over the age of 80 [1]. In recent years, universal definitions for HF have been introduced to further delineate specific phenotypes [2]. As the incidence of HF continues to rise with age, there are opportunities for nurse practitioners to use a nuanced approach in caring for older adults and to intervene focusing on early identification for the prevention and treatment of HF. Using the universal definitions along with HF stages and New York Heart Association (NYHA) classification can be beneficial in guiding care.

Pathophysiology

HF results from structural and/or functional changes in the heart and may be accompanied by systemic or pulmonary or systemic congestion and confirmed with an increased level of natriuretic peptide levels [2]. There are a multitude of cardiovascular and non-cardiovascular etiologies that should be considered

---

E-mail address: margaret.bowers@duke.edu

https://doi.org/10.1016/j.yfpn.2022.11.008
2589-420X/23/© 2022 Elsevier Inc. All rights reserved.

when evaluating a patient with HF. Cardiovascular diagnoses include CAD, valvular disease, hypertension, congenital heart lesions, arrhythmias, and non-cardiovascular diagnoses include thyroid disorders, anemia, iron overload, metabolic, diabetes mellitus, alcohol, cardiotoxic medication, peripartum, and infiltrative diseases [3,4].

There are two primary etiologies of HF, ischemic or idiopathic dilated cardiomyopathy, with reduced left ventricular pumping resulting in an increase in preload and reduced stroke volume. The second is a result of hypertrophic, hypertensive or restrictive cardiomyopathy with impaired ventricular filling. The terms systolic and diastolic HF have been updated to HF with reduced ejection fraction (HFrEF) and HF with preserved ejection fraction (HFpEF), respectively, to further describe the structural and functional changes in the heart.

Ischemia from coronary artery disease triggers a cascade of events that lead to activation of the renin-angiotensin-aldosterone system (RAAS) as well as stimulation of catecholamines ultimately resulting in fluid retention with associated natriuretic peptide levels and a reduction in cardiac output and can lead to HFrEF. This cascade of neurohormonal activation results in elevated pressures in the pulmonary vascular system with resultant congestion and/or increased right-sided pressures in the heart with subsequent systemic and hepatic congestion [4].

The increase in systemic vascular resistance associated with prolonged hypertension may result in left ventricular hypertrophy and impaired cardiac filling leading to the development of HFpEF with shifts in pressure/volume curves causing systemic and pulmonary congestion. Endothelial dysfunction triggers a cascade of cardiovascular responses including inflammation in the coronary microvasculature [5]. Hypertrophy of cardiac myocytes and inflammatory cytokines that increase oxidative stress all contribute to the development of HFpEF [5]. It is evident that the pathophysiology of both HFrEF and HFpEF are complex systems that have both cardiac and systemic effects.

Definitions and classifications

In 2021, universal definitions of HF were identified to provide improved clarity on differentiating patient populations and treatment approaches. According to Savarese and colleagues [6], normal EF in women is between 54% to 74%, and in men 52% to 72%. Table 1 provides a framework to facilitate a clinical approach however, there are factors beyond ejection fraction that need to be considered. Patients may have a combination of echocardiographic changes including a low ejection fraction and reduced diastolic filling. In this situation, the approach would be for a patient with HFrEF to consideration of factors that exacerbate HFpEF.

The American College of Cardiology (ACC) and American Heart Association (AHA) designed a classification system that associates disease pathophysiology and clinical status to describe disease progression and guide treatment [2] (Table 2).

Table 1
Universal heart failure definitions (data from 2/6)

HF with reduced ejection fraction (HFrEF)	EF ≤ 40%
HF with mildly reduced ejection fraction (HFmrEF)	EF 41% to 49%
HF with improved ejection fraction (HFimpEF)	Baseline EF ≤ 40% with a 10-point increase from baseline and subsequent measurement >40%
HF with preserved ejection fraction (HFpEF)	EF ≥ 50%

Data from Bozkurt B, Coats AJ, Tsutsui H, et al. Universal Definition and Classification of Heart Failure: A Report of the Heart Failure Society of America, Heart Failure Association of the European Society of Cardiology, Japanese Heart Failure Society and Writing Committee of the Universal Definition of Heart Failure [published online ahead of print, 2021 Mar 1]. J Card Fail. 2021;S1071-9164(21)00050-6; and Savarese, G., Stolfo, D., Sinagra, G. et al. Heart failure with mid-range or mildly reduced ejection fraction. Nat Rev Cardiol. 2022; 19: 100–116.

The NYHA functional class (Table 3) is dynamic and used to provide important information about an individual's ability to perform activities of daily living.

History

Although the etiology of HF is varied, in older adults, HFpEF is seen most often. Patient history may describe symptoms that are acute, chronic, or acute on chronic and the nurse practitioner should determine the phase of HF when triaging a patient. There are a variety of factors that make the diagnosis of HF in older adults challenging including multi-morbidities, cognitive impairment, frailty, and polypharmacy. In older adults, some of the signs and symptoms of decompensated HF may be masked by underlying conditions such as cognitive impairment related to dementia or stroke.

In patients with a prior diagnosis of HF, identifying the precipitant(s) of an acute exacerbation is a key aspect of managing symptoms. Common precipitants include ischemia, uncontrolled hypertension, arrhythmias (most often atrial fibrillation), anemia, acute infection, thyroid disorders, worsening

Table 2
American College of Cardiology and American Heart Association classification system for heart failure

ACC/AHA stage	
A	No structural heart disease or symptoms but at high risk for HF
B	Structural heart disease, elevated natriuretic peptides, or cardiac troponins. No signs or symptoms of HF.
C	Structural heart disease with current or prior HF symptoms.
D	Advanced HF with refractory symptoms

From Bozkurt B, Coats AJ, Tsutsui H, et al. Universal Definition and Classification of Heart Failure: A Report of the Heart Failure Society of America, Heart Failure Association of the European Society of Cardiology, Japanese Heart Failure Society and Writing Committee of the Universal Definition of Heart Failure [published online ahead of print, 2021 Mar 1]. J Card Fail. 2021;S1071-9164(21)00050-6; with permission.

Table 3
New York Heart Association classification

NYHA functional class	Symptoms
I	Able to complete ordinary activities without HF symptoms.
II	Slight limitations in physical activity due to HF symptoms.
III	Significant limitations in physical activity associated with HF symptoms.
IV	HF symptoms at rest. Unable to complete physical activity without HF symptoms

From Bozkurt B, Coats AJ, Tsutsui H, et al. Universal Definition and Classification of Heart Failure: A Report of the Heart Failure Society of America, Heart Failure Association of the European Society of Cardiology, Japanese Heart Failure Society and Writing Committee of the Universal Definition of Heart Failure [published online ahead of print, 2021 Mar 1]. J Card Fail. 2021;S1071-9164(21)00050-6; with permission.

kidney function, medications, such as nonsteroidal anti-inflammatory drugs (NSAIDs) that contribute to decompensation and non-adherence to medications or diet.

HF symptoms in older adults may be overlooked since they can also be a result of normal physiologic changes and/or comorbid conditions. These symptoms include dyspnea, fatigue, and a reduced exercise tolerance. It is crucial to determine the duration of these symptoms to be able to discriminate whether the patient is in acute HF or not. Common symptoms of HF include fatigue, dyspnea, orthopnea, PND, reduced exercise tolerance, and peripheral edema. More recently the term, bendopnea, has been used to describe the breathlessness that occurs within 30 seconds of bending forward and is often seen in older adults with chronic HF [7].

Cognitive impairment in an older adult impacts the ability to obtain a detailed history and input should be sought from family and caregivers. It is important to note that an altered mental status is also a sign of poor cerebral perfusion and may be indicative of an acute HF episode.

In addition to cognitive impairment, older adults may have challenges with vision, hearing, and physical limitations that affect their ability to perform self-care and manage complex medical regimens. Evaluating frailty in an older adult with HF is an important component of assessment. In a systematic review and meta-analysis by Yang and colleagues, frailty posed a higher risk of hospitalization and mortality in patients with chronic HF [8].

Assessment

Physical examination findings that may indicate HF include tachycardia, weak or thready peripheral pulses, elevated jugular venous pressure (JVP), laterally displaced point of maximal intensity reflecting cardiomegaly, extra heart sounds, S3 and/or S4, crackles, hepatomegaly, Hepatojugular reflux, abdominal or peripheral edema.

Initial workup in a patient presenting with symptoms indicative of HF in the ambulatory setting includes a variety of labs and imaging. A comprehensive metabolic panel includes evaluating both hepatic and kidney function, calcium and magnesium, complete blood count, thyroid stimulating hormone, urinalysis, lipid panel, iron studies, and BNP or NT-pro BNP. An electrocardiogram to determine if there are rhythm or ischemic changes and a chest x-ray to evaluate for cardiomegaly and/or pulmonary congestion. A transthoracic echocardiogram (TTE) provides information regarding structural changes in the heart including wall motion, valvular changes, ejection fraction, hypertrophy, and allows the clinician to provide targeted treatment.

Diagnosis

Once the history and clinical data are reviewed a diagnosis of HFrEF, HFmrEF, HFimpEF or HFpEF should guide treatment. This diagnosis does not occur in isolation and is often complicated by other cardiac diagnoses such as atrial fibrillation, coronary artery disease, and hypertension. There are non-cardiac common diagnoses that also compound the treatment of patients with HF such as diabetes mellitus, sleep apnea, kidney disease, and obesity.

Management

HF management requires a multifaceted approach including medications, devices, advanced therapies, goals of care including patient education. Nurse practitioners in primary care play a key role in medication management, establishing goals of care and reinforcing patient education. Collaboration with cardiology providers and HF specialists is important when discussion regarding implantable devices and advanced therapies needs to occur.

Medications

The evidence-based guidelines for HFrEF are well established however there are fewer options for patients with HFpEF. The four pillars of medication (Table 4), which have strong evidence to reduce hospitalizations and improve morbidity and mortality in HFrEF, are as follows: (1) angiotensin neprilysin inhibitor, angiotensin-converting enzyme inhibitor, or angiotensin receptor blocker, (2) beta-blocker, (3) mineralocorticoid receptor antagonist, and (4) sodium-glucose cotransporter 2 inhibitors.

A medication that has been added to the armamentarium of treatments for HFrEF is vericiguat, a soluble guanylate cyclase stimulator that is indicated for symptomatic patients with NYHA Class II-IV symptoms, an EF <45% who require outpatient intravenous diuresis or have been recently hospitalized [9]. This mechanism of action focuses on reducing inflammation, fibrosis, hypertrophy, and relaxation of smooth muscle cells [9]. The most common adverse effects associated with vericiguat are anemia, hypotension, and syncope. This medication is teratogenic and should not be used in pregnant women or those who are breastfeeding. Vericiguat should not be used in patients with hepatic impairment or a GFR < 15 mL/min/ 1.73 m [2].

In the Change the Management of Patients with Heart Failure (CHAMP) registry, in patients with HFrEF, lack of initiation and underdosing are

Table 4
Medications to reduce hospitalizations and improve morbidity and mortality in heart failure with reduced ejection fraction

Medication	Evidence-based dosing range minimum to maximum
Angiotensin neprilysin inhibitor (ARNi)	Sacubitril is combined with Valsartan 24/26 mg twice daily to 97/103 mg twice daily
Angiotensin-converting enzyme inhibitor (ACEi)	Captopril 6.25 mg 3 times daily to 50 mg three times daily
	Enalapril 2.5 mg twice daily to 20 mg twice daily
	Ramipril 1.25 mg daily to 10 mg daily
	Lisinopril 2.5 mg daily to 40 mg daily
Angiotensin receptor blocker (ARB)	Candesartan 4 mg daily to 32 mg daily
	Losartan 25 mg daily to 150 mg (divided doses)
	Valsartan 20 mg twice daily to 160 mg twice daily
Beta-blocker (BB)	Metoprolol succinate 12.5 mg daily to 200 mg daily
	Carvedilol 3.125 mg twice daily to 25 mg twice daily
	Weight ≥ 85 kg 50 mg twice daily
	Bisoprolol 1.25 mg daily to 10 mg daily
Mineralocorticoid receptor antagonist (MRA)	Spironolactone 12.5 mg daily to 50 mg daily
	Eplerenone 25 mg daily to 50 mg daily
Sodium-glucose cotransporter 2 inhibitor	Empagliflozin 10 mg daily
	Dapagliflozin 10 mg daily.
I_f channel inhibitor	Ivabradine 5 mg twice daily to 7.5 mg twice daily
Soluble guanylate cyclase stimulator	Vericiguat 2.5 mg daily to 10 mg daily
Vasodilators	Hydralazine 25 mg three times daily to 75 mg three times daily
	Isosorbide 20 mg three times daily to 40 mg three times daily
	Dinitrate
Digoxin	Lanoxin 0.125 mg daily to 0.25 mg daily

associated with a higher morbidity and mortality [10]. Clinicians may be hesitant to titrate medications in older adults due to concerns about hypotension and potential fall risk [10]. In a patient with HFrEF who does not require immediate decongestion, titration of guideline-directed medical therapy (GDMT) should be done on a weekly or biweekly schedule to achieve the target dose, and hemodynamic stability as tolerated by the patient. This is challenging for NPs managing a multitude of medical problems in primary care settings.

Patients with HFpEF who are symptomatic and have an EF ≥ 50% should be treated with diuretics to manage fluid overload. SGLT2 inhibitors should be considered since the benefit outweighs the risk. The addition of ARNi, MRA, and ARB may be considered however the evidence is not clear regarding the effectiveness of these treatments.

Polypharmacy
Patients with HF often have multiple comorbid conditions that require additional medications. Polypharmacy poses a significant challenge when HF

treatment may require a minimum of five medications. In addition to the number of medications prescribed, there must be a consideration for the financial burden associated with a large pill burden.

In addition to pill burden, there are certain medication classes that should be avoided when treating a patient with HF. NSAIDs are associated with an increased risk of hospitalization and interfere with the RAAS and may promote water and sodium retention and should be avoided [3]. For example, an older adult with severe osteoarthritis and HFrEF who requires pain management to enhance their quality of life should not use an NSAID, instead use acetaminophen and non-pharmalogic treatments. Non-dihydropyridine calcium channel blockers such as diltiazem and verapamil have been associated with HF exacerbations and possible HF hospitalizations and should be avoided in patients with HF.

Devices

A diagnosis of HF is associated with a high risk of sudden cardiac death therefore, implantable devices should also be considered to reduce mortality and/or improve HF symptoms [11]. For patients on GDMT for at least 3 months, 40 days, or more post-myocardial infarction with an EF <30% and greater than 1-year survival referral for an implantable cardioverter/defibrillator should be offered [3,11,12]. Referral for cardiac resynchronization therapy should be considered to improve HF symptoms in a patient with NYHA Class I-III, an EF ≤ 35% on GDMT, and electrocardiogram with a QRS duration of >150 milliseconds to improve symptoms.

Advanced therapies

Recognition of when a patient should be referred for advanced HF therapies can be easily recalled using the mnemonic, "I NEED HELP" (Table 5). Expanded indications for advanced HF therapies such as cardiac transplantation and ventricular assist devices no longer exclude older adults from being

Table 5
Mnemonic for indications of advanced heart failure

I	Intravenous inotropes
N	NYHA class IIIB/IV or persistently elevated natriuretic peptides
E	End-organ dysfunction
E	EF ≤ 35%
D	Defibrillator shocks
H	Hospitalizations >1 for HF in past 12 mo
E	Edema despite escalating diuretics
L	Low systolic blood pressure (≤90 mm Hg), high heart rate
P	Progressive intolerance requiring down-titration of GDMT

Data from Morris, A., Khazanie, P., Drazner, M., Albert, N., Breathett, K., Cooper, L., Eisen, H., O'Gara, P., Russell, S., and on behalf of the American Heart Association Heart Failure and Transplantation Committee of the Council on Clinical Cardiology; Council on Arteriosclerosis, Thrombosis and Vascular Biology; Council on Cardiovascular Radiology and Intervention; and Council on Hypertension. Circulation. 2021;144:e238-e250.

considered. Consultation with advanced HF clinicians is imperative when patients meet the criteria in Table 5.

Goals of care

A shared decision-making approach is recommended in addressing the complex factors that influence how a patient, their family, and caregivers manage an HF diagnosis. Managing symptoms and improving quality of life are hallmarks of HF treatment and in addition to these goals of care, individual patient priorities should be addressed at the outset of the diagnosis. At the onset of the diagnosis, patient and family education should focus on self-care. Specific topics to address include signs and symptoms of worsening HF, medication adherence, dietary sodium restriction, limiting fluid intake, weight monitoring, physical activity as tolerated, smoking cessation, and weight loss if indicated. Referral to cardiac rehabilitation provides a forum for monitored exercise as well as social support.

Patient values, goals, and preferences should be addressed at the onset of an HF diagnosis and be included in an annual wellness visit. The fact that an HF diagnosis is associated with a high mortality, clarifying end-of-life wishes, and addressing palliative care should be part of the goals of care discussion [13–15].

DISCUSSION

Implementing a triage strategy to correlate signs and symptoms of HF to determine the appropriate treatment setting is paramount when practicing in an outpatient clinic. Early recognition of overt and subtle signs of HF decompensation are vital to appropriate triage. What do you do when a patient presents "warm and wet," hemodynamically stable and well perfused but fluid overloaded? Using a simple framework noted in Fig. 1 can assist in this type of triage.

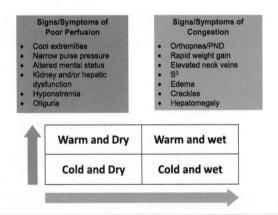

Fig. 1. Triage strategy to correlate signs and symptoms of heart failure.

Table 6	
Determining patient acuity to the appropriate setting of care	
Risk and disposition	Signs and symptoms
High risk/admit to hospital	Hemodynamically unstable—shock, poor perfusion
	Acute conditions—acute coronary syndrome, stroke, sepsis, significant arrhythmia
	Respiratory distress and/or hypoxia
	Anuria
Medium risk/consider hospitalization	New onset HF symptoms
	Hypotension without shock
	Tachycardia
	Hyponatremia
	Kidney or hepatic dysfunction
	Substantial BNP or pro-BNP elevation
	Elevated cardiac troponin without an acute coronary event
Lower risk/refer to HF specialty practice	Hemodynamically stable
	Responds well to IV diuretic with symptomatic improvement
	Stable kidney and hepatic function

In the situation noted above, doubling the diuretic dose for two to 3 days or the addition of a thiazide-like diuretic, metolazone, may facilitate decongestion and the patient can be safely treated in the ambulatory setting. The primary goal of managing HF is to manage patient symptoms. Improving both congestion and perfusion are factors that need to be considered to improve quality of life. The goal is for patients to be well perfused and without congestion, "warm and dry." Patients who are "warm and wet," are hemodynamically stable and may be safely managed in an outpatient setting with diuretic adjustment. Patients who are poorly perfused. "cold" need more advanced therapies which usually include referral to an advanced HF specialist and/or hospitalization.

Implication for advanced practice nurses

As the older adult population continues to increase and the prevalence of HF rises, nurse practitioners need to be prepared to provide evidence-based treatment for this population when they present with HF. Using a straightforward approach to determining patient acuity can facilitate treatment and transition to the appropriate setting of care (Table 6).

SUMMARY

Nurse practitioners in an ambulatory practice, have the opportunity to intervene early in the prevention, detection, and treatment of HF. As the population ages, primary care NPs will be facing an increased prevalence of this chronic condition. Understanding evidence-based HF treatment, setting goals of care and when to refer for advanced therapies are key aspects to consider in this patient population.

CLINICS CARE POINTS

- Changes in mental status, a sign of worsening heart failure may be difficult to evaluate in patients with cognitive impairment.
- Heart failure with preserved ejection fraction is highly prevalent in older adults and often associated with atrial fibrillation.
- Underdosing with guideline-directed medical therapy in patients with heart failure and reduced ejection fraction is associated with higher morbidity and mortality.
- Determining patient acuity with respect to hemodynamic stability, perfusion, and level of congestion should guide risk determination and whether or not the patient should be hospitalized.

Disclosure
The author has nothing to disclose.

References
[1] Liu E, Lampert B. Heart failure in older adults: Medical management and advanced therapies. Geriatrics 2022;7(36):1–11.
[2] Bozkurt B, et al. 2021 Universal Definition and Classification of Heart Failure A Report of the Heart Failure Society of America, Heart Failure Association of the European Society of Cardiology, Japanese Heart Failure Society and Writing Committee of the Universal Definition of Heart Failure. J Card Fail 2021;27(4):387–413.
[3] Heidenreich PA, Bozkurt B, Aguilar D, et al. 2022 AHA/ACC/HFSA Guideline for the Management of Heart Failure: A Report of the American College of Cardiology/American Heart Association Joint Committee on Clinical Practice Guidelines. J Am Coll Cardiol 2022;79(17):e263–421.
[4] Schwinger RHG. Pathophysiology of heart failure. Cardiovasc Diagn Ther 2021;11(1):263–76.
[5] Gevaert A, Boen J, Segers V, et al. Heart failure with preserved ejection fraction: A review of cardiac and noncardiac pathophysiology. Front Physiol 2019;10(638):1–14.
[6] Savarese G, Stolfo D, Sinagra G, et al. Heart failure with mid-range or mildly reduced ejection fraction. Nat Rev Cardiol 2022;19:100–16.
[7] Larina V, Poryadin G, Bogush N, et al. Clinical profile of elderly patients with chronic heart failure and bendopnea. Polish Arch Intern Med 2019;129(12):939–41.
[8] Yang X, Lupond J, Vidan M, et al. Impact of frailty on mortality and hospitalization in chronic heart failure: A systematic review and meta-analysis. J Am Heart Assoc 2018;7:e008251.
[9] Kassis-George H, Verlinden N, Fu S, et al. Vericiguat in heart failure with a reduced ejection fraction: Patient selection and special considerations. Ther Clin Risk Management 2022;18:315–22.
[10] Greene SJ, Butler J, Albert NM, et al. Medical Therapy for Heart Failure With Reduced Ejection Fraction: The CHAMP-HF Registry. J Am Coll Cardiol 2018;72(4):351–66.
[11] Hussein A, Wilkoff B. Cardiac implantable electronic device therapy in heart failure. Circ Res 2019;124:1584–97.
[12] Morris A, Khazanie P, Drazner M, et al. and on behalf of the American Heart Association Heart Failure and Transplantation Committee of the Council on Clinical Cardiology; Council on Arteriosclerosis, Thrombosis and Vascular Biology; Council on Cardiovascular Radiology and Intervention; and Council on Hypertension. Circulation 2021;144:e238–50.

[13] Allen LA, Stevenson L, Grady K, et al. American Heart Association; Council on Quality Care and Outcomes Research; Council on Cardiovascular Nursing; Council on Clinical Cardiology; Council on Cardiovascular Radiology and Intervention; Council on Cardiovascular Surgery and Anesthesia. Circulation 2012;125(15):1928–52.

[14] Ponikowski P, Voors AA, Anker SD, et al. 2016 ESC Guidelines for the diagnosis and treatment of acute and chronic heart failure: The Task Force for the diagnosis and treatment of acute and chronic heart failure of the European Society of Cardiology (ESC). Developed with the special contribution of the Heart Failure Association (HFA) of the ESC. Eur J Heart Fail 2016;18(8):891–975.

[15] Krishnaswami A, Beavers C, Dorsch M, et al. Innovations, Cardiovascular Team and the Geriatric Cardiology Councils, American College of Cardiology. Gerotechnology for older adults with cardiovascular diseases: JACC State-of-the-art review. J Am Coll Cardiol 2020;76(22):2650–70.

Advances in Family Practice Nursing 5 (2023) 67–75

ADVANCES IN FAMILY PRACTICE NURSING

A Life Course Approach to Understanding Urinary Incontinence in Later Life

Thanchanok Wongvibul, PhD Candidate, MSN, RN

College of Nursing, The Ohio State University, 1577 Neil Avenue, Columbus, OH 43201, USA

Keywords

• Life course • Urinary incontinence • Bladder health • Risk factors • Quality of life

Key points

• Risk factors for urinary incontinence (UI) are due to unmodifiable and potentially modifiable factors.

• Unmodifiable factors include age, gender, changes in bladder and pelvic floor function, medical conditions, menopause, and history of vaginal delivery, whereas potentially modifiable factors include smoking, alcohol intake, and obesity.

• Influences on bladder health begin during infancy and continue throughout the life span. Bladder anatomy and physiology change as individuals age may contribute to the various syndromes of UI.

• To help people with UI at all stages of life, it is very important to primarily target at preventing or treating the causes identified.

• To improve UI, a life-course approach to modify risk factors may mitigate symptoms later in life.

INTRODUCTION

Background and significance

Urinary incontinence (UI), the complaint of any involuntary leakage of urine, is a highly prevalent condition that affects 20% to 30% of the population during their lifetime [1]. The prevalence of UI is similarly reported in men and women aged older than 80 years. However, before that age, women are 2 to 3 times more likely than men to develop any type of UI [2]. This condition is a major problem in older adults, especially with those who have functional and

E-mail address: wongvibul.1@osu.edu

https://doi.org/10.1016/j.yfpn.2022.11.005
2589-420X/23/© 2022 Elsevier Inc. All rights reserved.

cognitive impairment [3]. Overall, UI can affect up to 30% of community-dwelling older adults and more than 50% of older adults who live in nursing home [2].

UI is a costly condition with annual expenditures similar to other chronic diseases. The cost of UI includes the direct costs of resources for the care or treatment of UI and the indirect costs, which are defined as the loss of productivity due to morbidity or disability [4]. In 2001, the annual direct cost of UI in the United States was estimated at US$16.3 billion, including US$12.4 billion for women and US$3.8 billion for men [5]. Additionally, UI can also lead to a decrease in quality of life (QOL) and stigmatization [6].

Older adults who experience UI can be reluctant to seek help due to embarrassment or a false belief that UI is a normal consequence of aging. However, rather than age itself, the increasing prevalence of UI is actually associated with additional factors and functional impairments associated with aging [7]. Risk factors for UI are due to unmodifiable and potentially modifiable factors. Unmodifiable factors include age, gender, changes in bladder and pelvic floor function, medical conditions, menopause, and history of vaginal delivery, whereas potentially modifiable factors include smoking, alcohol intake, and obesity [8,9].

The purpose of this article is to describe bladder functions as well as the associated factors of UI across the life span. A better understanding of UI serves as a platform to raise awareness among healthy individuals and health-care professionals about the significance of incontinence care and encourage researchers to develop appropriate interventions for reducing UI.

A life course approach to continence care

UI is a common but often underreported medical condition that significantly influences QOL and well-being [10]. The prevalence of UI normally increases because of the risk factors, such as changes in bladder function, education level, number of pregnancies, menopause, and chronic conditions that associated with aging [8,9]. As older adults are more likely to develop UI than any other group, understanding the risk factors associated with UI at the early stage is key to reduce the risk of developing UI and delay the progression of UI symptoms before they worsen once individuals get older. Adopting a life course approach will provide an insight into the impact of biological and behavioral factors on UI across the life span from childhood until old age. By screening individuals for risk factors, especially modifiable ones, and taking actions to minimize the effects of those factors at the early stage, these will potentially prevent or delay the development of UI later in life and lead to the improvement of QOL among individuals who are experiencing UI [9].

Bladder health and urinary incontinence across the life span

Influences on bladder health begin during infancy and continue throughout the life span. Bladder anatomy and physiology changes result in or contribute to the various syndromes of UI [8]. Moreover, bladder habits and dysfunctions at one stage of life may affect bladder health in subsequent stages [11].

Childhood

Influences on bladder health can begin as early childhood. At birth, the bladder capacity is small, and there is a lack of coordination between bladder muscles and sphincter muscles [11]. Without voluntary control, the bladder will empty at higher voiding pressure due to a failure of complete sphincteric relaxation [11]. Up to the age of 5 years, UI is considered as physiologic or normal circumstance. However, after 5 years of age, UI may be classified as pathologic condition due to the delay of neurologic bladder control, discoordinated voiding, infrequent voiding, or structural anatomic and neurologic deficit [12]. There is evidence showing that impaired bladder health during childhood is associated with the presence of lower urinary tract symptoms (LUTS) such as micturition frequency, nocturia, and urgency in adults [13]. Moreover, through hereditary or environmental factors, children of parents with a history of overactive active bladder symptoms including UI are also at increased risk for developing UI [11]. An appropriate toilet training program is needed for children aged beginning at 21 to 36 months [14]. Children need to master several different skills, such as recognizing signals of a full bladder and postponing urination until they can reach the toilet to achieve bladder control [14].

Adolescence

Although there is a lower prevalence of UI in adolescence, persistent UI in childhood is associated with an increased risk of daytime incontinence in adolescence and adulthood [15]. Besides the demographic and environmental factors, such as, family history and female gender, bladder conditions in adolescents are also related to behavioral and physical factors [11]. For example, bathroom restriction imposed by teachers within schools can be a risk factor for daytime UI in school-age children [15]. In addition, stress UI or a leakage of urine during moments of physical activity contributes to UI in adolescent female athletes in gymnastics, track and field, basketball, or other impact sports [16]. These exercises may lead to sufficient increase in intra-abdominal pressure, which causes changes in the urethral sphincteric unit, resulting in UI [16]. Adolescents, who carry UI to adulthood or old age, can be considered similar to those with a chronic illness due to the possible disruption of developmental changes, body image, and socialization [17]. Therefore, public awareness and early detection of UI among adolescents is critical to prevent and delay the development of UI.

Adulthood and old age

Age-related changes in structure and function of the urinary system can begin at the age of 20 years and become more common by the age of 40 years [18]. Normally around 10% of adults experience UI, and the incidence increases with age [19]. This condition is often dismissed as a normal part of aging. However, the increasing prevalence of UI is actually associated with additional comorbidities and functional impairments that accompany growing older [7]. Age-related changes affect the central nervous system that control bladder function and the bladder structures, such as decreased awareness of bladder filling, increased frequency of involuntary detrusor contractions, decreased power of bladder contractions, and decreased muscle tone in pelvic floor muscles contribute to the high prevalence of LUTS in older adults [11,20]. UI in older adults is commonly associated with the negative effects on physical and psychosocial dimensions of health-related QOL [21]. Physical consequences of UI include an increase in falls, functional decline, and nursing home admission [22]. Moreover, UI also triggers psychosocial distress, such as anxiety, embarrassment, social isolation, and depression [22].

Associated factors of urinary incontinence across the life span
Unmodifiable factors
Pregnancy and delivery. In addition to age-related physiologic changes, pregnancy is considered a strong risk factor for UI in women [23]. During pregnancy and delivery, factors including changes in hormonal and ureterovesical angles, anatomic defects developing after delivery, increased pressure on levator muscles and ligaments, and changes in connective tissues may lead to temporary or long-lasting UI [24]. The prevalence of UI increases from 55.1% in the first to 70.1% in the third trimester [25]. The mean prevalence doubles in the vaginal delivery group compared with the cesarean section group [11]. Most of the women who have UI during pregnancy normally return to full continence after delivery because the stretched muscles and tissues recover. However, women who had a vaginal delivery tend to have a higher likelihood of persistent UI after giving birth. There is evidence showing that UI after childbirth can last 12 years or longer [26]. In addition, higher body mass index (BMI), greater parity as well as older maternal age at first birth are also found to be strongly associated with persistent UI [26].

Menopause. Menopause is one of the natural and normal life stages of women. Estrogen, decreases as a result of menopause, causes vaginal atrophy, reduces supportive tissues surrounding the urethra, weakens pelvic muscles, and may consequently increase tendency for UI [27]. In addition, during this period, estrogen deficiency may also affect other hormones and metabolism, resulting in obesity, which is one of the risk factors of UI. The prevalence of UI in menopausal women ranges from 9% to 69% [27], and stress incontinence is more prevalent during the menopause [28].

Medical conditions. Numerous comorbidities, such as Parkinson disease, Alzheimer disease (AD), cerebrovascular disease, diabetes mellitus (DM), hypertension, obstructive sleep apnea, and normal-pressure hydrocephalus, are associated with UI [8]. DM can lead to alterations in detrusor muscle function, innervation, and function of the neuronal component due to microvascular damage, which results in urge incontinence [29]. Meanwhile, the causes of UI associated with AD may stem from cognitive and functional impairment of neurodegenerative processes, or the medical treatment [30]. The relationship between hypertension and UI is less established than that in other medical conditions but there is evidence showing that high-blood pressure accompanies bladder receptor dysfunction that influences the lower urinary system [31]. Beside these medical conditions, other prevalent risk factors of UI described in men are prostate cancer and its treatment [32]. UI is one of the most common and serious side effects that occurs with prostate cancer following treatments, such as radical prostatectomy, radiotherapy, and cryotherapy [33]. Persistent UI affects most patients following the radical prostatectomy due to damage occurring to the striated muscle fibers of the urinary sphincter mechanism and its innervation [34]. In addition, UI may also develop because of tumor progression following active surveillance or from bladder neck and sphincter involvement in advanced disease [34].

Potentially modifiable factors
Smoking
Tobacco is a contributing factor for stress incontinence. The risk of stress incontinence is positively correlated with both the current intensity of cigarette consumption and the lifetime exposure to cigarette smoking [35]. Smoking can affect the lower urinary system by altering the vascular or microvascular supply to the bladder and pelvic muscle. It can increase abdominal pressure secondary to pulmonary-related disease or coughing, which results in UI [31]. Moreover, smoking is the most important known risk factor for bladder cancer, which might increase the risk for UI because of tumor pressure in the spine or near the bladder [36].

Alcohol consumption
The association between alcohol consumption and UI is unclear. Several studies show a direct effect of alcohol on UI [37,38]. However, some studies reported greater urine loss in participants who drink alcohol [31]. Therefore, alcohol alone may not cause UI but it may be a trigger for those who are prone to bladder leaks. Because alcohol is a diuretic, it might increase urine production and detrusor instability [31]. In addition, it can also irritate the bladder and worsen symptoms of overactive bladder [39].

Obesity
Some studies show that obesity and overweight are directly associated with new onset UI or incident UI. For example, there was a clear dose–response effect of weight on UI with each 5-unit increase in BMI associated with about a 20% to 70% increase in the risk of UI [40]. However, the mechanism of the association of obesity and incontinence is imprecise. Excess body weight may increase abdominal pressure and results in increased bladder pressure and mobility of the urethra [33]. Moreover, insulin resistance and oxidative stress are other mechanisms that may cause vascular damage and lead to the pelvic floor and detrusor muscles impairment [33].

Management principles of urinary incontinence
Prevention is a key factor at all phases of life to decrease the prevalence of UI for older adults. The assessment of UI in older adults must include an evaluation of comorbidities, medications, functional, and cognitive impairment [8].

Generally, the evaluation of UI should be systematic and contain history, medical history, review of systems, social history, physical examination, investigations, and treatment expectations [19]. Providers should focus on the important elements including timing and frequency of UI symptoms, type, and severity of UI [19,41] Moreover, urodynamic studies can also determine the precise cause of UI and plan for an appropriate treatment [8].

The main treatments of UI are pharmacologic and nonpharmacological treatments [42]. Pharmacologic treatments include medications and hormone replacement to treat UI symptoms, whereas the nonpharmacological treatments include physical activity along with lifestyle and behavioral modifications [43]. Nonpharmacological treatments are first line because the benefits are associated with low risk of harm and limited expenses. Physical activities and lifestyle changes such as having proper nutrition, smoking cessation, reduced alcohol intake, fluid restriction, and weight loss are recognized as beneficial guidelines to reduce UI episodes [8]. In addition, other nondrug interventions for UI include scheduled voiding, prompted voiding (PV), bladder training, and pelvic floor muscle exercise (PFME) have also been shown to be effective in improving UI [19]. PV alone or PV with exercise is associated with modest and short-term improvements of UI in older adults [44]. Meanwhile, PFME through a trained practitioner helps relieve UI symptoms in women with stress and mixed UI [45].

Pharmacologic treatment may be considered if nonpharmacological therapy alone is not effective. For urge and mixed incontinence, Antimuscarinic drugs such as oxybutynin, tolterodine, solifenacin, darifenacin, tropism chloride, and fesoterodine can be prescribed for urge and mixed incontinence [19]. Choice of agent may depend on providers' experience and preference, individual preference, formulary coverage, and insurance coverage [19]. However, pharmacologic therapy must be approached very carefully in older adults. The basic prescribing principle, start low and go slow, avoids potential side effects [46]. Finally, if UI is resistant to both nonpharmacological and pharmacologic treatments, surgical techniques may be considered as a third option [47]. However, the clinicians should discuss adverse effects with patients before the surgery.

SUMMARY
UI is a condition, which can occur in both men and women across the life span. The prevalence of UI generally increases with age because age is often associated with factors that predispose older adults to UI. These factors include changes in bladder and pelvic floor function, medical conditions, number of pregnancies, and menopause. Other potentially modifiable factors include smoking, alcohol intake, and obesity. At each stage of life, treatment of UI should target at preventing or treating the causes identified. Therefore, a better understanding of UI through a life-course approach is helpful for health-care professionals to develop early interventions for reducing UI and improve QOL.

IMPLICATION FOR ADVANCED PRACTICE REGISTERED NURSES

A life-course approach is successful for modifying risk factors, such as encouraging exercises and bladder trainings, optimizing diet, smoking cessation, reducing alcohol intake, and controlling weight mitigate UI symptoms. Before the treatment of UI, it is very important for health-care professionals to carefully evaluate the history and classify symptoms. Nonpharmacological treatments should be provided before the initiation of pharmacologic treatment because the benefits are associated with low risk of harm and limited expenses. Specific needs, preferences, functional abilities, and cognitive function of older adults should be considered when selecting treatment. Adverse effects, resulting from a medication or other interventions should also be explained and discussed with the patients before starting the treatment.

CLINICS CARE POINTS

- Treatment for UI depends on the type of incontinence, its severity and the underlying cause.
- It is very crucial for health-care professionals to carefully evaluate the history and classify symptoms before treating UI in older adults.
- When selecting the treatment, specific needs, preferences, functional abilities, and cognitive function of older adults should also be considered.
- Nonpharmacological treatments, such as, physical exercise, lifestyle modification, and bladder training should be first recommended as self-care treatments. If these treatments do not work, other options, including medicines and surgery may be suggested.
- Adverse effects, resulting from a medication or other interventions should always be explained and discussed before starting the treatment.

References
[1] Du C, Lee W, Moskowitz D, et al. I leaked, then I Reddit: experiences and insight shared on urinary incontinence by Reddit users. Int Urogynecol J 2020;31(2):243–8.
[2] Cook K, Sobeski LM. Urinary incontinence in older adult. Pharmacology Self-Assessment Program. Available at: https://www.accp.com/docs/bookstore/psap/p13b2_m1ch.pdf. Accessed June 25, 2022.
[3] Tak EC, van Hespen A, van Dommelen P, et al. Does improved functional performance help to reduce urinary incontinence in institutionalized older women? a multicenter randomized clinical trial. BMC Geriatr 2012;12:51.
[4] Hu TW, Moore K, Subak L, et al. Economics of incontinence. Available at: https://www.ics.org/Publications/ICI_2/chapters/Chap14.pdf. Accessed April 21, 2022.
[5] Wilson L, Brown JS, Shin GP, et al. Annual direct cost of urinary incontinence. Obstet Gynecol 2001;98(3):398–406.
[6] Taylor DW, Cahill JJ. From stigma to the spotlight: a need for patient-centred incontinence care. Healthc Manage Forum 2018;31(6):261–4.
[7] DuBeau CE. Beyond the bladder: management of urinary incontinence in older women. Clin Obstet Gynecol 2007;50(3):720–34.

[8] Demaagd GA, Davenport TC. Management of urinary incontinence. P T 2012;37(6): 345–361H.

[9] Xue K, Palmer MH, Zhou F. Prevalence and associated factors of urinary incontinence in women living in China: a literature review. BMC Urol 2020;20(1):159.

[10] Biswas B, Bhattacharyya A, Dasgupta A, et al. Urinary incontinence, its risk factors, and quality of life: a study among women aged 50 years and above in a rural health facility of west bengal. J Midlife Health 2017;8(3):130–6.

[11] Ellsworth P, Marschall-Kehrel D, King S, et al. Bladder health across the life course. Int J Clin Pract 2013;67(5):397–406.

[12] Schultz-Lampel D, Steuber C, Hoyer PF, et al. Urinary incontinence in children. Dtsch Arztebl Int 2011;108(37):613–20.

[13] Fitzgerald MP, Thom DH, Wassel-Fyr C, et al. Childhood urinary symptoms predict adult overactive bladder symptoms. J Urol 2006;175(3 Pt 1):989–93.

[14] Rogers J. Daytime wetting in children and acquisition of bladder control. Nurs Child Young People 2013;25(6):26–33.

[15] Nieuwhof-Leppink AJ, Schroeder RPJ, van de Putte EM, et al. Daytime urinary incontinence in children and adolescents. Lancet Child Adolesc Health 2019;3(7):492–501.

[16] Greydanus DE, Patel DR. The female athlete. Before and beyond puberty. Pediatr Clin North Am 2002;49(3):553.

[17] Luo Y, Zou P, Wang K, et al. Prevalence and associated factors of urinary incontinence among Chinese adolescents in Henan province: a cross-sectional survey. Int J Environ Res Public Health 2020;17(17):6106.

[18] Chmielewski P, Strzelec B, Borysławski K, et al. Effects of aging on the function of the urinary system: longitudinal changes with age in selected urine parameters in a hospitalized population of older adults. Anthropological Rev 2016;79(3):331–45.

[19] Bettez M, Tu le M, Carlson K, et al. 2012 update: guidelines for adult urinary incontinence collaborative consensus document for the canadian urological association. Can Urol Assoc J 2012;6(5):354–63.

[20] Siroky MB. The aging bladder. Rev Urol 2004;6(Suppl 1):S3–7.

[21] Ko Y, Lin SJ, Salmon JW, et al. The impact of urinary incontinence on quality of life of the elderly. Am J Manag Care 2005;11(4 Suppl):S103–11.

[22] Goode PS, Burgio KL, Richter HE, et al. Incontinence in older women. JAMA 2010;303(21):2172–81.

[23] Jean-Michel M, Kroes J, Marroquin GA, et al. Urinary incontinence in pregnant young women and adolescents: an unrecognized at-risk group. Female Pelvic Med Reconstr Surg 2018;24(3):232–6.

[24] Kocaöz S, Talas MS, Atabekoğlu CS. Urinary incontinence in pregnant women and their quality of life. J Clin Nurs 2010;19(23–24):3314–23.

[25] Moossdorff-Steinhauser HFA, Berghmans BCM, Spaanderman MEA, et al. Urinary incontinence during pregnancy: prevalence, experience of bother, beliefs, and help-seeking behavior. Int Urogynecol J 2021;32(3):695–701.

[26] MacArthur C, Wilson D, Herbison P, et al. Urinary incontinence persisting after childbirth: extent, delivery history, and effects in a 12-year longitudinal cohort study. BJOG 2016;123(6):1022–9.

[27] Dinc A. Menopause and urinary incontinence. In: Milchev P, Lukpanovna N, Sancar B, et al, editors. Recent studies in health sciences. Sofia (Bulgaria): St. Kliment Ohridski University Press; 2019. p. 341–50.

[28] Kirss F, Lang K, Toompere K, et al. Prevalence and risk factors of urinary incontinence among Estonian postmenopausal women. Springerplus 2013;2:524.

[29] Izci Y, Topsever P, Filiz TM, et al. The association between diabetes mellitus and urinary incontinence in adult women. Int Urogynecol J Pelvic Floor Dysfunct 2009;20(8):947–52.

[30] Lee HY, Li CC, Juan YS, et al. Urinary incontinence in Alzheimer's disease. Am J Alzheimers Dis Other Demen 2017;32(1):51–5.

[31] John G. Urinary incontinence and cardiovascular disease: a narrative review. Int Urogynecol J 2020;31(5):857–63.

[32] Fernández-Cuadros ME, Nieto-Blasco J, Geanini-Yagüez A, et al. Male urinary incontinence: associated risk factors and electromyography biofeedback results in quality of life. Am J Mens Health 2016;10(6):NP127–35.

[33] Grise P, Thurman S. Urinary incontinence following treatment of localized prostate cancer. Cancer Control 2001;8(6):532–9.

[34] Parsons BA, Evans S, Wright MP. Prostate cancer and urinary incontinence. Maturitas 2009;63(4):323–8.

[35] Bump RC, McClish DK. Cigarette smoking and urinary incontinence in women. Am J Obstet Gynecol 1992;167(5):1213–8.

[36] The American Cancer Society. Bladder and bowel incontinence Updated February 1, 2020. Available at: https://www.cancer.org/treatment/treatments-and-side-effects/physical-side-effects/stool-or-urine-changes/bladder-incontinence.html#written_by. Accessed June 25, 2022.

[37] Lee AH, Hirayama F. Is alcohol consumption associated with male urinary incontinence? Low Urin Tract Symptoms 2011;3(1):19–24.

[38] Lee AH, Hirayama F. Alcohol consumption and female urinary incontinence: a community-based study in Japan. Int J Urol 2012;19(2):143–8.

[39] Dallosso HM, Matthews RJ, McGrother CW, et al. The association of diet and other lifestyle factors with the onset of overactive bladder: a longitudinal study in men. Public Health Nutr 2004;7(7):885–91.

[40] Subak LL, Richter HE, Hunskaar S. Obesity and urinary incontinence: epidemiology and clinical research update. J Urol 2009;182(6 Suppl):S2–7.

[41] Wilson JA, Waghel RC. The Management of urinary incontinence. 2016. Available at: https://www.uspharmacist.com/article/the-management-of-urinary-incontinence. Accessed June 25, 2022.

[42] Balk EM, Rofeberg VN, Adam GP, et al. Pharmacologic and nonpharmacologic treatments for urinary incontinence in women: A systematic review and network meta-analysis of clinical outcomes. Ann Intern Med 2019;170(7):465–79.

[43] Talley KMC, Wyman JF, Bronas U, et al. Defeating urinary incontinence with exercise training: Results of a pilot study in frail older women. J Am Geriatr Soc 2017;65(6):1321–7.

[44] Roe B, Flanagan L, Maden M. Systematic review of systematic reviews for the management of urinary incontinence and promotion of continence using conservative behavioural approaches in older people in care homes. J Adv Nurs 2015;71(7):1464–83.

[45] Singh N, Rashid M, Bayliss L, et al. Pelvic floor muscle training for female urinary incontinence: Does it work? Arch Gynecol Obstet 2016;293(6):1263–9.

[46] Kim S, Liu S, Tse V. Management of urinary incontinence in adults. Aust Prescr 2014;37:10–3.

[47] Downey A, Inman RD. Recent advances in surgical management of urinary incontinence. F1000Res 2019;8:F1000, Faculty Rev-1294.

Advances in Family Practice Nursing 5 (2023) 77–91

ADVANCES IN FAMILY PRACTICE NURSING

The Three-Generation Pedigree
Elucidating Family Disease Patterns to
Guide Genetic Screening, Testing, and Referral

Laura Hays, PhD, APRN, CPNP-PC

College of Nursing, University of Arkansas for Medical Sciences, 4301 West Markham Street Slot 529, Little Rock, AR 72205, USA

Keywords
- Family history • Genetic counseling • Gene/environment disease
- Advanced practice registered nurse • Clinical decision making • Pedigree
- FH taking • Genetic testing

Key points

- Family history pedigrees are three-generation pictoral diagrams of an individual's (the proband) biological relatives, with attached pertinent health information.

- Comprehensive family histories in pedigree form aid primary care providers identify patterns of disease and recognize individuals who may benefit from genetic services.

- Family histories are dynamic, and must be continually updated to remain accurate; collecting family histories must be intentionally prioritized in primary care practices.

- Advanced practice registered nurses are well-positioned in primary care settings to advantage the clinical utility of the three-generation pedigree, increasing health care quality and outcomes for individuals and populations.

INTRODUCTION

The completion of the Human Genome Project in the 1990s [1] propelled our abilities to decipher genetic influences on disease, allowing us to predict risk for certain individuals or populations according to their genotypes. The advanced science also allows identity of increased population or subpopulation rare genetic variant carrier status. Therefore opportunities for screening and testing

E-mail address: lhays@uams.edu

https://doi.org/10.1016/j.yfpn.2022.11.006
2589-420X/23/

based on enhanced risk stratification to diagnose disease before symptoms or pathologic changes occur are significantly increased. Although congenital genetic conditions and some genetic syndromes present in early life, there are many genetic influences on disease in older adulthood with familial implications. For example, in a database of two groups of related individuals with family histories of atenuated familial adenomatous polyposis ($n = 810$), age of diagnosis averaged 58 years [2]. In addition, those unaffected in these groups acquired a 69% risk of the cancer by aged 80 years [2].

It is vital that advanced practice registered nurses (APRNs) have the requisite knowledge to recognize warranted testing that optimizes early detection and diagnosis of genetic-influenced disease across the lifespan. A three-generation pedigree (3GP) is a graphic presentation of a client's family health history integrating genetic, environmental, and behavioral information. The 3GP is a key tool for collection and organization of data for making clinical decisions about genetic referral within the context of a client's medical and family history. The 3GP visual depiction of family structure helps practitioners more clearly see patterns of disease and identify actionable "red flags" in clients' records. See Box 1. The purpose of this paper is to educate nurses on the clinical utility of the 3GP and the practical aspects of how to incorporate the 3GP into clients' medical records.

Definition/Description

Pictoral recorded family histories date back centuries. Modern nomenclature and pedigree structure were adopted by the Pedigree Standardization Task Force of the National Society of Genetic Counselors in 1995 [3] and updated in 2008 [4]. This set of pedigree symbols, definitions, and abbreviations, along with pedigree line definition denoting relationships are recognized as the gold standard for publication by many health care journals and textbooks in the genetics/genomics field. This nomenclature is also the accepted format for AMA Manual of Style. The National Institutes of Health Cancer Institute's standard pedigree nomenclature, an adapted format, can be found in Fig. 1.

The client is represented in the pedigree as the *proband* and is the person around whom the familial relationships are oriented. Other family members are added, with attention to age at disease diagnoses, sex of family members affected, ancestral origin of grandparents and parents, consanguinuity, and any major environmental or occupational exposures [5]. Fig. 2 shows examples

---

Box 1: Red flags in 3GP that may warrant follow-up

- Age at onset of disease < expected
- # of relatives affected > expected
- Multiple primary cancers
- Unexplained sudden deaths in young healthy-appearing persons
- Patterns of disease (skip generations; mother-to-son, etc.)

Standard Pedigree Nomenclature

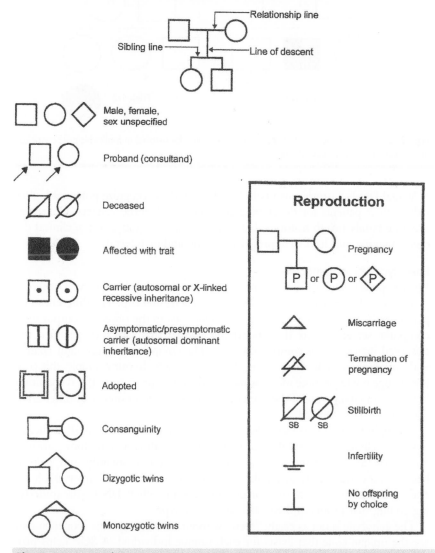

Fig. 1. NIH National Cancer Institute standard pedigree nomenclature. (*From* National Cancer Institute. National Institutes of Health (NIH). Available at https://nci-media.cancer.gov/pdq/media/images/613538.jpg.)

of the increased carrier risk to the proband (indicated by arrows) in family history scenarios of autosomal recessive conditions. A person with a sibling that is affected with an autosomal recessive condition has their own risk of being a carrier of the disease increased to 2/3. Having a niece or nephew affected with an autosomal recessive condition increases that person's carrier status risk to 1/2 [6].

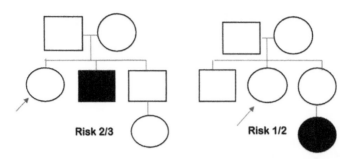

Fig. 2. Increased carrier risk to the proband (indicated by *arrows*) in family history scenarios of autosomal recessive conditions.

Visual family histories also help health providers recognize potential higher risk in their patients for developing genetically influenced cancers. Collecting accurate family health histories that increase risk recognition aid in clinical decision making and lead to appropriate testing and/or referrals.

Phenotype versus genotype

Phenotype is the whole of the expressed traits which can be observed, whereas genotype is the structure of an individual's genetic makeup. The difference in a person's phenotype versus genotype is analogous to the observed output on a computer screen versus the underlying coding that exists to produce the observed image on the computer screen. The computer coding might change without an observable alteration to the screen image. In our example, this coding change might become more pronounced (or less pronounced) if the lighting in the room changes, or if the humidity changes, or if a number of other environmental things change.

To apply the previous example to the clinical application of a 3GP, a client's observed clinical features, that is, height, weight, disease symptoms, are the output on the computer screen. These are easiest to identify and record, because they are readily available––just look at the screen! Conversely, a client's genotype is the sum of their genetic makeup––their DNA––the underlying coding that produces their observed phenotype.

The genotype is not as easily "seen" without extensive genetic sequencing to see the unique code that exists for each unique individual. A 3GP helps providers to see patterns of diseases and other syndromes in families using phenotype histories that hint at specific underlying genotypes and allow targeted genetic testing for those conditions, saving both time and cost to individuals and health systems. This was shown by identification of a novel form of progressive hereditary disease affecting bone ossification using 3GP analysis. Motivated by recognizing that phenotypic features of three generations of family members did not fit the typical disease manifestation of hereditary heterotropic ossification, Liu and Zhao [7] investigated further and found additional genetic mutations that may be associated with this disease in others.

Modes of inheritance

Genetic variance and disease may be inherited in a variety of ways. Previously we looked at examples of autosomal recessive inheritance. These are conditions that require the disease-causing variant to be inherited from both parents for the individual to be affected.

Consideration for providers of older adult health care is that certain populations are known to have high carrier rates of some recessive genetic variants, making the associated diseases more common in these populations compared with the general population. It is important for providers to know their practice populations and the populations that reside in their geographic areas. For example, Tay-Sachs disease is an autosomal recessive disease that affects individuals of Ashkenazi Jewish descent at higher frequencies than the general population. Ashkenazi Jewish individuals have a carrier rate of 1/30 for variants causing the disease, compared with 1/300 in the general public [6].

Diseases inherited by autosomal dominant mode are typically associated with pedigrees that have disease present at each generational level. These include Huntington's disease, BRCA-related cancers, and Marfan syndrome. Several other cardiovascular disorders are inherited in this fashion, including hereditary long QT syndrome and familial hypercholesterolemia.

X-linked inheritance can be recessive or dominant, and is most recognized in pedigree analysis by the presence of affected sons of affected mothers. X-linked diseases include red-green color blindness (recessive inheritance), and Rett syndrome (dominant inheritance).

Multifactorial disease inheritance is more complex and includes analysis of the complete pedigree—the graphic representation and the collected family history that provides information about phenotypic histories. Conditions such as cardiovascular disease and diabetes have myriad environmental and genetic influences. Using a 3GP web-based or software program with analytical capabilities is helpful for identifying increased patient risk based on pre-determined algorithms.

Use of analytical 3GP programs can identify increased proband risk for conditions such as Parkinson's disease, parkinsonism, or familial dementias. Knowing specific gene mutations involved in families affected with Parkinson's disease or parkinsonism provides valuable information about the potential effectiveness of levodopa for treatment of symptoms [8]. Treatment strategies for familial neurodegenerative dementias also continue to evolve and include gene-targeted and symptom-specific therapies [9].

Older adults: when is it "normal"?

Many conditions with genetic influences may be attributed to normal aging processes in older adults, therefore limiting treatments that might be beneficial. Among the top disease diagnoses in older adults are cardiovascular disease, hypertension, cancer, and diabetes, yet all of these conditions can have genetic components to inheritance. Genetic variation can impact not only diagnosis of disease, but also individuals' responses to treatments for disease. Identifying family patterns of disease allows all family members to receive appropriate screening, testing, treatment, or disease monitoring, regardless of age. See Box 2 for examples of some of the conditions associated with normal aging processes that have also been associated with genetic variation.

Population and extended pedigrees versus three-generation pedigrees

A population pedigree is similar to a 3GP, but focuses on a larger group or population. Population pedigrees can contain data from thousands of members of a population and are useful for research in anthropological genetics and association studies [10].

Extended pedigrees, which include multiple related households, allow researchers to investigate both the genetic effects and environmental effects of related and unrelated household members, as well as household and non-household related family members [10]. See Fig. 3 for a depiction of how investigators begin to comprise hypotheses based on consideration of both genetic and environmental exposures.

Extended pedigrees have been used to determine the estimated age of onset for rare diseases for which actionable screenings exist. These studies guide clinical practice guidelines for when to begin screening for disease when a client has a positive family history. Jonker and colleagues [11] preformed testing to obtain an accurate estimator for age of onset of asymptomatic stage in those with facioscapulohumeral muscular dystrophy, a rare genetic muscle disorder. They used data from 10 pedigrees with 155 individuals represented for their analysis. Their resulting formula is helpful for estimating onset of asymptomatic stage in high-risk families and could be applied to other families with rare genetic variants to know when it is clinically efficacious to begin screening [11].

Association studies can be conducted using extended pedigrees to identify genetic variants correlated with disease states or phenotypic traits. For example, the Danish Huntington's disease Registry is one of the oldest and most complete extended pedigrees collected for families with histories of the disease [12]. Gilling and colleagues [12] published a description of the registry which contains pedigree and sequencing information from 445 families with

---

Box 2: Disease diagnoses associated with older adulthood and genetic variation

- Cardiovascular disease
- Hypertension
- Cancer
- Type II diabetes
- Hypercholesteremia
- Sensory issues—some hearing loss, visual affects
- Balance issues—some related neurologic disease

Related/Non-related	Household/Non-household	
	H	**NH**
R	**R/H**	**R/NH**
NR	**NR/H**	**NR/NH**

Fig. 3. Investigating effects of gene/environmental impacts by looking at differences among related and non-related individuals in the same and different households.

history of Huntington's disease. They reported that mean age at testing was inversely correlated with CAG (Cytosine, Adenine, Guanine) repeat size. The average age of those with normal CAG repeat size was 62 years; however, the average age of those with expanded CAG repeat was 50 years [12]. For an individual with a family history of Huntington's disease, a pedigree identifying ages of family members at onset of disease symptoms would be valuable for knowing the likelihood for carrying and having inherited an expanded allele.

Precision medicine

Precision medicine, which incorporates the use of an individual's genomic data to predict disease susceptibility, disease prognosis, or response to treatment, is advanced through the identification of genomic variation and highly powered association testing within large diverse biobanks [13]. These biobanks are culminations of individual genome-wide association studies which are then archived, or banked, for further aggregate research use. For biobanked data to advantage high quality health care that is inclusive, fair, and equitable across populations, they must be representative of all races, ethnicities, and subpopulations, with rigorous methods for collection and annotation [13,14].

By scanning genetic markers across a large number of complete sequenced genomes, researchers can identify associations among marker variants and known disease [15]. This information is then used to predict disease risk in individuals with the genetic variation pre-symptomatically and drive prevention and care management plans. For example, knowing that an individual has genetic variation predictive of increased risk of malignant hyperthermia, an autosomal dominant condition which results in multi-organ systems failure if diagnosed late, would lead to additional precautions before initiating a procedure with anesthesia [16]. Operative anesthesia is known to trigger metabolic crises in individuals with this predisposition. An individual of any age with family history of metabolic crisis after anesthesia induction is therefore at increased risk of malignant hyperthermia, and could be identified with use of a 3GP.

History

A 3GP is advantageous for screening for conditions known to have high hereditary incidence. Many chronic conditions and cancers are considered to have multifactorial genesis; they are caused by combined influences of genes and environment with differing mixes of these ingredients for each client. For example, approximately 5% to 10% of all cancer cases have a genetic basis [17]. Having a family history of disease is itself an independent risk factor for many common chronic conditions.

Specifically, 10% of those diagnosed with melanoma have positive family histories for the malignancy [18,19]. Because of this, some recommendations for melanoma management include referral of family members for genetic counseling who meet specific criteria [20]. Considerations for older adults include that most hereditary melanoma cases result from variants in the CDKN2A gene. Individuals with variants in this gene also have an 18% lifetime risk of pancreatic cancer and therefore are recommended to undergo annual magnetic resonance imaging and/or endoscopic ultrasound of the pancreas beginning at 45 years of age [20].

Campacci and colleagues [17] used a primary screening 5-item questionnaire to identify women at risk for hereditary cancer predisposition syndromes from a convenience sample of 20,000 women from an outpatient population presenting for routine mammogram or cervical cancer screening at a large cancer hospital in Brazil over 12 months. From this sample, 1938 women were identified as at risk. The group then drew pedigrees for the women at risk and analyzed the pedigrees revealing that 465 of the families met at least one clinical criteria for referral to genetic cancer services [17]. Two-hundred seventy-three of those families were referred for further testing for hereditary breast and ovarian cancer, and 195 for Lynch syndrome [17].

Bailly and colleagues [21] also used 3GPs to gain a better clinical picture of patients with idiopathic dilated cardiomyopathy at an academic hospital in Johannesburg, South Africa, and to see whether there was evidence of familial risk related to their disease. This form of cardiomyopathy with no known cause is believed to be hereditary in up to 50% of cases [22]. Identifying and screening family members at high risk of having the disease can lead to earlier diagnosis and treatment even before their symptoms manifest. Fifty probands with the condition were recruited and their 3GPs were completed; pedigrees were categorized as positive, intermediate, or negative for presence of familial disease. Of the 50 pedigrees created, 14 were categorized as positive, and 9 were considered intermediate risk and were able to be further examined [21].

Pediatric providers can also optimize the use of 3GPs to see patterns of depressive and other psychiatric disorders in families. Van Dijk and colleagues [23] used secondary data from the Adolescent Brain Cognitive Development study ($n = 11,200$) with cross-sectional information on children's psychiatric functioning and parent's accounts of their and the grandparents' depression histories [24]. They found that risk of depressive and psychiatric disorders even at prepubertal ages increased with the addition of each affected previous generation. This finding did not differ with socioeconomic status, sex, or race/ethnicity [23].

Edelman and colleagues [25] tested the implementation of a 3GP electronic tool in prenatal settings to assess clients' genetic risk particularly focused on ancestry and carrier status of cystic fibrosis and hemoglobinopathies. Their objective was to improve the incidence and quality of recording a 3GP in clients' medical records. Six-hundred eighteen medical records were reviewed pre- and post-study implementation at four sites in the United States. Differences in ancestry were found between the phases; these changes were verified correctly documented in the second phase, indicating improved documentation post-study. In addition, an average of 7.6 genetic clinical decision support risk factors were identified post-study, along with 2.8 obstetric risk factors as a result of the improved post-study 3GP records [25].

Issue management
Challenges to use/limitations and potential solutions
One of the greatest challenges to broad use of the 3GP is the inability of electronic medical records (EMRs) to communicate across health care systems. For example, if a client completes a 3GP with her primary care provider and then sees specialty providers for women's health care, dermatologic care, dental care, or ophthalmologic care, that 3GP history does not always transfer to each additional provider. Nations with centralized health care records have distinct advantages with dynamic family records that can be added to from multiple family members across single systems.

Mirosevic and colleagues [26] recently evaluated available tools to aid family history taking in primary care settings. De Hoog and colleagues' [27] systematic review identified 18 tools to support family history taking in primary care, but reported that no family history collection tool was able to integrate information into a patient EMR. From 2014 to 2022, nine additional tools were identified by Mirosevic's team; however, just one of those had the ability to transfer information into a patient's EMR.

Some US states have implemented virtual health records such as Arkansas's State Health Alliance for Records Exchange (SHARE) network [28]. This health information exchange allows a client's health information to be shared in a standardized electronic format among participating doctors, nurses, specialists, health services professionals, and public health authorities in a secure format in real-time, protected by federal and state privacy and security laws. There are currently more than 3500 participating Arkansas facilities, including hospitals, medical practices, behavioral health facilities, long-term post-acute facilities, pharmacies, and dentists [28]. A 3GP record shared within this state-wide health information exchange would be accessible by providers across disciplines, saving clinical time and resources and significantly boosting clinical decision support.

Another limitation to use of the 3GP is the time an in-depth pedigree requires. One way to mitigate this might be to use a prescreening tool to determine when to prioritize the additional time needed for a graphical 3GP. One such prescreener was developed by Walter and colleagues [29] and contains six questions validated against a 3GP for determining risk for four common chronic conditions: diabetes, ischemic heart disease, breast cancer, and colorectal cancer [29]. A shorter prescreener like this could be a first step to 3GP implementation for all patients in busy primary care settings to identify client risk and implement prevention measures. Having patient-facing 3GP programs that could be completed at patients' conveniences before provider appointments would also address this issue.

Enhanced data input
Some have created condition-specific tools that are compatible with broader pedigree building software to aid assessment in their own fields. For example, Feero and colleagues [30] developed a tool to compute risk assessment for colorectal cancer in conjunction with the US Surgeon General's My Family Health Portrait. This tool was developed, in part, in response to the 2014 National Colorectal Cancer Roundtable which reported ill-equipped EMR systems unable to adequately store family history data for clinical risk assessments. They aimed to predict risk rather than development of disease with this study and used 150 patient-entered pedigrees from the ClinSeq cohort [31] as their sample [30]. Although this study supported analytical validity of the tool, future work needs to validate its clinical utility with diverse patient populations.

Kennelly and colleagues [32] point out the importance of accurate family histories for informing risk management of familial cancer syndromes. By carefully assessing family history of disease and applying diagnostic criteria such as the Amsterdam II [33] or revised Bethesda guidelines [34], an individual's lifetime colorectal cancer risk may be estimated at greater than 60% in some cases [32]. Other family history tools use diagnostic criteria from the National Comprehensive Cancer Network (NCCN) [35].

Another group tested the use of an animated virtual counselor versus the US Surgeon General's My Family Health Portrait online tool when constructing a 3GP for individuals of vulnerable populations [36]. They followed the 3GP collections with live genetic counselor interviews and found that the virtual tool overcame literacy barriers and resulted in greater completion (virtual tool 97%; My Family Health Portrait 51%), and greater accuracy ($P < .0001$) [36]. The virtual character VICKY (Virtual Counselor for Knowing Your family history) has now been updated and tested in Spanish [37].

DISCUSSION
Most countries have public health newborn screening programs that screen infants for wide panels of rare genetic diseases shortly after birth. These programs are designed to diagnose infants with rare diseases treatable presymptomatically, avoiding devastating health effects or death, and significantly reducing societal costs. Using a family history tool to identify and provide targeted interventions for patients at higher risk of disease provide similar benefits

to patients by early diagnosis and treatment. Indeed, one of the early leading calls for an organized research agenda to evaluate the use of family histories came from the Center for Disease Control and Prevention's 2002 workshop--Family History for Public Health and Preventive Medicine: Developing a Research Agenda [38]. Members of that workshop questioned whether a multigeneration pedigree could be effective as a public health-oriented tool because of its time-intensive nature and the need for patients to gather information, perhaps sharing the questions with relatives at home. Web-based, patient-facing tools would effectively address those issues. The workshop members also imagined that a family history tool used in a large public health setting would need to be limited in the number of diseases it could efficiently analyze [38]. By 2022, Mirosevic and colleagues [26] found that computerized tools could efficiently assess up to 98 separate diseases.

The US Surgeon General declares Thanksgiving Day as National Family History Day each year. Traditionally a day of large family gatherings in the United States, families are encouraged to use this day to discuss and document their family health histories [39]. Health care providers can take advantage of this declaration to cite additional evidence of the importance of talking about family health histories and encourage their patients of all ages to initiate these family discussions. Gerontologic providers, in particular, can impress upon their patients the value of the gift of family health histories to their children and grandchildren. In many cases, these gifts of shared information may result in benefit to the benefactor as well.

The NIH National Institute on Aging's infographic (Fig. 4) illustrates how an individual's risk to develop both early-onset and late-onset Alzheimer's disease is increased if their DNA contains certain gene variants. It is important to remember that simply having a genetic variant that increases risk for a disease or condition does not mean that an individual will certainly develop that disease or condition. For example, the *APOE* gene is associated with an increased risk of developing Alzheimer's disease [40]. This gene is inherited from both biological parents and variation may occur in different ways, resulting in different phenotypic effects.

One more rare variation of the *APOE* gene, the *APOEε2* allele, confers increased protection rather than risk for the disease. The more detrimental *APOEε4* allele is associated with increased risk of Alzheimer's [41]. Remembering that an individual inherits two *APOE* alleles, an individual with one *APOEε4* allele may have an increased risk of developing Alzheimer's disease by 3.7 times; an individual inheriting two *APOEε4* alleles (one from both parents) may have increased risk by 12 times. Conversely, having one protective *APOEε2* allele may reduce an individual's risk of disease development by 40% [41].

Limitations

An accepted limitation of genetic screening or testing is the ethical premise that a treatment or cure should be requisitely available. Population screening has historically adhered to the Wilson and Junger criteria established in 1968,

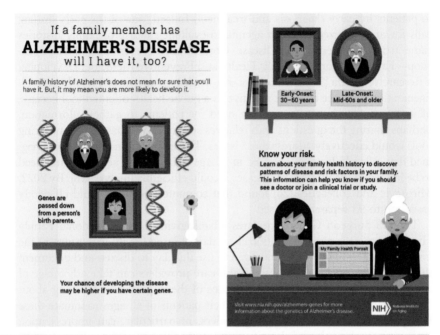

Fig. 4. NIH National Institute on Aging's infographic on Alzheimer's genetics. (*From* National Institute of Aging. National Institutes of Health (NIH). If a Family Member Has Alzheimer's Disease, Will I Have It, Too? Available at https://www.nia.nih.gov/health/infographics/if-family-member-has-alzheimers-disease-will-i-have-it-too#:~:text=A%20family%20history%20of%20Alzheimer's,if%20you%20have%20certain%20genes.)

which states that there should be an accepted treatment with established facilities for diagnosis and treatment before a public screening policy is initiated [42]. In their practices, practitioners should present all information and potential implications of genetic testing to their patients before any testing and allow the patients to reach informed decisions about what is in their best interests.

In addition, clinicians should exercise discretion by not over-reaching when applying genetic risk to complex cases that have potential for multifactorial influences. For example, a history of dying by suicide increases the risk for other family members' suicide deaths; however, it is unclear whether this is because of genetic influences, or because of acquired behavioral or shared experiential histories [43].

SUMMARY

A family history pedigree, a 3GP of a person's biological relatives with attached pertinent health information, is a standard tool used to more readily recognize patients who may benefit from genetics services. The depiction of both relationships and disorder traits advantage the pedigree over a simple genealogy for identifying patterns of disease expression and risk of disease inheritance.

APRNs are positioned as primary care, gerontology, well-woman care, and well-child care providers and prescribe preventive health services and referrals for genetic testing and services. In addition, they treat patients in specialty settings such as cancer, dermatology, and cardiology clinics, among others. Understanding the clinical utility of the 3GP in practice allows greater recognition of patterns of familial disease and subsequent increased patient disease risk.

CLINICS CARE POINTS

Genetics and genomics considerations should be parts of comprehensive physical examinations by providers across the lifespan. Although focus has historically been placed on pediatric genetics diagnoses, the science of genomics has evolved to include the gerontological population as well.

Evidence-based pearls and pitfalls for point of care

When a potentially significant family history is identified, consider the following actions:

- *Talk with the patient.* Assess their knowledge of the condition or disease of concern. If there is a pattern of disease in the family, the patient may already have greater than expected lay knowledge of the disease.
- *Consider the needs of the extended family.* New knowledge gleaned from a patient's family history has implications for others in the family. Specific patterns of inheritance may identify other family members with increased risk for the disease. If the condition has both genetic and environmental contributors, preventive strategies are appropriate to offer the family.
- *Order appropriate screening or confirmatory testing for the condition.* This may include screening for certain cancers at earlier ages, or ordering disease-specific testing in collaboration with genetic specialists, if indicated.
- *Place referrals to genetic specialty services and for genetic counseling.* A primary purpose for constructing a 3GP is facilitating patients' timely referrals to genetic services.

Disclosure

The author has no conflicts of interest to disclose. The author received no funding for the development of this article other than her faculty employment at the University of Arkansas for Medical Sciences College of Nursing.

References

[1] Lander ES, Linton LM, Birren B, et al. Initial sequencing and analysis of the human genome. Nature 2001;409(6822):860–921.

[2] Burt RW, Leppert MF, Slattery ML, et al. Genetic testing and phenotype in a large kindred with attenuated familial adenomatous polyposis. Gastroenterology 2004;127(2):444–51.

[3] Bennett RL, Steinhaus KA, Uhrich SB, et al. Recommendations for standardized human pedigree nomenclature. pedigree standardization task force of the national society of genetic counselors. Am J Hum Genet 1995;56(3):745–52.

[4] Bennett RL, French KS, Resta RG, et al. Standardized human pedigree nomenclature: update and assessment of the recommendations of the national society of genetic counselors. J Genet Couns 2008;17(5):424–33.

[5] Bennett RL. Family health history: the first genetic test in precision medicine. Med Clin North Am 2019;103(6):957–66.

[6] Langlois S, Wilson RD. Carrier screening for genetic disorders in individuals of Ashkenazi Jewish descent. J Obstet Gynaecol 2006;28(4):324–32.

[7] Liu Y, Zhao Xd. A Three-generation pedigree of multifocal heterotopic ossification with bilateral involvement. Orthopedics 2021;44(1):e139–45.

[8] Jia F, Fellner A, Kumar KR. Monogenic parkinson's disease: genotype, phenotype, pathophysiology, and genetic testing. Genes (Basel) 2022;13(3); https://doi.org/10.3390/genes13030471.

[9] Kwok JB, Loy CT, Dobson-Stone C, et al. The complex relationship between genotype, pathology and phenotype in familial dementia. Neurobiol Dis 2020;145:105082.

[10] Williams-Blangero S, Blangero J. Collection of pedigree data for genetic analysis in isolate populations. Hum Biol 2006;78(1):89–101.

[11] Jonker MA, Vart P, Rodriguez Girondo M. Estimating the age at onset distribution of the asymptomatic stage of a genetic disease based on pedigree data. Stat Methods Med Res 2020;29(8):2344–59.

[12] Gilling M, Budtz-Jørgensen E, Boonen SE, et al. The Danish HD Registry-a nationwide family registry of HD families in Denmark. Clin Genet 2017;92(3):338–41.

[13] Carress H, Lawson DJ, Elhaik E. Population genetic considerations for using biobanks as international resources in the pandemic era and beyond. BMC Genomics 2021;22(1):351.

[14] Annaratone L, De Palma G, Bonizzi G, et al. Basic principles of biobanking: from biological samples to precision medicine for patients. Virchows Arch 2021;479(2):233–46.

[15] NIH N. Genome-Wide Association Studies Fact Sheet. https://www.genome.gov/about-genomics/fact-sheets/Genome-Wide-Association-Studies-Fact-Sheet Updated 8/17/2020. Accessed August 28, 2022.

[16] Ellinas H, Albrecht MA. Malignant Hyperthermia Update. Anesthesiol Clin 2020;38(1):165–81.

[17] Campacci N, de Lima JO, Carvalho AL, et al. Identification of hereditary cancer in the general population: development and validation of a screening questionnaire for obtaining the family history of cancer. Cancer Med 2017;6(12):3014–24.

[18] Read J, Wadt KA, Hayward NK. Melanoma genetics. J Med Genet 2016;53(1):1–14.

[19] Christodoulou E, van Doorn R, Visser M, et al. NEK11 as a candidate high-penetrance melanoma susceptibility gene. J Med Genet 2020;57(3):203–10.

[20] Halk AB, Potjer TP, Kukutsch NA, et al. Surveillance for familial melanoma: recommendations from a national centre of expertise. Br J Dermatol 2019;181(3):594–6.

[21] Bailly C, Henriques S, Tsabedze N, et al. Role of family history and clinical screening in the identification of families with idiopathic dilated cardiomyopathy in Johannesburg, South Africa. S Afr Med J 2019;109(9):673–8.

[22] Ntusi NB, Badri M, Gumedze F, et al. Clinical characteristics and outcomes of familial and idiopathic dilated cardiomyopathy in Cape Town: a comparative study of 120 cases followed up over 14 years. S Afr Med J 2011;101(6):399–404.

[23] van Dijk MT, Murphy E, Posner JE, et al. Association of multigenerational family history of depression with lifetime depressive and other psychiatric disorders in children: results from the adolescent brain cognitive development (ABCD) Study. JAMA Psychiatry 2021;78(7):778–87.

[24] Dick AS, Lopez DA, Watts AL, et al. Meaningful associations in the adolescent brain cognitive development study. Neuroimage 2021;239:118262.

[25] Edelman EA, Lin BK, Doksum T, et al. Implementation of an electronic genomic and family health history tool in primary prenatal care. Am J Med Genet C Semin Med Genet 2014;166c(1):34–44.

[26] Miroševič Š, Klemenc-Ketiš Z, Peterlin B. Family history tools for primary care: A systematic review. Eur J Gen Pract 2022;28(1):75–86.

[27] de Hoog CL, Portegijs PJ, Stoffers HE. Family history tools for primary care are not ready yet to be implemented. A systematic review. Eur J Gen Pract 2014;20(2):125–33.

[28] Arkansas_Office_of_Health_Information_Technology. SHARE State health alliance for records exchange. Web International; 2022. Available at: https://sharearkansas.com/about/about-share/ Arkansas Department of Health; Arkansas Department of Health Information Technology. Accessed July 4 2022, 2022.

[29] Walter FM, Prevost AT, Birt L, et al. Development and evaluation of a brief self-completed family history screening tool for common chronic disease prevention in primary care. Br J Gen Pract 2013;63(611):e393–400.

[30] Feero WG, Facio FM, Glogowski EA, et al. Preliminary validation of a consumer-oriented colorectal cancer risk assessment tool compatible with the US Surgeon General's My Family Health Portrait. Genet Med 2015;17(9):753–6.

[31] Biesecker LG, Mullikin JC, Facio FM, et al. The ClinSeq Project: piloting large-scale genome sequencing for research in genomic medicine. Genome Res 2009;19(9):1665–74.

[32] Kennelly RP, Gryfe R, Winter DC. Familial colorectal cancer: Patient assessment, surveillance and surgical management. Eur J Surg Oncol 2017;43(2):294–302.

[33] Vasen HF, Watson P, Mecklin JP, et al. New clinical criteria for hereditary nonpolyposis colorectal cancer (HNPCC, Lynch syndrome) proposed by the International Collaborative group on HNPCC. Gastroenterology 1999;116(6):1453–6.

[34] Umar A, Boland CR, Terdiman JP, et al. Revised Bethesda Guidelines for hereditary nonpolyposis colorectal cancer (Lynch syndrome) and microsatellite instability. J Natl Cancer Inst 2004;96(4):261–8.

[35] Gupta S, Provenzale D, Llor X, et al. NCCN Guidelines Insights: Genetic/Familial High-Risk Assessment: Colorectal, Version 2.2019. J Natl Compr Canc Netw 2019;17(9):1032–41.

[36] Wang C, Paasche-Orlow MK, Bowen DJ, et al. Utility of a virtual counselor (VICKY) to collect family health histories among vulnerable patient populations: A randomized controlled trial. Patient Educ Couns 2021;104(5):979–88.

[37] Cerda Diez M DEC, Trevino-Talbot M, et al. Designing and Evaluating a Digital Family Health History Tool for Spanish Speakers. Int J Environ Res Public Health 2019;16(24):4979.

[38] Yoon PW, Scheuner MT, Khoury MJ. Research priorities for evaluating family history in the prevention of common chronic diseases. Am J Of Prev Med 2003;24(2):128–35.

[39] Announcement: National Family History Day - November 24. MMWR Morb Mortal Wkly Rep 2016;65(46):1305.

[40] Serrano-Pozo A, Das S, Hyman BT. APOE and Alzheimer's disease: advances in genetics, pathophysiology, and therapeutic approaches. Lancet Neurol 2021;20(1):68–80.

[41] Reiman EM, Arboleda-Velasquez JF, Quiroz YT, et al. Exceptionally low likelihood of Alzheimer's dementia in APOE2 homozygotes from a 5,000-person neuropathological study. Nat Commun 2020;11(1):667.

[42] Andermann A, Blancquaert I, Beauchamp S, et al. Revisiting Wilson and Jungner in the genomic age: a review of screening criteria over the past 40 years. Bull World Health Organ 2008;86(4):317–9.

[43] Mishara BL, Weisstub DN. Genetic testing for suicide risk assessment: Theoretical premises, research challenges and ethical concerns. Prev Med 2021;152(Pt 1):106685.

Advances in Family Practice Nursing 5 (2023) 93–106

ADVANCES IN FAMILY PRACTICE NURSING

Peripheral Arterial Disease in Primary Care

Kara Elena Schrader, DNP, FNP-C[a],*,
Kristin Castine, DNP, ANP-BC[b],
Pallav Deka, MS, PhD, AGACNP-BC[c]

[a]Michigan State University College of Nursing, 1355 Bogue Street, A 129 Life Sciences, East Lansing, MI 48824, USA; [b]Health Programs, Michigan State University College of Nursing, 1355 Bogue Street, A106 Life Sciences, East Lansing, MI 48824, USA; [c]Michigan State University College of Nursing, 1355 Bogue Street, C247 Bott Building, East Lansing, MI 48824, USA

Keywords
• Peripheral artery disease • Primary care • Older adult • Atherosclerosis

Key points

• Peripheral artery disease is underrecognized by health care providers and the public.

• Delayed diagnosis can result in serious complications including critical limb ischemia, amputation, and death.

• The most common pathologic cause of peripheral artery disease is atherosclerosis and is more prevalent in older adults.

• Peripheral artery disease is the third leading cause of morbidity related to atherosclerosis.

• Early identification of risk and institution of guideline-directed medical therapy is essential for the prevention of complications related to peripheral artery disease.

INTRODUCTION

Peripheral artery disease (PAD) is defined as stenosis of the peripheral arteries due to atherosclerosis that reduces perfusion to the extremities [1]. In the United States, an estimated 8.5 million Americans aged 40 years and older have PAD [2]. Persons with PAD have a high risk of cardiovascular (CV)-related morbidity and mortality such as carotid artery disease, coronary artery disease (CAD), and cerebral artery disease [3]. In addition, increased age is

*Corresponding author. *E-mail address:* schrad29@msu.edu

https://doi.org/10.1016/j.yfpn.2022.11.007
2589-420X/23/© 2022 Elsevier Inc. All rights reserved.

associated with higher prevalence, doubling every decade with the highest prevalence in ages 60 to 80 years [2,4]. Owing to the growing older population numbers, the American Heart Association (AHA) estimates that by 2050 an estimated 19 million people in the United States will have PAD [5].

An important role of the primary care provider (PCP) is disease prevention. Promoting CV health across the lifespan reduces the risk of atherosclerotic cardiovascular disease (ASCVD). PAD is a disease of the circulatory system and falls within the broad diagnosis of ASCVD [1,2]. Many of the risk factors for ASCVD are preventable and should be discussed during primary care visits. Early identification and treatment of disease states such as diabetes, CAD, hyperlipidemia, and hypertension (HTN) are crucial in the prevention of poor outcomes related to these conditions. It is vital for the PCP to identify persons at risk for PAD and to institute early treatment to prevent serious complications [4]. This article will provide Nurse Practitioners (NP) practicing in primary care with the knowledge and tools to identify persons, specifically older adults (OAs), at risk for PAD of the lower extremities (LE) and to institute guideline-directed medical therapy (GDMT) for early-stage disease.

BACKGROUND AND SIGNIFICANCE

Atherosclerosis is the most common cause of PAD and most often occurs in the LEs [1,3]. PAD follows CAD and stroke as a leading cause of morbidity related to atherosclerosis [3]. Mortality rates are high in persons with PAD with an estimated one-third of patients dying within 5 years of diagnosis [5]. Despite the seriousness of complications, PAD is underrecognized [3,4]. Patients with PAD can present with or without symptoms and can progress to serious complications such as arterial ulcers, gangrene, and amputation [1,3,4]. Knowledge of the symptoms and management of PAD is lacking among many health care professionals (HCPs), which delays diagnosis and adequate treatment [3]. In addition, most of the public is unaware of the symptoms and complications of PAD [3,6]. Delay in diagnosis and treatment can occur in the OA due to LE pain being attributed to arthritis or degenerative disease, which are also common in normal aging [3,4]. PAD is often asymptomatic until late in the disease that also results in delayed diagnosis and treatment [4].

RACIAL DISPARITIES

Racial disparities exist with a 30% higher lifetime risk of developing PAD in the African American (AA) population regardless of socioeconomic status [7–10]. This population is less likely to receive revascularization and therefore experience a greater risk of amputation for which there are higher rates of morbidity and mortality [5,7,8,11]. This disparity results in poorer outcomes for some ethnic populations [5]. Implicit bias and structural racism have been identified as probable reasons for decreased access to appropriate treatment [5,7,9–11].

QUALITY OF LIFE

Quality of life (QoL) is affected in the OA with PAD [9,12]. QoL measures in OA are associated with borderline and low ankle brachial index (ABI) [9]. In symptomatic PAD patients, this decline in QoL can be attributed to the inability to be physically active, a barrier that also negatively impacts mental health [9,12].

HEALTH CARE COST

Complications resulting in hospitalizations for PAD can lead to a heavy cost burden on the individual and the health care system. The estimated cost burden of complications requiring hospitalization related to PAD is over 6 billion dollars per year [13]. The most severe complication of PAD is critical limb ischemia (CLI) which often results in amputation and contributes to much of the cost burden. Cost varies depending upon the treatment strategy. During a US study of the cost burden for Medicare beneficiaries, Mustapha and colleagues (2018) discovered the cost of endo-revascularization and surgical revascularization were comparable ($49,700 and $49,200, respectively), whereas amputation was significantly higher ($55,700) [14].

THE AMERICAN HEART ASSOCIATION PAD NATIONAL ACTION PLAN

In 2022, the AHA created *The PAD National Action Plan* based on the gap in public and provider knowledge. The strategic goals for this plan focuses on public and HCP awareness [5,6]. The aim of this initiative is to reduce serious complications and improve QoL for people living with PAD [5,6]. Six goals were created to improve awareness, diagnosis, and treatment of PAD (Box 1).

PATHOPHYSIOLOGY

PAD is considered an obstructive atherosclerotic disease with similar pathology to that of CAD and cerebrovascular disease [4,15]. The development of an atherosclerotic plaque inside an artery leads to stenosis of the artery, resulting in reduced blood flow to distal areas [15] (Fig. 1). The process of atherosclerotic stenosis is initiated by an injury to the endothelial lining of the arteries from factors such as smoking, HTN, hyperlipidemia, hyperglycemia, and chronic inflammation [16]. In the initial stages of plaque formation, perfusion to distal locations may be mildly impaired and the stenosis may not be severe enough to experience symptoms [17]. In those individuals that are symptomatic, the most common symptom is pain in the calf while walking and exercising and relieved with rest [16]. This is known as intermittent claudication and is a result of the increase in demand for oxygen in distal tissues due to stenosis, resulting in ischemia [15,17]. As the plaque grows over time, claudication can occur at lower levels of exertion. At this stage, an individual may report the inability to walk as far as they previously did before they experienced pain [16].

The peripheral artery most affected by atherosclerosis is the superficial femoral artery [17]. Although less prevalent, disease of the common femoral

Box 1: Six goals of the PAD National Action Plan

1. Reach people with PAD and those at risk for PAD by improving public awareness of symptoms and diagnosis.
2. Enhance professional education for multidisciplinary health care professionals who care for people with PAD.
3. Activate health care systems to provide enhanced programs for the detection and treatment of PAD, with a focus on understanding and addressing patient-centered outcomes.
4. Reduce the rates of nontraumatic LE amputations related to PAD through public outcome reporting and public health interventions.
5. Increase and sustain research to better understand prevention, diagnosis, and treatment of PAD.
6. Coordinate advocacy efforts to shape national policy and improve health outcomes.

Data from The American Heart Association PAD National Action Plan. Available at https://www.heart.org/-/media/Files/Health-Topics/Peripheral-Artery-Disease/PAD-NAP-ExecSummary.pdf.

and popliteal arteries is more debilitating, causing pain of intermittent claudication to occur with shorter walking distances [17]. With advancing disease in any location, symptoms of reduced blood flow can occur such as dependent rubor and changes to the appearance of the leg and/or foot [17]. These changes present as loss of hair, thinning of skin, and possible atrophy of the muscles [17]. Severe stenosis leads to compromised perfusion and tissue death referred to as CLI for which the risk of amputation is high [16,17].

RISKS FACTORS
The risk factors for developing PAD are the same as the risks associated with ASCVD and include hyperlipidemia, HTN, diabetes, smoking, and family history of PAD [3,4,15] (Table 1). Recent studies have shown a genetic influence for the development of PAD.18 However, the three most common risk factors are aging, smoking, and diabetes [3,4,15]. NPs have skills to assist in reducing modifiable risk factors for PAD by using behavior change strategies. It is vital that NPs identify those at risk for PAD, complete a thorough assessment, and begin preventative strategies focused at reducing complications associated with this condition as soon as possible.

Assessment
To assess for PAD in OAs, an evaluation should begin with a thorough health history [4,18]. The history should contain information on current health status including chronic conditions such as CAD, carotid disease, diabetes, HTN, hyperlipidemia, and other co-morbidities that increase the risk of PAD. Adults over 40 who smoke are at an especially high risk of PAD. Therefore, a social history should include determination of smoking status and alcohol consumption. It is also important to assess nutritional intake, physical activity level, and ascertain whether LE pain occurs with ambulation. Review of systems should

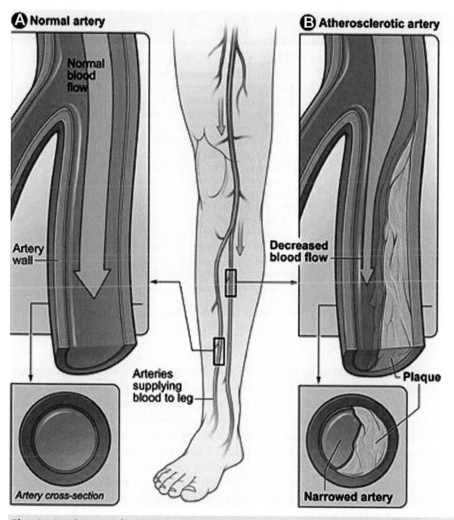

Fig. 1. Development of atherosclerotic plaque leading to stenosis (A, B). (*From* National Heart. Lung, and Blood Institute. National Institutes of Health (NIH). Peripheral Artery Disease – Causes and Risk Factors. Available at https://www.nhlbi.nih.gov/health/peripheral-artery-disease/causes.)

cover specifics about skin or nail changes and peripheral edema. Concluding the interview by asking about other concerns may provide additional clues to a potential PAD diagnosis.

Physical assessment to diagnose PAD starts with an overall impression of the general appearance, review of vital signs, and body mass index (BMI). Mental status assessment is essential in OA to identify changes in orientation or executive function which may influence health status. Carotid arteries, heart, and

Table 1
Risk factors for developing peripheral artery disease

Risk factor	Impact
Aging: non-modifiable	• Atherosclerosis increases with age [3] • A ged 65 and older is an independent risk factor [3] • Can occur without any other associated risks [3]
Smoking: modifiable	• Smoking doubles the risk of developing PAD [4] • The risk related to smoking is cumulative based upon the age one begins to smoke and the number of years of smoking [4] • Smoking in combination with any of the other risk factors increases lifetime risk fivefold [7]
Diabetes: modifiable	• The longer the duration of diabetes, the higher the risk of developing PAD [4] • High prevalence of diabetes in OA • R isk of claudication is two- to threefold greater than compared with those without diabetes [4] • May or may not have symptoms initially [4] • Higher risk of PAD complications [4] • Diabetic foot ulcers are significantly related to PAD by decreasing healing which increases the risk of amputation [4]
Genetics: non-modifiable	• Currently, four variants have been identified that influence thrombotic activity specific to PAD [20]

lung sounds need to be auscultated and assessed for deviations from normal. Abdominal assessment should include auscultating for aortic and renal bruits [4]. An inspection of the skin is necessary to identify changes in pigmentation and appearance, hair distribution, breaks in skin integrity (sores, ulcers, rashes, skin tears), and the presence of edema [4]. Skin texture, along with temperature, also provides valuable information. Pulses should be palpated downward, ideally starting at the femoral artery noting presence and strength along with comparing right to left side. Auscultation for femoral bruits is important to detect interference in arterial flow [4,18]. In addition, functional assessment with a validated tool should be conducted with OA [19].

Diagnosis

The calculation of the ABI can provide information that allows the classification of the extent of the arterial disruption with suspected PAD [4]. The ABI is determined using a blood pressure cuff and a Doppler. The systolic blood pressure (SBP) in the upper extremities and bilateral ankle regions (dorsalis pedis and posterior tibial) are calculated with the patient in a supine position (Fig. 2). The highest of the ankle pressures are divided by the highest of the extremity readings. The resultant number is then compared with an interpretation chart (Table 2). Readings less than or equal to 0.9 require action and intervention [4].

Aging, along with chronic conditions such as diabetes and kidney disease, may impact ABI calculations due to physiologic arterial changes that occur

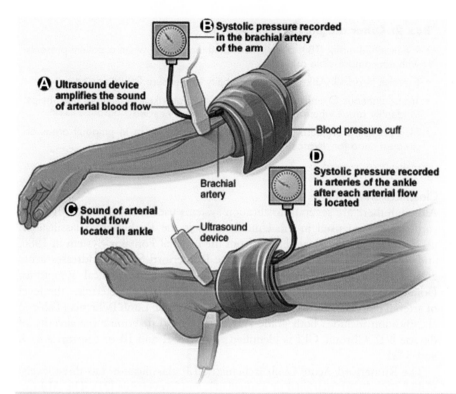

Fig. 2. Ankle-brachial testing (ABI). (*From* National Heart (A-D). Lung, and Blood Institute. National Institutes of Health (NIH). Atherosclerosis – Diagnosis. Available at https://www.nhlbi.nih.gov/health/atherosclerosis/diagnosis.)

with these conditions. This is important to remember when trying to diagnose PAD. As a result of aging, and disease-based physiologic changes, utilization of other diagnostic methods may be necessary and include TBI, exercise treadmill ABI, transcutaneous oximetry test (TcPO2), and skin profusion pressure (SPP) [4,18]. Patients with PAD who do not improve with GDMT may require further testing such as duplex ultrasound, computed tomography angiography (CTA), magnetic resonance angiography (MRA), or invasive angiogram, especially if revascularization is being considered [4]. (Box 2).

Table 2		
Interpretation of ankle-brachial index [4]		
ABI score	Interpretation	Next step
< or = 0.9	Abnormal	Begin management
0.91 to 0.99	Borderline	Exercise ABI (if suspect)
1.0 to 1.4	Normal	Check for other causes
> 1.4	Noncompressible	Perform Toe-brachial index (TBI)

Box 2: Other diagnostic methods [3]

- Toe-brachial index (TBI): allows for evaluation of PAD when a patient presents with noncompressible arteries
- Exercise treadmill ABI: provides the ability to measure limitations objectively
- Transcutaneous Oximetry Test (TcPO2): measures taken at multiple sites; helps to identify areas where revascularization is most needed
- Skin perfusion pressure (SPP): along with TcPO2, helps to pinpoint areas of greatest need for revascularization

Classification

Although there are several classification systems used to assess PAD, the most common system used in the United States is the Rutherford Classification [21,22]. This system was adapted from the original Fontaine System in 1986, and further revised in 1997 [21,22]. The Rutherford System addresses acute and chronic presentations separately and relies upon clinical symptoms, Doppler, ABI assessment, and pulse volume readings to determine the level of arterial involvement [21]. The Rutherford Chronic Limb Ischemia (Table 3) classification includes both grade and categories to determine the severity of disease [21]. Chronic CLI is identified at grades II and III or categories 4, 5, and 6 [21].

The Rutherford Acute Limb Ischemia (ALI) classification has three levels: viable, threatened (marginal or immediate), and irreversible [21]. The ALI categories are used by vascular specialists to determine surgical treatment.

Management in primary care

The AHA and the American College of Cardiology (ACC) guidelines for the management of PAD stress early detection through the determination of ABI and use of duplex ultrasound or angiogram to confirm a diagnosis [4]. Use of oral medications, revascularization, endovascular intervention (when required), and regular interval assessment by a PCP may all be part of the management plan [4]. Any necessary surgical interventions, such as a femoropopliteal-tibial bypass, would require a referral and evaluation by a vascular surgeon.[4]

The goal of PCPs is to improve arterial circulation and avoid the progression of vascular disease. This is especially important to prevent amputations and avoid CV risks, which impact QoL for individuals living with PAD. From a primary care standpoint, preventative measures include promoting smoking cessation (when indicated), structured aerobic exercise, healthy diet (ie, Mediterranean), and optimal chronic disease management [4,17,23–25].

Lifestyle changes

Smoking cessation

Cigarette smoking remains the leading modifiable risk factor to prevent the progression of PAD [4,26]. Every patient encounter needs to include a

Table 3
Rutherford clinical categories of chronic limb ischemia

Grade	Category	Clinical description	Objective criteria
0	0	Asymptomatic	Normal treadmill
	1	Mild claudication	Completes treadmill exercise[a]; AP after exercise >50 mm Hg but at least 20 mm Hg lower than resting value
I	2	Moderate claudication	Between categories 1 and 3
	3	Severe claudication	Cannot complete standard treadmill exercise[a] and AP after exercise is < 50 mm Hg
II	4	Ischemic rest pain	Resting AP < 60 mm Hg; ankle or metatarsal PVR flat or TP < 30 Hg
III	5	Minor tissue loss: nonhealing ulcer, focal gangrene with diffuse pedal ischemia	Resting AP < 60 mm Hg, ankle, or metatarsal PVR flat or barely pulsatile; TP < 40 mm Hg
	6	Major tissue loss-extending above the TM level, functional foot no longer salvageable	Same as category 5

Abbreviations: AP, ankle pressure; PVR, pulse volume recording; TM, transmetatarsal; TP, toe pressure.
[a]Five minutes at 2 mph on 12% incline.
From Rutherford RB, Baker JD, Ernst C, et al. Recommended standards for reports dealing with lower extremity ischemia: revised version [published correction appears in J Vasc Surg 2001 Apr;33(4):805]. J Vasc Surg. 1997;26(3):517-538. https://doi.org/10.1016/s0741-5214(97)70045-4; with permission.

discussion on smoking status and steps to reduce or eliminate smoking. The conversation should include the avoidance of second-hand smoke as well [25,27]. Assistance should be offered using nicotine replacement therapy (patch, gum, lozenge, etc.), such as varenicline or bupropion (Wellbutrin) [27]. Dose adjustments should be made for the OA with renal impairment [27]. The Centers for Disease Control and Prevention (CDC) program 1 to 800-QUITNOW can also be beneficial to assist with smoking cessation [27].

Exercise/physical activity
Strong evidence supports the use of supervised structured aerobic exercise programs to maintain functional status for OA diagnosed with PAD [4]. Providers should explain the importance of aerobic exercise in the development of collateral circulation to improve perfusion and alleviate symptoms. These programs require supervision by a qualified professional and should be at least 12 weeks in length [4,28]. A face-to-face visit with the provider managing the PAD treatment is needed before referral for Supervised Exercise Therapy (SET). The provider must provide information regarding ASCVD and PAD risk factor reduction (education, counseling, behavioral interventions, and outcome assessments) [28].

The Centers for Medicare and Medicaid (CMS) may reimburse outpatient SET for OA with symptomatic PAD if specific components are met [28] (Box 3). Ideally, training should occur at least 3 times a week for 30 to 60 min each time (a total of 36 sessions) [4,28]. Sessions should include alternating periods of walking and rest to combat claudication. It is important to encourage OA to start with a shorter duration (10 min) of activity and gradually increase over time to meet the recommendations. With time, training should accommodate for improvements with changes in intensity and duration of activity. Warm-up and cool-down activities before and after sessions are also important to avoid any injuries. The PCP should inquire about adherence to physical programs/activities when it is self-directed and encourage OA to remain active [4].

Nutrition
Focus on a healthy food intake is important for the prevention or management of PAD symptoms [24,25]. Evidence supports embracing a Mediterranean diet high in plant-based foods, olive oil, and nuts with lean protein and limited processed foods [24,25]. This type of diet has the potential to improve PAD outcomes and overall CV health [24,25]. For the OA, meal guidance from the US Department of Agriculture's MyPlate for the OA may also be of benefit. Referral to a nutritionist can be considered to assist the OA with understanding the components of this diet and aid in meal planning.

Pharmacology
Medication management for symptomatic PAD should include an antiplatelet such as clopidogrel (Plavix®) or aspirin [4]. This recommendation is strongly supported in the research literature [4]. Both of these medications have been

---

Box 3: CMS criteria for SET

The SET program must:

- Consist of sessions lasting 30 to 60 min comprising a therapeutic exercise-training program for PAD in patients with claudication (up to 36 sessions over a 12-week period)
- Be conducted in a hospital outpatient setting, or a provider's office
- Be delivered by qualified auxiliary personnel necessary to ensure benefits exceed harms, and who are trained in exercise therapy for PAD, and
- Be under the direct supervision of a physician, physician assistant, or nurse practitioner/clinical nurse specialist who must be trained in both basic and advanced life support techniques

Medicare coverage depends on plan.

Adapted from Centers for Medicare & Medicaid Services. Supervised Exercise Therapy (SET) for Symptomatic Peripheral Artery Disease (PAD). Decision Summary. May 2017. https://www.cms.gov/medicare-coverage-database/view/ncacal-decision-memo.aspx?proposed=N&NCAId=287.

found to be effective in reducing ASCVD events such as myocardial infarction or stroke [4]. Oral anticoagulants have not been shown to provide benefits and carry the additional risk of hemorrhage [4,29].

Patients with PAD experiencing claudication may find some relief from cilostazol (Pletal®) [4,29]. This medication has been found to lessen symptoms of claudication and improve ambulation [1]. Side effects, such as lightheadedness and palpitations, may impact adherence to the regimen and increase fall risk. Further, cilostazol should be avoided in OA with heart failure (HF), a common condition in this age group [4,29].

Chronic disease management

There is strong evidence to support the addition of a statin in the medication regimen for any patient with PAD [4]. The low-density lipoprotein (LDL) goal should be 70 mg/dL or less, as per the current AHA/ACC guidelines [2,30]. In addition, OA with comorbid PAD and HTN require antihypertensive medication to prevent further CV-related issues [1]. There is no evidence to support the use of one antihypertensive medication over another as it relates to improving outcomes in PAD [4,30]. Target BP readings need to be within the recommended range per HTN management guidelines [4,31]. Current guidelines indicate the range should be typically less than 130/80 mm Hg, with adjustments made for age and comorbidities [4,31]. In OA 65 years and older with limited life expectancy, engaging in shared decision-making regarding BP goals is recommended [31]. Diabetes is the number one risk of complications related to PAD [32]. Management of the disease is essential to prevent serious complications such as amputation. It is essential that PCPs use the most current ADA guidelines to set targets for glycated hemoglobin (A1c). In the OA, age, functional status, health status, and life expectancy need to be considered when setting A1C targets [32] (Table 4).

Referral

When nonsurgical interventions fail to prevent the progression of PAD, a referral to a specialist, such as a vascular surgeon, may be required [4]. To achieve the goal of minimizing tissue loss, endovascular or surgical revascularization may be indicated to promote improvement in claudication [4]. Procedures can range from angioplasty and stents to surgical bypass [4]. A thorough discussion of the risks and benefits should be conducted by the specialist before any procedure to ensure informed, mutual decision-making [4].

Table 4
Chronic disease management goals in peripheral artery disease

Chronic disease	Target
Hypertension	≤ 130/80 mm Hg [4,31]
Diabetes	A1C 7.0% to 7.5% [32]
Hyperlipidemia	LDL<70 mg/dL [30]

Management summary
Management of PAD in primary care should begin with a focus on lifestyle changes and strategies that can prevent disease progression. Discussions related to management should focus on the prevention of serious complications [26]. GDMT includes smoking cessation (if applicable), physical activity, and appropriate nutrition. Specific prevention strategies should also include the management of associated comorbidities [3,26]. Medications such as anti-platelets and cilostazol can reduce symptoms associated with intermittent claudication. Re-evaluation should occur at least every 6 months, or sooner when indicated [26].

Implications for nurse practitioner practice
PAD affects over 8.5 million Americans over the age of 40 and the number is expected to rise. OA and adults over 40 who smoke are at the highest risk of developing PAD. PAD is considered an ASCVD condition for which there are evidence-based guidelines to prevent the progression of the disease. NPs can improve care by identifying risk factors for PAD, assessing for symptoms, and early initiation of GDMT to prevent progression and complications.

SUMMARY
OA are at particular risk for developing PAD but are underdiagnosed. Late diagnosis leads to poor outcomes, reduced QoL, and higher cost burden. Racial disparities also exist resulting in less aggressive treatment that leads to higher morbidity and mortality in the AA population. Further education is warranted for HCPs and increasing public awareness to improve the identification of symptoms for early diagnosis and treatment. Asking every patient about leg pain with ambulation is a proactive that question can glean valuable information. Prevention of PAD is a goal every NP should strive to achieve.

CLINICS CARE POINTS

- Providers should consider PAD as a differential for complaints of LE pain, especially in the OA.
- Early diagnosis can reduce complications related to PAD.
- Ankle Brachial Index is used to classify the extent of PAD and to determine treatment strategies.
- GDMT includes smoking cessation, nutitional modifications, physical activity and management of associated chronic illnesses.

Disclosure
The authors have nothing to disclose.

References
[1] National Heart. Lung, Blood Institute. What is peripheral artery disease? Updated March 24, 2022. Available at: https://www.nhlbi.nih.gov/health/peripheral-artery-disease. Accessed October 29, 2022.

[2] Tsao CW, Aday AW, Almarzooq ZI, et al. Heart disease and stroke statistics-2022 update: a report from the American heart association. Circulation 2022;145(8):e153–639.

[3] Criqui MH, Matsushita K, Aboyans V, et al. Lower extremity peripheral artery disease: contemporary epidemiology, management gaps, and future directions: A scientific statement from the American Heart Association. Circulation 2021;144(9):e171–91 [published correction appears in Circulation. 2021 Aug 31;144(9):e193].

[4] Gerhard-Herman MD, Gornik HL, Barrett C, et al. 2016 AHA/ACC guideline on the management of patients with lower extremity peripheral artery disease: executive summary: a report of the american college of cardiology/american heart association task force on clinical practice guidelines. J Am Coll Cardiol 2017;69(11):1465–508.

[5] American Heart Association. PAD roundtable report. a vascular disease thought leaders' summit report 2019. Available at: https://www.heart.org/-/media/Files/Health-Topics/Peripheral-Artery-Disease/PAD-Roundtable-Report–Final.pdf Published 2019. Accessed October 29, 2022.

[6] The American Heart Association. PAD National Action Plan: Executive Summary. Available at: https://www.heart.org/-/media/Files/Health-Topics/Peripheral-Artery-Disease/PAD-NAP-ExecSummary.pdf. Accessed October 2022.

[7] Minc SD, Goodney PP, Misra R, et al. The effect of rurality on the risk of primary amputation is amplified by race. J Vasc Surg 2020;72(3):1011–7.

[8] Arya S, Binney Z, Khakharia A, et al. Race and social economic status independently affect risk of major amputation in peripheral artery disease. J Am Heart Assoc 2018;7(2): e007425.

[9] Wu A, Coresh J, Selvin E, et al. Lower extremity peripheral artery disease and quality of life among older individuals in the community. J Am Heart Assoc 2017;6(1):e004519.

[10] O'Donnell TF, Powell C, Deery SE, et al. Regional variation in racial disparities among patients with peripheral artery disease. J Vasc Surg 2018;68(2):519–26.

[11] Mustapha J, Fisher BT, Rizzo JA, et al. Explaining racial disparities in amputation rates for the treatment of peripheral artery disease (PAD) using decomposition methods. J Racial Ethnic Health Disparities. 2017;4(5):784–95.

[12] Golledge J, Leicht AS, Yip L, et al. Relationship between disease specific quality of life measures, physical performance, and activity in people with intermittent claudication caused by peripheral artery disease. Eur J Vasc Endovasc Surg 2020;59(6):957–64.

[13] Kohn CG, Alberts MJ, Peacock WF, et al. Cost and inpatient burden of peripheral artery disease: Findings from the National Inpatient Sample. Atherosclerosis 2019;286:142–6.

[14] Mustapha JA, Katzen BT, Neville RF, et al. Determinants of long-term outcomes and costs in the management of critical limb ischemia: a population-based cohort study. J Am Heart Assoc 2018;7(16):e009724: 1-11.

[15] Creager MA, Loscalzo J. Arterial Diseases of the Extremities. In: Jameson J, Fauci AS, Kasper DL, et al, editors. Harrison's principles of internal medicine. 20th edition. McGraw Hill; 2018. Available at: https://accessmedicine.mhmedical.com/content.aspx?bookid=2129&sectionid=192030522. Accessed October 29, 2022.

[16] Libby P, Buring JE, Badimon L, et al. Atheroscler Nat Rev Dis Primers 2019;5(56):1–18; https://doi.org/10.1038/s41572-019-0106-z.

[17] Gasper WJ, Iannuzzi JC, Johnson MD. Occlusive disease: femoral & popliteal arteries. In: Papadakis MA, McPhee SJ, Rabow MW, et al, editors. Current medical diagnosis & treatment 2022. McGraw Hill; 2022. Available at: https://accessmedicine.mhmedical.com/book.aspx?bookID=3081. Accessed August 21, 2022.

[18] Smith DK, Arnold MJ, Larson J. How to refine your approach to peripheral arterial disease. J Fam Pract 2020;69(10):500–6.

[19] McDermott MM. Medical management of functional impairment in peripheral artery disease: A review. Prog Cardiovasc Dis 2018;60:586–92.

[20] Klarin D, Lynch J, Aragam K, et al. Genome-wide association study of peripheral artery disease in the Million Veteran Program. Nat Med 2019;25(8):1274–9.

[21] Hardman RL, Jazaeri O, Yi J, et al. Overview of classification systems in peripheral artery disease. Semin Intervent Radiol 2014;31(4):378–88.

[22] Rutherford RB, Baker JD, Ernst C, et al. Recommended standards for reports dealing with lower extremity ischemia: revised version. J Vasc Surg 1997;26(3):517–38 [published correction appears in J Vasc Surg 2001 Apr;33(4):805].

[23] Kullo IJ, Rooke TW. Peripheral Artery Disease. N Engl J Med 2016;374(9):861–71.

[24] Mattioli AV, Coppi F, Migaldi M, et al. Relationship between Mediterranean diet and asymptomatic peripheral arterial disease in a population of pre-menopausal women. Nutr Metab Cardiovasc Dis 2017;27(11):985–90.

[25] Ruiz-Canela M, Estruch R, Corella D, et al. Association of Mediterranean diet with peripheral artery disease: the PREDIMED randomized trial. JAMA 2014;311(4):415–7.

[26] Sutton M, Kreider K, Thompson J, et al. Improving outcomes in patients with peripheral arterial disease. J Vasc Nurs 2018;36(4):166–72; https://doi.org/10.1016/j.jvn.2018.06.005.

[27] Center for Disease Control and Prevention (CDC). Smoking & tobacco use: how to quit. 2022. Available at: https://www.cdc.gov/tobacco/patient-care/clinical-tools/index.html June 17, 2021. Accessed October 29.

[28] Centers for Medicare & Medicaid Services. Supervised exercise therapy (SET) for symptomatic peripheral artery disease (PAD). decision summary. 2017. Available at: https://www.cms.gov/medicare-coverage-database/view/ncacal-decision-memo.aspx?proposed=N&NCAld=287. Accessed September 21, 2022.

[29] Pletal (cilostazol) [package insert]. Rockville, MD: Otsuka Pharmaceutical, Inc; 2015. Available at: https://www.accessdata.fda.gov/drugsatfda_docs/label/2017/020863s024lbl.pdf. Accessed October 27, 2022.

[30] Arnett DK, Blumenthal RS, Albert MA, et al. 2019 ACC/AHA guideline on the primary prevention of cardiovascular disease: Executive summary. Circulation 2019;140:e563–95.

[31] Carey RM, Whelton PK. 2017 ACC/AHA hypertension guideline writing committee. prevention, detection, evaluation, and management of high blood pressure in adults: synopsis of the 2017 american college of cardiology/american heart association hypertension guideline. Ann Intern Med 2018;168(5):351–8.

[32] American Diabetes Association. Standards of medical care in diabetes – 2022 abridged for primary care providers. Clin Diabetes 2022;40(1):10–38.

Women's Health

Advances in Family Practice Nursing 5 (2023) 107–118

ADVANCES IN FAMILY PRACTICE NURSING

Assessment and Management of Pelvic Organ Prolapse for the Rural Primary Care Provider

Lisa S. Pair, DNP, CRNP, WHNP-BC, FAUNA[a],*,
William E. Somerall Jr, MD, MAEd[b]

[a]The University of Alabama at Birmingham, 1720 2nd Avenue South, NB 536, Birmingham, AL 35294-1210, USA; [b]The University of Alabama at Birmingham, 1720 2nd Avenue South, NB 534, Birmingham, AL 35294-1210, USA

Keywords
- Pelvic organ prolapse • Pelvic prolapse • Vaginal prolapse
- Pelvic organ prolapse women • Pelvic organ prolapse treatment

Key points
- Pelvic organ prolapse (POP) is a common female condition resulting in loss of pelvic floor support in the anterior, posterior, or apical areas of the vagina.
- Conservative management consists of lifestyle management, pelvic floor muscle therapy, and the use of a vaginal support device (pessary), which can reduce symptoms.
- The primary care provider can assess patients with POP and begin conservative management to address the symptoms and improve the patient's quality of life.

INTRODUCTION

Pelvic organ prolapse (POP), a common condition of the female genital tract, is estimated to occur in about 50% of women [1,2]. POP occurs because of the loss of muscular and fascial support of the pelvic floor. Depending on where the loss of support occurs, the anterior vaginal wall, posterior vaginal wall, partial or complete uterine prolapse, or a combination of any of the above can develop. Frequently, the woman will present with complaints of pelvic pressure, fullness, heaviness, or vaginal bulging at or through the vaginal introitus

---

*Corresponding author. 5604 Ridgeview Drive, Trussville, AL 35173.
E-mail address: lpair@uab.edu

https://doi.org/10.1016/j.yfpn.2022.11.001
2589-420X/23/

[1]. Many times, there is difficulty with voiding, defecation, urinary continence, or sexual function. The purpose of this article is to provide information for assessment, diagnosis, and nonsurgical, conservative management of POP for the primary care provider.

It is important that primary care providers work to improve health access for those patients whose social conditions, such as distance-to-travel or transportation, creates issues when specialty care services are not available locally. In addition, about 50% of patients referred to specialty clinics received initial management before referral [3]. Frequently, primary care providers are familiar with urinary incontinence (UI) symptoms and treatment but less so for POP. Thus, primary care providers can benefit with education regarding assessment and management of POP before referral.

PELVIC ORGAN PROLAPSE
Anterior wall prolapse (cystocele) is the most common POP occurring 2 times more often than posterior wall prolapse (rectocele) and 3 times more often than apical prolapse of the uterus or apical vaginal wall following hysterectomy (enterocele) [1]. Anterior wall defects occur due to weakness of bladder support that eventually creates a bulge into the anterior vagina because of disruption of the anterior endopelvic fascia and the *levator ani* muscles. Posterior wall defects are also caused by the separation of the *levator ani* muscles in the midline separating the vagina and rectum that creates a bulge into the lower vagina (Fig. 1). Apical wall defects (enterocele) occur because of a weakness of the apical vaginal support allowing the uterus, if present, and abdominal contents (viscera) to prolapse into the upper vagina (Fig. 2). The degree of prolapse may be minimal and cause few symptoms to complete prolapse of pelvic structures into the vagina extending beyond the vaginal introitus [1]. Of women presenting with symptoms of POP, 13% reported only stress incontinence, 5% reported only urge incontinence, whereas 76% reported a combination of both stress and urge incontinence [4].

TRANSGENDER SURGERY AND PELVIC ORGAN PROLAPSE
Transgender individuals will obtain health services from primary care providers. Transgender and gender nonconforming individuals are those who gender identity differs from the gender assigned at birth [5]. Gender dysphoria is defined as significant psychological distress between their gender identify and their sex assigned at birth. It is important for providers to understand the current gender-affirming surgery available to individuals suffering with gender dysphoria because pelvic floor dysfunction can result from surgical reconstruction. Female-to-male gender-affirming surgery currently incorporates 3 approaches to creating a neophallus (surgically constructed penis) for which there is currently no consensus on best approach [6]. Most individuals will undergo complete hysterectomy with bilateral salpingo-oophorectomy (removal of uterus, fallopian tubes, and ovaries). In addition, they will undergo vulvectomy or colpocleisis (surgical procedure suturing the vaginal walls together);

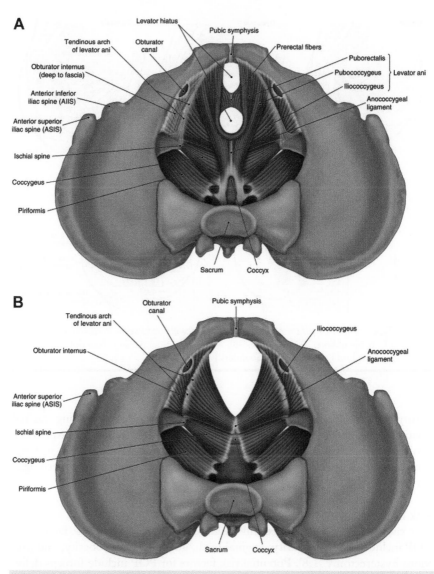

Fig. 1. Superior views of the muscles of the pelvic floor; female pelvis. (**A**), Superficial view. (**B**), Deeper view. (*From* Muscolino, J. Chapter 18: Tour #8—Palpation of the Pelvic Muscles. In: The Muscle and Bone Palpation Manual with Trigger Points, Referral Patterns and Stretching, 3rd Edition. 2022:438–461; with permission.)

both of which eliminates the vagina [5]. As a result, POP is not experienced in this population. With male-to-female gender-affirming surgery, there is a consensus on best surgical approach [6]. The surgical goals can include surgically designed vulva, vagina (neovagina), and shortened urethra. Because of

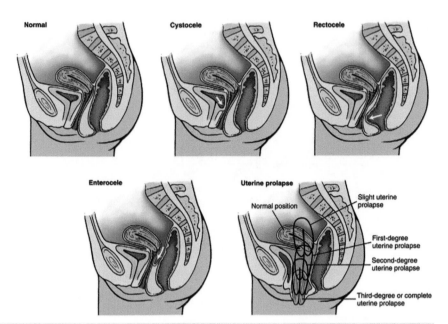

Fig. 2. Types of genital organ prolapse. *(Reprinted with permission from* Monahan, F.D., Drake, D.T., & Neighbors, M. [eds.]. [1998]. *Medical-surgical nursing: Foundations for clinical practice* [2nd ed.]. Philadelphia: Saunders.)

a surgically created vagina, these individuals must undergo lifelong vaginal dilation to maintain sexual penetration. In addition, individuals may experience prolapse of the neovagina, which usually occurs approximately 4% in long-term follow-up [7]. These individuals need to be referred to a urogynecologist for care.

Risk factors for pelvic floor prolapse

The cause of POP is complex and multifactorial. Established risk factors for POP include increased parity, vaginal birth, advancing age, obesity, and previous hysterectomy [1,8]. Potential risk factors for POP include forceps delivery, high infant birth weight (>4500 g), prolonged second stage of labor, age less than 25 years at first delivery, family history of POP, occupations requiring heavy lifting, smoking, constipation, and connective tissue disorders [1,9,10].

Women who present to clinic may or may not have symptoms of pelvic prolapse. Upon physical examination, about 40% to 50% have evidence of prolapse on visual inspection but only 3% have symptoms [1,11]. The lack of a chaperone and time can provide a challenge to primary care providers in assessing and managing patients with POP. Many patients struggle with access to specialty care and desire management by their primary care provider whenever possible. Providing care close to the patient is associated with greater positive outcomes [12].

History

The primary goal of the history is to determine which prolapse-related symptoms the patient may experience and their effect on quality of life [8,13]. The vaginal, bladder, and bowel symptoms associated with POP most reported include

- vaginal bulging
- pelvic pressure and discomfort
- increased voiding frequency
- nocturia
- UI
- difficulty voiding
- hesitancy
- slow stream
- straining or changing positions to void
- constipation
- incomplete emptying resulting in straining
- accidental bowel leakage

If the patient has bladder symptoms, a 3-day bladder diary may be helpful to assess for urinary frequency, leakage, fluid intake, and pad use. An example of a bladder diary can be found as Addendum A [14].

In addition, it is important to assess for lifestyle factors and health conditions that are associated with the above symptoms. Such conditions such as obesity, smoking, occupational or recreational factors associated with heavy lifting, and neurological conditions such as Parkinson disease, multiple sclerosis, and cognitive impairment can affect optimal management of symptoms.

Screening tools may be instrumental for busy clinicians. Screening tools help clarify possible discrepancies between the provider and the patient's perception of how severe the symptoms are. There is no universal standard for using screening tools for patients who present with POP. However, there are validated screening tools that can assist in evaluating patient reported outcomes [15]. The Pelvic Floor Distress Inventory measures the patient's bother from POP; The Pelvic Floor Impact Questionnaire measures the life effect of POP and other symptoms; and The International Consultation on Incontinence Questionnaire and Vaginal Symptoms assesses the severity and effect of POP and the patient's vaginal symptoms [15].

Physical examination

Assessment begins with measurement of body mass index and a urine sample. The urine is assessed for blood, protein, leukocytes, nitrites, glucose, and ketones. The abdominal examination will assess for pelvic masses and distended bladder. The vaginal examination allows for the evaluation of POP, urinary leakage, strength of pelvic floor muscles, and the estrogenic effect of the vagina.

Pelvic organ prolapse staging
Physical assessment of the vagina involves using a speculum that will aid in visualizing whether the anterior vaginal wall, posterior vaginal wall, or the apex of the vagina or uterus is descending into and out of the vagina. The hymenal ring is the landmark used to grade the extent of the prolapse (Figs. 3 and 4). A stage 2 prolapse is described when any part of the vagina descends to −1 cm above the hymen. Anything −2 cm above the hymen is considered a stage 1 prolapse. Any prolapse of the vaginal or uterus that extends greater than +1 cm outside the hymen is considered stage 3 prolapse. Any prolapse that completely everts outward is considered stage 4 prolapse [16]. (Table 1) Pelvic floor muscle strength is assessed using a digital assessment of the pelvic floor muscle contraction [15,17]. The provider inserts the middle and index fingers 4 to 6 cm into the vagina and rotates the fingers to a vertical position. The patient is asked to contract her pelvic floor muscles and to hold the contractions for as long as possible and the provider scores the results using the modified Oxford scale [18]. See Table 2.

Vaginal mucosa
In addition to grading the prolapse stage, it is important to assess for excoriation or skin irritation from the pressure of the prolapsed vagina and/or uterus against the perineum or other tissue [19]. The vagina is also assessed for genitourinary syndrome of menopause (GSM), which may be seen in postmenopausal women not on hormone therapy. Optimizing vaginal support and health with localized estrogen increases vaginal epithelial thickness and may decrease the sensation and symptoms of POP and reduce vaginal wall erosion and discharge [20,21]. In addition, estrogen may improve continence in those with urinary issues. There are other options for those who desire to limit the use of estrogen in women. The use of vaginal dehydroepiandrosterone inserts and oral ospemifene are nonestrogen options for GSM [20].

Hidden or occult incontinence
One of the main issues with POP is that the prolapse itself can kink the urethra, which can affect voiding [19,22]. Patients may report no UI or incomplete bladder emptying because the prolapse itself is kinking the urethra preventing the symptoms of UI. It is important for providers to assess for adequate emptying and the possibility of occult UI in their assessment of patients with POP.

Because the urethra may be kinked, the evaluation for incomplete emptying is done by elevating the prolapse into an anatomical position thereby unkinking the urethra [19,22]. The patient is encouraged to bear down while supporting the vagina. The provider may need to use a ring forceps to support the vagina for this assessment. If the patient does not leak with Valsalva, then a cough is performed. This is often called an "empty bladder" stress test. The bladder is assessed for optimal emptying either via straight catheterization or bladder scan. This assessment confirms the patient is emptying completely. A postvoid residual of 150 cc or less is considered adequate voiding [19].

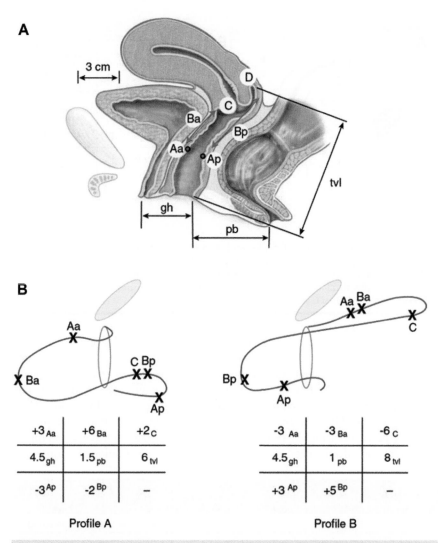

Fig. 3. Pelvic organ prolapse quantification (POP-Q) system for staging pelvic organ prolapse. Aa, point (**A**) anterior; Ap, point A posterior; Ba, point (**B**) anterior; Bp, point B posterior; C, cervix or vaginal cuff; D, posterior fornix (if cervix is present); gh, genital hiatus; pb, perineal body; tvl, total vaginal length. (*From* Victor Nitti: Vaginal Surgery for the Urologist. Saunders: Elsevier, 2012.)

Management
Conservative management for POP should be considered as the first-line management and can be initiated by primary care providers [17]. Studies have shown that prolapse is not likely to progress for up to 2 to 3 years [8,15,23,24]. Lifestyle modifications and physical therapy may improve POP symptoms. Because obesity is a risk factor for POP, implementing weight-

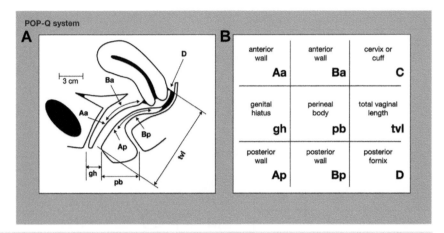

Fig. 4. POP-Q scoring system. (*From* Dwyer L, Kearney R. Conservative management of pelvic organ prolapse. Obstet Gynaecol Reprod Med 2021;31:35–41.https://doi.org/10.1016/j.ogrm.2020.12.003; with permission. *From* Bump RC, Mattiasson A, Bo K, et al. The standardization of terminology of female pelvic organ prolapse and pelvic floor dysfunction. Am J Obstet Gynecol 1996; 175:10.)

loss strategies may assist with symptom relief. Lifestyle interventions include dietary changes such as increased fluid intake and dietary fiber to manage constipation or pharmacologic management of constipation. In addition, reducing prolapse strain by limiting heavy lifting with either exercise or occupation and cessation of smoking, which decreases cough, have been found to reduce POP symptoms [25]. Physical therapists who specialize in pelvic floor therapy can provide pelvic floor muscle training (PFMT), which may improve the strength, duration, and effectiveness of the pelvic floor [18,25]. Indications for a pessary

Table 1
Pelvic organ prolapse staging

Stage	Description	Measurement from hymenal ring
Stage 1	Most distal prolapse is more than 1 cm above the hymen	Less than −1 cm
Stage 2	Most distal prolapse is between 1 cm above and 1 cm below the hymen	Most distal prolapse is −1 cm, level with hymen or +1 cm
Stage 3	The most distal prolapse is more than 1 cm below the hymen but no further than 2 cm less than total vaginal length (TVL)	≥ +2 but less than TVL −2 cm
Stage 4	The most distal prolapse protrudes to at least TVL −2 cm	≥ TVL −2 cm

Data from Madhu C, Swift S, Moloney-Geany S, Drake MJ. How to use the Pelvic Organ Prolapse Quantification (POP-Q) system? Neurourol Urodyn. 2018;37(S6):S39-S43. https://doi.org/10.1002/nau.23740

Table 2
Modified oxford scale for pelvic floor muscle strength

Grade	Description
0	No PFM contraction detected
1	Detects only a flicker of a contraction
2	Detects weak tension in PFM but no lift or squeeze
3	Detects lifting of posterior vaginal wall with contraction and squeezing on the base of the finger, inner pulling of the perineum inner
4	Detects elevation of the posterior vaginal wall against resistance and drawing in of the perineum
5	Detects a strong contraction against a strong resistance

Adapted from Rodrigues MP, Paiva LL, Mallmann S, Bessel T, Ramos JGL. Can the inability to contract the pelvic floor muscles influence the severity of urinary incontinence symptoms in females?. Int Urogynecol J. 2022;33(5):1193-1197. https://doi.org/10.1007/s00192-021-04880-1.

trial include POP symptoms, evident prolapse on examination, medical contra-indications for surgery, and the patient's desire for a pessary trial.

Vaginal support device (pessary)
A vaginal pessary is a silicone removable device that is fitted to the patient's prolapse and placed into the vagina to support POP. Patients have reported 90% effective treatment of symptoms and 75% satisfaction with pessary use [26]. Patients who may not be able to use a pessary are those with an active vaginal infection, possible noncompliance with follow-up, and sexually active patients who are unable to remove and reinsert their pessary. However, these are not absolute contraindications because once the vaginal infections have cleared, follow-up strategies are resolved, and sexually active patients may opt for partner assistance, pessary use can be considered.

The vaginal pessary is a silicone device that comes in various sizes and shapes. The most common pessaries used for POP are the ring with and without support, the cube pessary, the Gellhorn pessary, and the oval pessary with and without support [27,28] (Fig. 5). The pessary fits behind the symphysis pubis and the apex of the vagina. The provider measures this distance and selects a pessary size that fits within this measurement. There should be finger space between the pessary and the vaginal wall [21]. Starting with a ring, with or without support, is the first choice for most patients. The degree of POP will determine if the provider should use a pessary with support (pessary with a diaphragm) or not. If the pessary fits well, the patient may or may not feel its presence. However, the pessary should never cause discomfort. The pessary should remain inside the vagina with Valsalva and cough. Patients who are sexually active will need to be taught to insert and remove the pessary on their own. Those who are not sexually active can still be taught to self-manage or they can return to clinic for provider removal, assessment of vaginal mucosa for irritation and reinsertion every 6 to 12 weeks [27,28]. If the patient has incontinence, the vaginal pessary may not be optimal because once the prolapse is reduced, whatever incontinence the patient experienced before the pessary

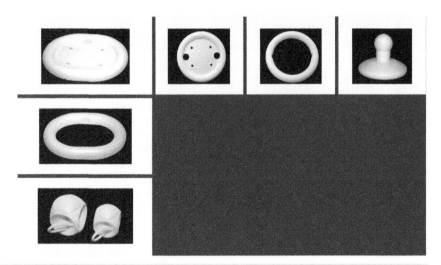

Fig. 5. Types of vaginal pessaries. (Used with permission from MedGyn.)

fitting may increase with pessary use. The patient should be referred to a specialist if this occurs [19,22].

Genitourinary syndrome of menopause

Patients with GSM may benefit with pharmacologic treatment with estrogen before pessary fitting. It is common for providers to treat GSM with vaginal estrogen for a month and then return for pessary fitting [20,27]. This allows time to order the pessary if needed. The use of vaginal estrogen may help keep the vaginal tissues optimally healthy, which may help limit vaginal wall irritation from the pessary.

Follow-up

Many patients can self-manage their pessaries. Most will insert the pessary in the morning, wear during the day, and remove at night. The cube pessary is the only pessary that must be removed regularly (every few days). The other pessaries can remain in place for up to 6 to 12 weeks. It is recommended that return visits occur early (6 weeks) in the beginning of pessary use. The frequency of evaluation can decrease when return visits show no vaginal mucosal issues with pessary use [27,28]. Many patients use vaginal pessaries for years. Occasionally, if the patient develops vaginal mucosal irritation or excoriation, the pessary is removed for a month to allow healing to occur. Use can resume once healing has occurred [27,28]. This break in use is not a cause for concern with long-term pessary use if healing is allowed. The provider should assess the vaginal mucosa, patient compliance, address any patient questions or concerns, and the patient's desire to continue with pessary use at follow-up visits. In most states, it is within the scope of practice for registered nurses to fit pessaries with training. The clinic manager should check with the state board of nursing for specific state practice rules.

Summary of initial management from primary care provider
- Screen for POP and UI and bowel issues [17]
- Rule out abdominal, bladder, and bowel pathologic conditions
- Initiate lifestyle management (weight loss, fluid adjustment, diet adjustment)
- Consider referral for PFMT
- Consider vaginal pessary trial

Patients should be referred to a urogynecology practice if the patient declines PFMT or vaginal pessaries, and if the provider is unable to fit the patient with a pessary that will stay in, the pessary results in UI symptoms that the patient does not desire to monitor. Moreover, patients can be fitted with a vaginal pessary at the urogynecology practice and follow-up visits can occur with their primary care provider.

CLINICS CARE POINTS

- Providing conservative management for POP can provide access to care for many rural patients
- Screen for POP, UI, and bowel issues
- Rule out abdominal, bladder, and bowel pathologic conditions
- Initiate lifestyle management (weight loss, fluid adjustment, diet adjustment)
- Consider referral for pelvic floor muscle therapy
- Vaginal support device (pessary) is considered the first-line treatment of POP

DISCLOSURE

The authors have nothing to disclose.

References

[1] Barber MD, Maher C. Epidemiology and outcome assessment of pelvic organ prolapse. Int Urogynecol J 2013;24(11):1783–90.
[2] Bohlin KS, Ankardal M, Nüssler E, et al. Factors influencing the outcome of surgery for pelvic organ prolapse. Int Urogynecol J 2018;29(1):81–9.
[3] Prentice A, Bazzi AA, Aslam MF. Treatment patterns of primary care physicians vs specialists prior to subspecialty urogynaecology referral for women suffering from pelvic floor disorders. World J Methodol 2019;9(2):26–31.
[4] Ellerkmann RM, Cundiff GW, Melick CF, et al. Correlation of symptoms with location and severity of pelvic organ prolapse. Am J Obstet Gynecol 2001;185(6):1332–8.
[5] Hughes M, Nikolavsky D, Ginzburg N. Transgender surgery and outcomes: focused for the FPMRS provider. Female Pelvic Med Reconstr Surg 2020;26(4):259–62.
[6] Zurada A, Salandy S, Roberts W, et al. The evolution of transgender surgery. Clin Anat 2018;31(6):878–86.
[7] Buncamper ME, van der Sluis WB, van der Pas RSD, et al. Surgical outcome after penile inversion vaginoplasty: a retrospective study of 475 transgender women. Plast Reconstr Surg 2016;138(5):999–1007.
[8] Pelvic Organ Prolapse: ACOG Practice Bulletin, Number 214. Obstet Gynecol 2019;134(5):e126–42.

[9] Schulten SFM, Claas-Quax MJ, Weemhoff M, et al. Risk factors for primary pelvic organ prolapse and prolapse recurrence: an updated systematic review and meta-analysis. Am J Obstet Gynecol 2022;227(2):192–208.

[10] Weintraub AY, Glinter H, Marcus-Braun N. Narrative review of the epidemiology, diagnosis and pathophysiology of pelvic organ prolapse. Int Braz J Urol 2020;46(1):5–14.

[11] Wu JM, Vaughan CP, Goode PS, et al. Prevalence and trends of symptomatic pelvic floor disorders in U.S. women. Obstet Gynecol 2014;123(1):141–8.

[12] English E, Rogo-Gupta L. Impact of distance to treatment center on care seeking for pelvic floor disorders. Female Pelvic Med Reconstr Surg 2017;23(6):438–43.

[13] Iglesia CB, Smithling KR. Pelvic organ prolapse. Am Fam Physician 2017;96(3): 179–85.

[14] NIDDK. National Institute of Diabetes and Digestive and Kidney Diseases. Available at: https://www.niddk.nih.gov/search?s=all&q=Your+Daily+Bladder+Diary. Accessed September 28, 2022.

[15] American Urogynecologic Society Best Practice Statement: Evaluation and counseling of patients with pelvic organ prolapse [published correction appears in female pelvic med reconstr surg. Female Pelvic Med 2018;24(3):256.

[16] Madhu C, Swift S, Moloney-Geany S, et al. How to use the pelvic organ prolapse quantification (POP-Q) system? Neurourol Urodyn 2018;37(S6):S39–43.

[17] Basu M. Assessment of the urogynaecology patient in primary care and when to refer. Post Reprod Health 2020;26(2):57–62.

[18] Rodrigues MP, Paiva LL, Mallmann S, et al. Can the inability to contract the pelvic floor muscles influence the severity of urinary incontinence symptoms in females? Int Urogynecol J 2022;33(5):1193–7.

[19] Somerall WE Jr, Pair LS. Importance of urologic assessment for pelvic organ prolapse with occult incontinence: a case study. Urol Nurs 2020;40(5):245–57.

[20] The NAMS 2020 GSM Position Statement Editorial Panel. The 2020 genitourinary syndrome of menopause position statement of The North American Menopause Society. Menopause 2020;27(9):976–92.

[21] Shaw CG, O'Shea M, Trotter K. Pessary use in pelvic organ prolapse. Womens Healthc 2021;9(5):46–8.

[22] Cohn JA, Smith AL. Management of occult urinary incontinence with prolapse surgery. Curr Urol Rep 2019;20(5):23.

[23] Gilchrist AS, Campbell W, Steele H, et al. Outcomes of observation as therapy for pelvic organ prolapse: a study in the natural history of pelvic organ prolapse. Neurourol Urodyn 2013;32(4):383–6.

[24] Miedel A, Ek M, Tegerstedt G, et al. Short-term natural history in women with symptoms indicative of pelvic organ prolapse. Int Urogynecol J 2011;22(4):461–8.

[25] Giannini A, Russo E, Cano A, et al. Current management of pelvic organ prolapse in aging women: EMAS clinical guide. Maturitas 2018;110:118–23.

[26] Zeiger BB, da Silva Carramão S, Del Roy CA, et al. Vaginal pessary in advanced pelvic organ prolapse: impact on quality of life. Int Urogynecol J 2022;33(7):2013–20.

[27] Pair LS, Somerall WE Jr. Overview of pessary fitting, use, and management for pelvic organ prolapse. Urol Nurs 2021;41(6):335–42.

[28] Harvey MA, Lemieux MC, Robert M, et al. Guideline No. 411: vaginal pessary use. J Obstet Gynaecol Can 2021;43(2):255–66.e1.

Advances in Family Practice Nursing 5 (2023) 119–135

ADVANCES IN FAMILY PRACTICE NURSING

ELSEVIER
MOSBY

Care for Women with Past Trauma Using Trauma-Informed Care

Patricia M. Speck, DNSc, CRNP, FNP-BC, AFN-C, DF-IAFN, FAAFS, DF-AFN, FAAN[a,*], LaQuadria S. Robinson, MSN, CRNP, PMHNP-BC[b], Karmie Johnson, DNP, CRNP, PMHNP-BC, CNE[c], Lauren Mays, DNP, CRNP, FNP-BC[d]

[a]Department of Family, Community, & Health Systems, UAB, The University of Alabama at Birmingham School of Nursing, 1720 Second Avenue South, South Birmingham, AL 35294-1210, USA; [b]Psychiatric Health Nurse Undergraduate Programs, Department of Family, Community, & Health Systems, UAB, The University of Alabama at Birmingham School of Nursing, 1720 Second Avenue South, South Birmingham, AL 35294-1210, USA; [c]Nursing Family, Community & Health Systems, UAB, The University of Alabama at Birmingham School of Nursing, 1720 Second Avenue South, South Birmingham, AL 35294-1210, USA; [d]Department of Family, Community, & Health Systems, UAB, The University of Alabama at Birmingham School of Nursing, 1720 Second Avenue South, South Birmingham, AL 35294-1210, USA

Keywords
• Trauma • Trauma-informed care • Stress • Stress response • Allostasis • Allostatic load

Key points
• Violence is prevalent in all societies globally where women are vulnerable to sexual violence.
• Women's healthcare providers have the opportunity to recognize, identify, and create unique interventions that are person centered, and trauma informed.

Continued

INTRODUCTION
Introduction to trauma-informed care
Trauma and mental illness have a complex relationship; trauma increases the risk of one's mental health deteriorating into a mental disorder, and those with mental illness are at higher risk for experiencing trauma [1]. Normal reactions

Corresponding author. E-mail addresses: pmspeck@uab.edu; pmspeck@gmail.com

https://doi.org/10.1016/j.yfpn.2022.11.002
2589-420X/23/© 2022 Elsevier Inc. All rights reserved.

Continued

- Trauma-informed care principles are necessary skills for organizations and providers to understand, where the outcome is creation of strategies to promote safety, peer support, trustworthiness/transparency, collaboration/mutuality, and cultural, historical, and gender issues.
- Although the occasional pharmacologic intervention is necessary, evidence-based nonpharmacologic interventions exist to mitigate acute and chronic exacerbations of trauma reactions.

to trauma may include anxiety, sadness, guilt, hopelessness, and reduced self-efficacy. These and other psychological symptoms often require behavioral health services, including psychiatry and psychology, that view the diagnostic criteria for disorders using a medical approach, such as pharmacologic interventions and specific behavioral therapies. Explained in the companion article, a client's presentation is not part of a pathology [2]. Rather medically identified adaptive behaviors and emotions are part of a normal adaptive process for overcoming trauma [3]. With enough experience overcoming familiar traumas, traumatized persons develop skills at overcoming similar traumas, called resiliance. Naïve to new or more serious traumas, for example, rape or war displacement, some overcoming skills assist in adjustments to the new trauma, but not all. Overcoming serious trauma for some becomes difficult, if not impossible. Reactions of caring healthcare providers to emotional symptoms and behaviors may be harmful if the patient perceives being put in a category or provider judgment, for example, diagnosis proffered is perceived as an abnormal label, followed by pharmacologic intervention. Oftentimes, recommendations to follow the plan are rejected, and often the consequence to *declining a medical recommendation* is documented as "refused" or "against medical advice." Seeking the expertise of mental health services, whose focus is often to mitigate worsening outcomes while increasing function, is an approach that does not recognize the client's unique perspective and personal attempts at healing. The judgements from healthcare providers are perceived as uncomfortable physiologically, and for some, they choose to not return for care, becoming *never served* [4]. An alternate approach for person-centered care by healthcare providers is the implementation of trauma-informed care (TIC). Over the last 25 years, evidence is mounting that the TIC framework is a hopeful, strengths-based approach [5,6] for providing healthcare. Caring used at all levels of healthcare is based in positive psychology [7] and hope theory [8], specifically to build self-efficacy and personal confidence using TIC principles so the person flourishes. Flourishing is "defined as optimal living based on one's values, happiness, interests, important relationships, and sense of meaning" (p. 7) [9]. The outcome is the result of a process and mirrors Maslow's developmental approach, empowering survivors of trauma to survive, and through overcoming, then thrive and eventually flourish, which is the embodiment of resilience.

A trauma-aware organization uses teams that include community and customers to assist in creating an environment that is inclusively welcoming, collaborating with and empowering survivors to set their own goals, based on their personal life's journey and current developmental stage. Structuring organizations with trauma-informed person-centered care that is based in positive psychology and hope theories, the trauma-aware orgnization first creates a safe environments for all, where traumatized patients benefit. Workplaces with trauma-informed staff are attuned to the impact of trauma on survivors and workers improve skill and understanding through continuing education, clinical supervision, and quality improvement. Team members must also be educated on secondary trauma and provided opportunities to improve recognition of situational traumas in the workplace to increase their own skills at overcoming and building resilience through learning activities focusing on coping strategies [1,10]. In the event of past traumas, these organizations have support services to assist members of the organizations, as they remember and are triggered to face their own trauma experiences. Essential is providing services without assigning blame or shame to the need for support.

As healthcare organizations explore their contribution to patient traumas, open dialogue about the perception of offense is necessary to address historical events. Failure to use TIC to explore perceptions of personal lived experiences diminishes any possibility of creating a trauma-informed organization or in assisting members in understanding the reasons for and the possible actions necessary to mitigate long-term health consequences of the trauma impact in patients and the organization. Whether the organization or the persons being served, open dialogue is essential in a culturally humble and kind organization. Minimally, systems that promote provision of TIC are aware of 4 basic principles [11].

1. *Realize* the prevalence of traumatic events and the widespread impact of trauma
2. *Recognize* the signs and symptoms of trauma
3. *Respond* by integrating knowledge about trauma into policies, procedures, and practices
4. *Resist retraumatization* actively

TIC is a framework that recognizes the impacts of trauma on health and well-being and offers a solution to deploying care to optimize patient outcomes [1,11]. A trauma-aware workplace supports supervision and program practices that educate all direct service staff members on secondary trauma, encourages the processing of trauma-related content through participation in peer-supported activities and clinical supervision, and provides them with professional development opportunities to learn about and engage in effective coping strategies that help prevent secondary trauma or trauma-related symptoms [1,10]. TIC is founded on 6 key principles [1].

1. Safety
2. Trustworthiness and transparency

3. Peer support
4. Collaboration and mutuality
5. Empowerment
6. Cultural, historical, and gender issues

As organizations implement structural TIC in care delivery, a safe workplace is legislated [12], with a variety of tools available to organizations [10] who seek guidance from the experts. The World Health Organization is currently considering a validated trauma-informed protocol for healthcare providers responding to human trafficking globally (personal conversation September 29, 2022 with Deb O'Hara-Rusckowski). TIC principles embody a culture and atmosphere that are *aware*, *sensitive*, and *responsive*. To be successful, healthcare personnel identify and reflect on their comfort level before working with traumatized populations of patients by taking training classes that are continuous and interactive [13]. TIC interventions incorporate the understanding of the impact of trauma on individuals' psychological and physical reactions that occur immediately or often are delayed [1,11] and are dependent on their developmental stage and age. Often the trauma affects the patient's behavior and emotional response, useful to previously survive, and is now occasionally used during all aspects of the evaluation and examination with the potential to create barriers to the purpose of the visit. Seeking permission for all activities, using open communication that encompasses person-centered and TIC principles creates a safe environment that helps to build trust in an unfamiliar environment over time and cultivates an atmosphere of respect without judgement [14]. A heightened sensitivity from provider education and training helps identify signs and symptoms of trauma and triggers for the patient during the encounter, requiring viewing trauma as *formative* [15] and a well-developed and reptilian reaction to stimuli, however inadvertent. To decrease apprehension and the likelihood of retraumatization, recognition and openness by the provider demonstrates acceptance and person-directed care, allowing for clear guidance and instructions that are nonjudgmental in demeanor [16]. Other examples of provider-initiated TIC interventions are given in Table 1.

Evidence is emerging that there is more to do. In four (4) publications, the evidence of significant trauma is increasing, especially for women, often related to sexual trauma.

- 30% of adult women experience at least one physical assault by a partner [21].
- 15% to 50% of women have been victims of rape [21].
- 20% of female children are sexually abused by the age of 13 years [21].
- 41% of female veterans reported a history of military sexual trauma [22].
- 63.9% of primarily white, non-Hispanic individuals with some college education had experienced at least one adverse childhood experience (ACEs) [23].
- 12.5% of white, non-Hispanic individuals had experienced 4 or more ACEs [23].
- 83.2% of a more diverse sample of adults who had completed high school confirmed those findings, with respondents reporting at least one standard- or community-level adversity [24].

Table 1
Provider-initiated trauma-informed care interventions

TIC principle	Evidence of retraumatization	Suggested interventions
Safety	Organization and healthcare workers are not safe, judge, and are not to be trusted	Introductions and asking what the patient wants to be called and "see them" as people Encouraging choices, for example, where to sit in the clinical setting Asking permission to inquire about sensitive areas during interview or history taking, before touching Explain reason for and seek permission to touch Allow time to clarify and expand on concepts and processes misunderstood before evaluation/examination
Peer support	Feelings of being alone, without support	Provide referrals for patient to share with others who have similar lived experiences Creates accountability rooted in compassion Builds self-efficacy through positive psychology of providing the path to recovery posttrauma
Trustworthiness and transparency	Documentation is often laden with judgment, may meet mandatory reporting (MR) requirements	Establish trust through transparency about process and privacy Acknowledge distress, stopping until distress diminished, and permission is given to continue Change documentation, instead of writing "refused treatment," write "declined recommendations" and show to the patient If mandatory reporting, discuss with patient about the MR law and your role, and follow-up with patient

(continued on next page)

Table 1
(continued)

TIC principle	Evidence of retraumatization	Suggested interventions
		Use engaged open body positions, people's first language, respect their choices, remain in the moment as an active listener and without judgment
Collaboration and mutuality	Decisions are often directed, without input from patients, diminishing voice, and choice in personal care	Provider serves as educator and facilitator of care, collaborating with a team to offer comprehensive approaches to care
		Foster a mutual and a collaborative effort in decision-making
		Use *TeachBack* to engage the patient
		Opportunity for questions, expression of fears about their choices improves the shared decision-making that occurs as a team with a common goal of health of the patient
		Maximize high accountability on the patient's behalf for taking control care
		Provides a voice and choice for the patient, the ultimate arbitrator of their personal health
Cultural, historical, and gender issues (CHGI)	Feelings of lack of understanding of CHGI, without sensitivity to personal needs related to CHGI	Personal reflection about stereotypes; intrinsic and extrinsic bias is necessary to provide culturally humble care to persons who experience societal marginalization, either today or historically
		Promote recovery with engagement in all situations regardless of level of vulnerability
		Active support of individual health beliefs and practices related to CHGI

Data from Refs. [1,9,13,16–20].

- 37.3% of diverse respondents reported four (4) or more standard or community-level adversity [24].
- 33.2% of Philadelphia adults experienced emotional abuse and 35% experienced physical abuse during their childhood [24,25].
- 35% of adults grew up in a household with a substance-abusing member; 24.1% lived in a household with someone who was mentally ill [24,25].
- 12.9% lived in a household with someone who served time or was sentenced to serve time in prison [24,25].

Recognizing the prevalence of trauma, particularly ACEs in childhood and the additional ACEs identified by subsequent literature, is also a vital component of providing healthcare. Using a TIC approach to remain sensitive, nonjudgmental, and respectful in all encounters, regardless of emotions or behaviors demonstrated in Table 2, is a strategy to serve all populations equitably.

Vulnerable populations: women

Women's healthcare encounters are particularly vulnerable for persons who have experience with sexual trauma and as explained earlier, have cumulative negative impact and avoidance with repeated experiences. White coat hypertension is a common phenomenon in primary care visits thought to be associated with the sympathetic nervous system [26] and may be associated with early previous medical trauma and subsequent fear. Prior experiences of sexual trauma result in common gynecologic presentations and conditions and include chronic pelvic pain, sexually transmitted infections, and unintended pregnancies. Women with prior traumatic births, such as obstetric emergencies, unexpected complications, or poor neonatal outcomes, may also have negative healthcare connotations [27]. Acknowledging these experiences and empowering individuals to address their fears and concerns gives them a voice in their healthcare. Providers cognizant of and using the 6 key principles of TIC have tools to avoid retraumatization.

Vulnerable populations: healthcare providers

Vicarious trauma affects care providers, creating a stress reaction related to the exposure to others' traumatic experiences [1]. Awareness about one's own traumas, particularly early childhood traumas, and good self-care strategies improve the ability to continue care of the most vulnerable (and are topics for another article).

Mental health and recovery

Trauma creates a stress reaction, increasing the risk and symptom severity of mental illness [28]. Often, trauma precedes the mental health exacerbation, creating a bidirectional relationship where mental illness increases the risk of experiencing trauma and trauma increases the risk of developing psychological symptoms and mental disorders [1,22].

Understanding one's lived experiences allows providers to evaluate adaptive behaviors after trauma, along with the individual's interpretation of the trauma,

Table 2
Trauma-informed care practice considerations in recognizing and caring for patients with trauma

Flow of care	Examples of behaviors and/or misperceptions	TIC principle suggested interventions
Environmental and organizational considerations	Impatient, withdrawn, threatening, angry, belligerent, escalating, hypervigilance	Safety Seek safe environment that respects client's sociocultural perspective All organization/staff aware of and incorporate TIC Choices of available environmental comforts
Triage Vital signs	Pulling away from touch Avoidance of oral thermometer	Voice/Choice Establish rapport Seeking permission before touching; explain procedure; provide options and autonomy to choose from available options
History taking Intake	"I don't know." "Can we just skip over this?" Resistance Poor historian	Collaboration/Mutuality Patient-centered care allows patients to direct activities, declining services Seek permission to ask all sensitive questions Normalize discussion of trauma history
Physical examination	Eyes cast down shaking Fear	Trustworthiness Seek permission to validate concern, acknowledge the physical response, provide warm blanket Seek permission before touching, allowing the patient to maintain control of his or her body
Special consideration w/ genital examination	Dissociation behaviors Modesty/immodesty Additional people in room Nondisclosure of transitions	Cultural, Historical, Gender Stop evaluation; seek permission to engage in examination, for example, eye contact, comforting voice, use of mirrors to explain what you are doing, asking for questions Provide supplies for cleanup, allow privacy,

(continued on next page)

Table 2
(continued)

Flow of care	Examples of behaviors and/or misperceptions	TIC principle suggested interventions
		and rejoin when dressed
Treatment Planning Disposition	Passivity Detachment disinterest Rush to leave	Empowerment Collaboration with patients about treatment decisions; provide options for treatment preferences; change judgmental documentation Encourage statements of concern about process or treatment plan, ask what could have been done better and work together to optimize health Consider SDoH in treatment planning Assess the needs and goals of the patient during treatment planning Discuss referrals, including trauma-focused behavioral health interventions
Follow-up return visits	Not returning to clinic Not following through with referrals Variable adherence to treatment plan	Peer and Community Support Connect with community services to support continued engagement once barriers identified Develop an interprofessional network of TIC providers Ask about referral experience with interprofessional partners Ask if client has found other community resources helpful

Abbreviation: SDoH, social determinants of health.
© Speck, Johnson, Robinson, and Mays, 2022 *Used with permission; Data from* Refs. [9,17].

rather than categorize behaviors as pathologic (eg, diagnostic labeling). Today, rather than asking *What is wrong with the person?*, ask *What happened to the person?* Understanding the trauma enigma discussed fully in this article allows the provider to explore the adaptive behaviors and physical (biological, physiologic, and developmental) expressions, behaviors, and symptoms following the person's lived traumatic experience to determine the severity or chronicity of their trauma. In fact, their symptomatic and behavioral variations are normal reactions (and adaptations) to abnormal (and traumatic) events [3]. Once providers become aware of the significant (and toxic) traumatic experiences in clients' lives, by viewing the behavioral and emotional presentations as adaptive, identification and classification of the presenting symptoms and behaviors often shift from a "pathology" mindset (ie, defining clients strictly from a diagnostic label, implying that something is wrong with them) to one of the adaptations for overcoming obstacles with new skills and plans for the future as their personal response to surviving trauma. Embracing the belief that trauma-related reactions are adaptive, provider relationships shift to hopeful (positive psychology) [9], strengths-based approaches (principles of person-/family-centered care, empowerment, relational care, and innate health and healing) [6] that build on the belief that responses to traumatic experiences reflect originality, innovation, creativity, self-preservation, determination, fortitude, and endurance. Providers have the opportunity to capture these talents in a structured inquiry, with the goals of: (1) to empower, (2) build self-efficacy, and (3) increase confidence in the patient's and one's own life trajectory.

Provider interventions

Occasionally, the sensations of trauma are overwhelming, requiring medical intervention to extinguish anxiety and fear [29], beyond the scope of this writing. For the provider, recognizing when the patient is a danger to self or others is an opportunity to rapidly intervene. Affirmation about the person's value to self, significant supporters, and society at large is a strengths-based positive psychological promotion. The method is essential to build self-efficacy and eventual confidence to self-regulate fear using Pavlovian stimulus to extinction methods [6,9,29–31]. The ability to change the brain's response, also known as neuroplasticity, "is the 'hope' of the nervous system." [30] Strengths-based methods, theories that focus on symptoms, and methods that focus on activities and interventions in Table 3 provide a path for many in overcoming trauma and avoiding medical pathologic diagnoses, all while they are building overcoming skills, moving toward resilience.

DISCUSSION

TIC is an approach to the care of individuals that uses a strengths-based approach with underpinnings of positive psychology, hope theory, solutions-based and trauma-focused cognitive-based approaches to trauma. The purpose is to normalize reactions to abnormal events, mitigating judgements, self-blame, and shame and focus on the strengths self-identified as useful in their journey to

Table 3
Strengths-based and cognitive methods for overcoming trauma

Method	Activities and goals	Intervention

Positive psychology [7]
Focused on the well-being, strengths, and most favorable functioning of an individual, and flourishing.
	Key concepts:
	PERMA/PERMAH
	• Positive emotions
	• Engagement
	• Relationships
	• Meaning to life
	• Accomplishment
	• Strength and values
	• Health
	• Grit
	• Gratitude
		Health promotion
		• Movement
		  • Healthy diet
		  • Sleep
		  • Journaling
		Evidence-based well-being interventions
		• Positive emotions
		• Gratitude for positive experience
		• Intentional choices of activities

Snyder's hope theory [8] Snyder's hope theory suggests that thought processes are the crux of hope. People with high hope often have multiple pathways toward their goals and the agency necessary to build motivation, whereas those with low hope typically do not.	Assumptions: • People walk path leading to desired outcome • People stay motivated when walking these paths • Hope is cognitive and affective elements • Theory includes goals, paths, and freedom of choice Goals: • Defined as "the object of a person's ambition or effort" • An aim or desired result • Goals are transformative in anchoring and directing hope	Pathways: Indicates that a person can generate plausible routes toward achieving their goals Includes having a plan for managing and overcoming any obstacles that show up on these pathways Planning multiple pathways can make a goal seem more attainable Agency: Determines "can do" attitude in a person who thinks they can use their pathways to achieve their goals

(continued on next page)

Table 3
(continued)

Method	Activities and goals	Intervention
SMART approach [32] (Strength-Focused and Meaning-Oriented Approach to Resilience and Transformation)	Assumptions: • Holds a holistic view of health • Uses facilitative strategies • Promotes dynamic coping	Builds the motivation necessary to work toward your goals with a sense of self-belief and trust in your pathways Eastern spiritual teachings Physical techniques • Yoga • Mediation • Psychoeducation (that promotes meaning reconstruction)
Trauma-focused cognitive behavioral therapy (TF-CBT)	Assumptions: PTSD is a result of negative emotions connected to the memories for the traumatic event and how the person thinks about the traumatic event	Three therapies 1. TF cognitive processing therapy (CPT): CPT focuses on unrealistic and/or unhelpful thoughts a person has about their traumatic experience and/or how the trauma has affected their beliefs about themselves, others, and the world. 2. Common elements treatment approach (CETA): CETA focuses on specifically targeting the symptoms of posttraumatic stress, anxiety, and/or depression in people affected by their traumatic experiences.

3. Prolonged exposure (PE): PE focuses on reducing the intense negative emotions that are caused by memories or being reminded of the trauma. The main negative emotions that go with remembering are fear and shame.

CHANGE happens using positivity and allowing each participant to demonstrate how they manage their own:
- Attitudes about their dignity
- Capacities
- Rights
- Quirks
- Challenges

Work practice theory [33]

Guiding principles
- Everyone is unique
- What receives attention becomes reality
- Words create reality
- Change is continuous
- Support with authenticity
- Teller of own experience
- Dream of future building on what you know and experience
- Be flexible and with capacity
- Be collaborative and adaptive
- Values differences

Solution-focused brief therapy [34–36]

Assumptions:
- Change is constant and certain
- Emphasis should be on what is changeable and possible
- Clients must want to change
- Clients are the experts in therapy and must develop their own goals

SFBT targets clients' default solution patterns, evaluates them for efficacy, and modifies or replaces them with problem-solving approaches that work

(continued on next page)

Table 3
(continued)

Method	Activities and goals	Intervention
	• Clients already have the resources and strengths to solve their problems • Therapy is short-term • The focus must be on the future—a client's history is not a key part of this type of therapy	
Strengths-based case management [5]	Case management model Steps away from the medical clinical perspective of care	Encourages building and nurturing informal support networks Identifying and accessing formal community services and institutional resources

recovery. When trauma is the earliest experience, oftentimes, the person has *feelings* about the environment, people, and interactions. The healthcare provider role is to use TIC to facilitate their journey using TIC principles to introduce a smorgasbord of formative information and summative solutions to the issues faced by those served. Then, their reflections about their personal options empower, which is essential to their recovery. TIC promises to revolutionize provider behaviors and methods, encourage their reflections about significant personal traumas, and finally provide pure person-centered care.

SUMMARY

Healthcare providers are indispensable in the identification of stress related diseases and the identification of patients with the lived experience of trauma. They may be the first person to offer person-centered TIC. Not only does the healthcare provider have the opportunity to see the person humanely, but they also have opportunity to encourage them, focused at their stage of development through empowerment strategies, to build self-efficacy and share their knowledge about how their feelings relate to their personal physiology of trauma. They also have the opportunity to help the person recognize that the path to a health is possible with activities based in positive psychology and hope theory where recognition, identification, and evidence-based interventions help the person walk toward a life of thriving with self-efficacy and flourishing with confidence as they hope and plan, set goals, and attain a higher level of wellness.

CLINICS CARE POINTS

- Trauma is universal and a substantial number of women experience past trauma, including sexual trauma where TIC provides 6 principles to improve engagement of patients and organization members alike.
- Healthcare providers have an opportunity to understand the world view of women and the history of the women's movement in the United States, increasing understanding about the significant quality-of-life issues suffered following family and sexual violence.
- Person-centered care allows the patient to determine what is important to them.
- Knowledge and collaboration with community support services is essential in comprehensive wrap-around services for patients with trauma experiences.
- Nurses are able to implement TIC in systems, families, and individual encounters, where patient-centered care is a focus and encounters are seen as accepting and compassionate for the person and their lived journey.

Disclosure

P.M. Speck: husband and son own patents and a medical device company, not mentioned and will not influence the content of the submission. K. Johnson, L.S. Robinson, and L. Mays: they proclaim they have no conflict of interest.

References

[1] Substance Abuse and Mental Health Services Administration. SAMHSA's Concept of Trauma and Guidance for a Trauma-Informed Approach. Substance Abuse and Mental Health Services Administration. Available at: https://scholarworks.boisestate.edu/cgi/viewcontent.cgi?article=1006&context=covid.

[2] Speck PM, Johnson K, Robinson LS, et al. Caring for Women with Past Trauma: The Physiology of Stress and Trauma. Adv Fam Pract Nurs 2022 (in press);(Women's Health Section).

[3] Frankl VE. From Death-Camp to Existentialism [Man's Search for Meaning]. Lasch I. 1946 [1959].

[4] Speck PM, Connor DP, Small E, et al. Never-served populations: addiction, risk, and health in drug court clients in Memphis TN. Washington, DC: American Public Health Association; 2006 2007 presented at.

[5] Fukui S, Goscha R, Rapp CA, et al. Strengths Model Case Management Fidelity Scores and Client Outcomes. Psychiatr Serv 2012;63(7):708–10.

[6] Gottlieb LN, Gottlieb B. Strengths-Based Nursing: A Process for Implementing a Philosophy Into Practice. J Fam Nurs 2017;23(3):319–40; https://doi.org/10.1177/1074840717717731.

[7] Seligman M, Csikszentmihalyi M. Positive Psychology: An Introduction. Am Psychol 2000;55:5–14; https://doi.org/10.1037/0003-066X.55.1.5.

[8] Snyder CR. Hope theory: rainbows in the mind. Psychol Inq 2002;13(4):249–75; https://doi.org/10.1207/S15327965PLI1304_01.

[9] Duncan AR, Jaini PA, Hellman CM. Positive psychology and hope as lifestyle medicine modalities in the therapeutic encounter: a narrative review. Am J Lifestyle Med 2021;15(1):6–13; https://doi.org/10.1177/1559827620908255.

[10] U. S. Department of Labor. Workplace violence: prevention programs. occupational safety and health administration. Available at: https://www.osha.gov/workplace-violence/prevention-programs. Accessed September 9, 2022.

[11] Substance Abuse and Mental Health Services Administration. Trauma-Informed Care in Behavioral Health Services. Treatment Improvement Protocol (TIP) Series 57. vol HHS Publication No. (SMA) 13-4801. US Deparment of Health and Human Services; 2014. p. 342.

[12] U. S. Department of Labor. Workplace violence: OSHA standards. occupational safety & health administration. Available at: http://www.osha.gov/SLTC/workplaceviolence/standards.html. Accessed September 9, 2022.

[13] Bassuk EL, Latta RE, Sember R, et al. universal design for underserved populations: person-centered, recovery-oriented and trauma informed. J Health Care Poor Underserved 2017;28(3):896–914; https://doi.org/10.1353/hpu.2017.0087.

[14] Fleishman J, Kamsky H, Sundborg S. Trauma-informed nursing practice. OJIN: Online J Issues Nurs 2019;24(2).

[15] Butler LD, Critelli FM, Rinfrette ES. Trauma-informed care and mental health. 2011.

[16] Bruce MM, Kassam-Adams N, Rogers M, et al. Trauma providers' knowledge, views, and practice of trauma-informed care. J Trauma Nurs 2018;25(2):131–8.

[17] Dowdell EB, Speck PM. Foundations for trauma informed care in nursing practice. Am J Nurs 2022;122(4):(pre-publication).

[18] Sanchez RV. The elopement process of adult survivors of sex trafficking during adolescence rutgers. State University of New Jersey; 2021.

[19] Blanch A, Filson B, Penney D, et al. Engaging women in trauma-informed peer support: a guidebook. Alexandria, VA: National Center for Trauma-Informed Care; 2012.

[20] McPeters SL, Bryant PH, Speck PM. The quagmire of social determinants of health for the legal nursing consultant: evaluating failure to thrive. J Leg Nurse Consulting 2021;32(3):10–25.

[21] Agency for Healthcare Research and Quality. Trauma informed care. U.S. department of health & human services. Available at: https://www.ahrq.gov/ncepcr/tools/healthier-pregnancy/fact-sheets/trauma.html. Accessed 2022, September 9.

[22] Barth SK, Kimerling RE, Pavao J, et al. Military sexual trauma among recent veterans: correlates of sexual assault and sexual harassment. Am J Prev Med 2016;50(1):77–86.

[23] Felitti VJ, Anda RF, Nordenberg D, et al. Relationship of childhood abuse and household dysfunction to many of the leading causes of death in adults. The Adverse Childhood Experiences (ACE) Study. Am J Prev Med 1998;14(4):245–58.

[24] Public Health Management Corporation, Merritt MB, Cronholm P, et al. Findings from the Philadelphia Urban ACE Survey. Institute for Safe Families. Available at: https://www.rwjf.org/en/library/research/2013/09/findings-from-the-philadelphia-urban-ace-survey.html. Accessed 2022, September 9.

[25] Skiendzielewski K, Forke CM, Sarwer DB, et al. The intersection of adverse childhood experiences and neighborhood determinants of health: An exploratory spatial analysis. Psychol Trauma 2022; https://doi.org/10.1037/tra0001320.

[26] Hanevold CD. White Coat Hypertension in Children and Adolescents. Hypertension 2019;73(1):24–30.

[27] American College of Emergency Physicians. Caring for patients who have experienced trauma: ACOG committee opinion, number 825. Obstet Gynecol Apr 1 2021;137(4): e94–9.

[28] Spitzer C, Vogel M, Barnow S, et al. Psychopathology and alexithymia in severe mental illness: the impact of trauma and posttraumatic stress symptoms. Eur Arch Psychiatry Clin Neurosci 2007;257(4):191–6.

[29] Kredlow MA, Fenster RJ, Laurent ES, et al. Prefrontal cortex, amygdala, and threat processing: implications for PTSD. Neuropsychopharmacology 2022;47(1):247–59.

[30] Miller-Karas E. Building resilience to trauma: the trauma and community resiliency models. Routledge; 2015.

[31] Fanselow MS. Fear and anxiety take a double hit from vagal nerve stimulation. Biol Psychiatry 2013;73(11):1043–4.

[32] Chan CLW, Chan THY, Ng SM. The strength-focused and meaning-oriented approach to resilience and transformation (SMART). Soc Work Health Care 2006;43(2–3):9–36.

[33] McCashen W. The strengths approach : a strengths-based resource for sharing power and creating change/by Wayne MaCashen. St Luke's Innovative Resources; 2005.

[34] Kim JS. Examining the Effectiveness of Solution-Focused Brief Therapy: A Meta-Analysis. Res Social Work Pract 2008/03/01 2007;18(2):107–16.

[35] Iveson C. Solution-focused brief therapy. Adv Psychiatr Treat 2002;8(2):149–56.

[36] De Shazer S, Berg IK, Lipchik EVE, et al. Brief Therapy: Focused Solution Development. Fam Process 1986;25(2):207–21.

Advances in Family Practice Nursing 5 (2023) 137–149

ADVANCES IN FAMILY PRACTICE NURSING

Care for Women with past Trauma

The Physiology of Stress and Trauma

Patricia M. Speck, DNSc, CRNP, FNP-BC, AFN-C, DF-IAFN, FAAFS, DF-AFN, FAAN[a],*,
LaQuadria S. Robinson, MSN, CRNP, PMHNP-BC[b],
Karmie Johnson, DNP, CRNP, PMHNP-BC, CNE[b],
Lauren Mays, DNP, CRNP, FNP-BC[b]

[a]Department of Family, Community, & Health Systems, UAB, The University of Alabama at Birmingham School of Nursing, NB-443A, 1720 Second Avenue South, Birmingham, AL 35294-1210, USA; [b]Department of Family, Community, & Health Systems, UAB, The University of Alabama at Birmingham School of Nursing, 1720 Second Avenue South, Birmingham, AL 35294-1210, USA

Keywords
- Trauma • Trauma-informed care • Stress • Stress response • Allostasis
- Allostatic load

Key points
- Trauma is linked to long-term health outcomes, where focusing singly on disease treatment guarantees missed opportunities to identify and intervene.
- The physiology posttrauma is predictable, strengthened by the years of bench science contributing to understanding of the long-term health consequences of trauma.
- Trauma and subsequent stress is the overarching term influencing shifts in neuroendocrine impact, where the body recognizes distress, eustress, and becomes numb with continuous stress.

INTRODUCTION
Persons with trauma backgrounds, particularly persons with sexual and physical abuse, disproportionately and significantly correlate with elevated medical

*Corresponding author. 1720 Second Avenue South, Birmingham, AL 35294-1210. E-mail addresses: pmspeck@uab.edu; pmspeck@gmail.com

https://doi.org/10.1016/j.yfpn.2023.01.006
2589-420X/23/

utilization of health care systems [1]. Adverse childhood experiences have association with behavioral, affective and cognitive, and personal domains that include posttrauma mental health disorders [1–3]. Posttraumatic stress disorders are common among trauma victims, where repeated adverse childhood experiences create a cocktail of toxicity, not amenable to typical psychological treatments [2]. The evidence supports significant poor physical health outcomes from trauma, including subsequent suffering, not well understood or asked about by health care providers in clinical settings. Persons with complex trauma symptoms then receive medical treatment of their diseases in isolation without addressing the root cause of trauma-induced stress diseases or subsequent behavioral choices. These same persons with complex trauma transfer epigenetic changes to their offspring who have similar health outcomes [4–7]. The physical symptoms from trauma and vagal nerve activation often result in substance use disorder or other adaptive disruptive behaviors that guarantee physical and behavioral symptoms with high health care utilization. The data collected reveal existing social determinants of health [8–11], but do not address which came first: trauma impact on the person or social determinants impact on the person. This article reviews the published literature to explain trauma and subsequent stress, and continuous suffering from trauma that results in epigenetic modification for subsequent generations and disease formation that shortens the lifespan.

TRAUMA AND STRESS

Serious or persistent trauma overwhelms an individual or community and often ignites the fight, flight, or freeze reaction at the time of the events, and frequently produces a sense of fear, vulnerability, and helplessness [12]. Fright, however, is a sudden realization of danger [13] and a precursor to fight, flight, or freeze reaction.

Individual trauma results from an event, series of events, or set of circumstances that is experienced by an individual as physically or emotionally harmful or life threatening and that has lasting adverse effects on the individual's functioning and mental, physical, social, emotional, or spiritual well-being [12].

The physiologic response following psychological trauma (as opposed to physical trauma, although similar) is predictable. There is significant evidence about the long-term aftermath of trauma (eg, chronic psychological and physical injury and pain) and reflections of suffering [14,15], which is beyond the scope of this article. Much is known about the short-term impact of trauma, occurring when the perception of an event overwhelms the brain with cascades of hormones [6]. The interpretation of a sensation is influenced by previous sensations and exposure to environmental (cultural) responses, which informs the individual's perception of trauma. Conscious thought assigns available language heard from persons in the environment to describe the event in the context of one's personal and community culture, and thereby constructs interpretation through transcription and retranscription of the sensory and emotional feelings [13,16]. Often these memories are not reliable and based on snapshots of events.

Activation of the vagal nerve and the release of the hormone adrenaline, also known as epinephrine, is the first sensation following trauma. The physical alert is felt as impending doom and defines the emotion [17,18]. The body responds with alarm, increasing the heart rate and blood flow centrally and to the brain and heightens the five senses (vision, hearing, taste, smell, and touch). The result is blood flow constriction, thereby reducing oxygenation to peripheral limbs (cold hands and feet) and unnecessary organ systems, such as the digestive, urinary, or reproductive systems [19]. Selye describes the physiologic response as general adaptation syndrome (GAS) to stress [17,20]. The GAS has three stages: (1) alarm, (2) resistance, and (3) exhaustion [21–23], as noted in Fig. 1.

The GAS alarm phase is met with shock and disbelief. In the seconds necessary for activation of cognition, naive exposure to the shock results in brief countershock (fight, flight, or freeze), unless trained to respond (eg, emergency responders and soldiers). Regardless of the traumatic experience, such as a significant death or environmental disaster, the recovery process begins with often uncontrollable ruminations, which eventually leads to a series of adaptations [24], often called overcoming. Experience in responding to and overcoming similar traumas is necessary for resilience (skilled responses) when confronted with another similar traumatic experience. The process of rumination singly, without intervention, results in a new stress response and memory adaptation (retranscription) in the context of environment [13]. Experience in overcoming the stressful event, such as a previous significant loss, generates a complex psychological and emotional response to the specific stress that involves environmental sensory triggers, which perpetuate the stressor [13]. Without personal and positive adaptation, the stress persists, exposures to similar stressors increase repeated stimulus responses, and result in maladaptation [25] to inward (self-loathing) or outward (behavioral aggression) anger, and shame. In persons bereaved with complicated depression, shame and guilt had association with psychopathology [26]. Regardless, the persistent physiologic responses to traumas lead to exhaustion and early death [6,27–32].

The earliest theories explaining the stress response by the bench scientists are now modified through useful biologic measures [22]. Still for the clinician, understanding the unique behavioral reactions to trauma in the context of GAS stages, listening to the trauma perceptions unique to the person experiencing traumatic events, is revealing and provides a foundation for targeted pavlovian extinction interventions to reverse maladaptation [18]. These adaptive (or maladaptive) behaviors often reveal a life-journey with significant childhood trauma known as adverse childhood experiences [27], developmental and adolescent limited situational behaviors with health risks, and perilous choices [33]. It is postulated that the earlier the trauma and maladaptation, where "early life adversity may become biologically embedded over time to negatively impact cognitive function in later adulthood" [29]. The implication is

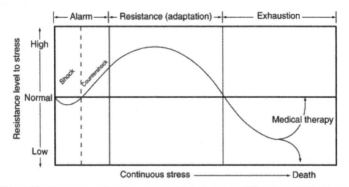

Fig. 1. General adaptation syndrome. (*From* Brown AC, Waslien CI. STRESS AND NUTRI-TION. In: Caballero B, ed. Encyclopedia of Food Sciences and Nutrition (Second Edition). Academic Press; 2003:5628-5636; with permission.)

that without intervention, the outcome (trauma perception interpretation) has significant numbing and intractable hardening of behavioral risk and beliefs about self-efficacy and confidence to change. Without knowledge of the lived experiences, the health care provider labels by using medical interpretations of a patient's sensory descriptions, behaviors, and socialized dependency (eg, adoption of victim status) or overt empowerment (eg, self-efficacy to overcome) as noted in Fig. 2.

Once labeled, health care provider judgment about the person and their situation, coupled with stereotypical beliefs and intrinsic and extrinsic bias, results in biased choices in diagnosis and treatment [34], with directives that support the socialized dependency that marginalizes the patient [34], possibly contributing to the structural disadvantage of all vulnerable populations [16]. Many respond to the marginalization and judgment by choosing to become never served in the health care system, not counted in large data systems, and only returning to seek health care in emergency situations when all other options are exhausted [35,36]. Nevertheless, the body does not forget, and the trauma is expressed in intrinsic body memories and physical indicators [37]. As such, the body often responds similarly when familiar stimuli are present, creating a continuous loop for confirming adaptation behaviors. The continual cascading of stress hormones in the resistance stage of GAS leads to the exhaustion stage of GAS. The patient then exhibits these sensations through behaviors that are off-putting, running their gauntlet using rude to superconciliatory tactics to push potential threats away. These patients are so uncomfortable in the setting, they do not return for care, becoming never served [36].

TRAUMA AND BIOLOGY

During the initial autonomic nervous system (ANS) response to traumatic stress, norepinephrine transmits into the amygdala, activating the sympathetic

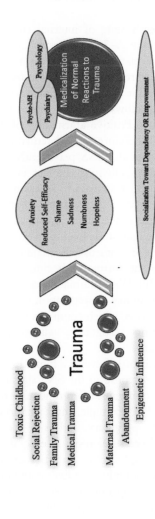

Fig. 2. Trauma across the lifespan and contributions of the health care response. (*Courtesy of Patricia M. Speck, DNSc, Birmingham, AL.*)

nervous system (SNS) (eg, fight, flight, or freeze) [38]. The amygdala signals the hypothalamic-pituitary-adrenal axis. The hypothalamic-pituitary-adrenal axis triggers the pituitary gland, initiating the release of cortisol, a hormone that regulates the biology of the stress response [39]. If the threat is no longer present, the prefrontal cortex sends a signal back to the amygdala to stop releasing the hormone cortisol. When the body has a healthy communication circuit, the amygdala and the prefrontal cortex communicates effectively and returns to homeostasis.

Homeostasis is the organism's state of internal stability while balancing nonspecific environmental change [5–7,40]. Allostasis is the process of maintaining homeostasis. There are many types of stressors in daily life. Typical stressors are familiar, non–life threatening, and pose temporary adjustments, requiring adaptation to nonspecific change. Experience with unique stressors, such as a public presentation, allows for rapid return to homeostasis when the environmental stressor ends. Positive affirmation of the performance improves allostasis processes and therefore a rapid return to homeostasis.

Allostatic loading occurs when the SNS persistently responds to stressful stimuli, exhausting the organism. Obvious changes occur immediately with fight or flight (or a fleeting freeze) responses in reaction to the adrenalin hormonal release. The allostasis process is necessary to return to homeostasis. When persistent threats from the environment create stress, the allostasis process is overwhelmed, now called allostatic load, preventing the return to baseline homeostasis [19]. With the homeostasis maintenance disruption, the environmental change signals the formative beginning of organ adaptation before disease and failure [19,30]. With traumatic stressors, such as an abusive family member, the result is hormonal dysregulation of metabolic, physiologic, emotional, or psychological process, which continues with each environmental encounter, and with each sensory recognition validating the physiologic and biologic preparation for trauma.

The hormones adrenalin and cortisol create a hypoxic environment through constriction of blood flow. In response to the SNS signaling, these hormones diminish the size and function of organs, often rendering diminished or prefailure functioning [20,21,28]. For example, hypertension functionally is a constriction of blood flow to periphery and is a stress-related response. When persistent, the increased pressures result in early death from circulatory malfunction (eg, heart disease and stroke). Another example is blood sugar regulation. With persistent SNS stimulus, the liver continues to release glucose into the circulatory system in anticipation of needed energy for fight or flight, and with diminished pancreas function (part of the digestive system with reduced blood flow), weight gain and metabolic changes eventually result in type 2 diabetes. Gallbladder failure or hypertonic digestive system in the absence of stones or disease is another example of hypoxic cellular demise, and contributes to the nonspecific digestive complaints (eg, colic or irritable bowel syndrome, respectively) following chronic stress-related events. The SNS stimulus is particularly important in the population of pregnant women, who may have contributing adverse childhood experiences and/or current multiple stresses in their family or intimate relationships (eg, drug use, financial insecurity, violence, or issues associated with the social determinants of health). Discovery of risk and initiation of Pavlovian extinction interrupters in SNS stimulation [18] is essential for women experiencing pregnancy induced hypertension or gestational diabetes.

The biologic mechanisms of the stress response system arise from the ANS, controlling organ function and hormonal regulation [17,41]. The ANS has two divisions: sympathetic and parasympathetic branches. The SNS responds to vagal nerve stimulation, operating independently, and responding to sensory, that is, what is seen (eyes), heard (ears), sniffed (nose), tasted (mouth), and/ or touched (skin) by stimuli in the environment, and interpreted as threatening. Fright, as the initial shock, brings awareness of danger and triggers the vagal nerve, which releases adrenalin and results in a cascade of hormones controlling organ responses. The interpreted sensation is fight, flight, or freeze. After the stimulus is gone, the parasympathetic nervous system initiates hormone release to mitigate the SNS, explained in Fig. 3.

Unfortunately, when the SNS is continuously stimulated through prolonged exposure to repeated trauma, the hormonal response results in excessive activation of the amygdala, which in turn signals the prefrontal cortex, which is now loaded with additional cortisol. The result is hyperarousal of the organism and the sensory systems. The mechanism of persistent SNS activation leads to a reduction in oxygenation, and eventually, a reduction in size and functioning of the hippocampus and prefrontal cortex, and all other organs denied blood flow through constriction. Additionally, the cellular structures predicting long life (eg, telomeres) shorten tips in concert with organs, foreshadowing accelerated aging and a shortened life [9,42,43]. Continued and unmitigated hyperarousal results in hypoxic fear through physical sensations that contribute to personal perceptions of symptoms. These symptoms include anxiety, insomnia, depression, short-term memory attenuation, and hypervigilance [38], among others.

Biologic, psychological, social, and spiritual exhaustion is one outcome that portends disease development [19]. The now persistent environmental stressor and the subsequent threats from the intrinsic body and sensory memory results in hypervigilance for early recognition and mitigation of any similar threat. Once sensory memory diminishes, generalized or no memory of events prevents reaction, a common outcome for persons continually stressed who report being numb and profoundly sad. Often persons with extensive traumas create self-pain to validate that they are alive (cutting) or place jewelry on erectile tissue for continual stimulation (nipples, clitoris).

In summary, stress-related diseases are numerous. One often overlooked area for disease development is in the epigenetic transfer of diseases to offspring of persons with trauma [44–46]. Epigenetic studies now reflect multiple generations of disease inheritance [5,47,48]. Although the person today cannot change history experienced by ancestors, awareness of the epigenetic transfer of instructions for the DNA chromosome in infant development and

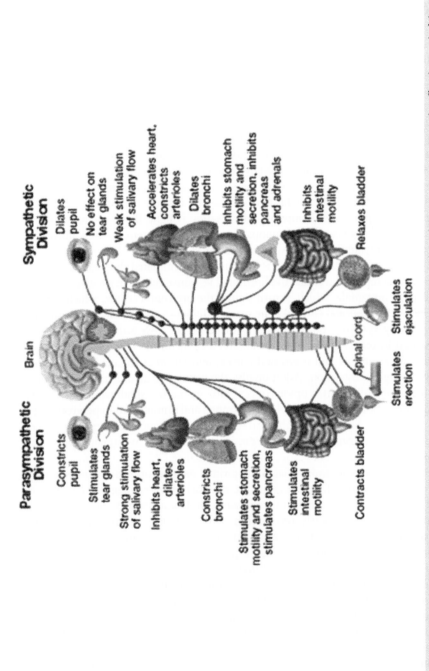

Fig. 3. Autonomic nervous system. (*From* Frith J, Newton J. Autonomic dysfunction in chronic liver disease. Liver international : official journal of the International Association for the Study of the Liver. 05/01 2009;29:483-9. https://doi.org/10.1111/j.1478-3231.2009.01985.x; with permission.)

generational familial disease (eg, cancers, diabetes, hypertension, or hypercholesterolemia, among others) [47–52] is an opportunity to enhance known strategies and interventions that prevent and mitigate disease development.

DISCUSSION

Humans are complex with ancient responses related to potential threats. Biologic reactions and organ failure in response to chronic stimulation by the ANS have nearly 100 years of evidence explaining what happens when traumatic stress is persistent. These reflexive actions in the body have the potential to cause disease, shorten life, and pass the trauma to offspring through epigenetic messaging.

The toxic and complex environments discussed in this paper explain unmitigated stress from traumas as the external threat to homeostasis and allostasis. When interrupted or persistent, allostatic loading creates a hypoxic condition from stress that promotes the death of organs and biologic processes that create consequential disease over time. Evidence now supports specific interventions for the interruption of allostatic loading as a pavlovian response to stress, explained in the article on trauma-informed care elsewhere in this issue. These interventions are psychological and nonpharmacologic for persons with early or persistent traumas wanting to learn overcoming skills necessary for the management of symptoms related to repeated or future traumatic experiences.

For the provider treating persons with complex emotions and sensations following trauma (eg, persistent feelings of shame and self-blame) trauma-focused cognitive behavioral therapy is an option. For others, positive strengths-based interventions offer self-directed healing for many childhood and adult experiences with trauma. For those with overcoming skills (eg, self-efficacy and confidence), exploring their lived experience with stress and trauma is the social connection necessary for a path forward. Although the literature focuses on medicalization or pathology of posttrauma outcomes, most traumatized persons recover without intervention. Using mental health recovery outlined in wraparound services, and methods of "self-discovery, integration of experiences and active self-management of well-being" [53] is a strategy supporting adversarial or trauma-related growth. For them, the combination of social support (positive affirmations), good hygiene (nutrition, exercise, sleep), and alchemy (faith) are key elements in later life recoveries, even though the physical health continues to suffer [10,54].

SUMMARY

Trauma is a life-altering event, contributing to shortened longevity, regardless of when and how often the significant trauma occurs. The continuum of reactions to trauma and stress covers the lifespan and is influenced by the developmental stage and phase of the individual. The earlier the trauma (eg, passed from previous generations or during gestation), the person responds by trying to control the physiologic and biologic changes occurring in their body. For preverbal, it might be maternal-fetal conditions, resulting in fetal demise or early birth [55], or after birth, increased crying and irritability in early infancy [4], where maternal and infant stress affects attachment and development [56]. For school-aged children, behavior obstinance, physical combativeness, or anger. For adolescents, adoption of risk behaviors and experimentation threatens their life, where suicide is increasing. By adulthood, trauma outcomes include substance use disorders, with persistent behaviors to control their environment, or adoption of extreme views to belong. The medicalization of trauma reactions and the treatments are a significant portion of the initial path to full recovery, especially when symptoms become barriers to introspection. When there is significant mental (anxiety, mood disorders, and others) or medical health outcomes (seizures, dementias, stress-related diseases), pharmacologic interventions include treatments that promote adherence and healthy living. Medical intervention cannot cure or even maintain mental health alone using traditional pathologic medicalization, and medication management. Once the emergent behaviors or feelings are addressed, it is prudent to include nonpharmacologic interventions for persons who have desires to explore the sensory feelings and memories of their lived experiences, inclusive of trauma and stress, exploring the stepwise acceptance of the personal meaning of the lived experiences.

Health care providers are indispensable in the identification of stress-related diseases and the identification of patients with the lived experience of trauma. They may be the first person to offer trauma-informed person-centered care, discussed elsewhere in this issue [57]. Not only does the health care provider have the opportunity to treat the person humanely and with compassion, but they also have opportunity to create safe environments that encourage empowerment strategies of building self-efficacy, sharing their knowledge about the physiology and biology of the ANS and how ANS contributes to the person's sensations and emotional feelings. They also have the opportunity to help the person recognize that the path toward health is possible with activities to help the person walk toward a life of thriving with self-efficacy and flourishing with confidence as they hope and plan, set goals, and attain a higher level of wellness.

CLINICS CARE POINTS

- Trauma is universal.
- Gender-based trauma, including sexual trauma, is a significant interruption in homeostasis. Health care providers have an opportunity to understand the world view of women and the history of the women's movement in the United States.
- Physiology, biology, and psychology posttrauma is predictable and informs the health care provider about the person's readiness to participate in nonpharmacologic health care in overcoming trauma and stress outcomes.
- Understanding the significant quality-of-life challenges, including suffering, following family and sexual violence influences social outcomes, possibly including social determinants of health.

DISCLOSURE

P.M. Speck: Husband and son own patents and a medical device company, not mentioned and will not influence the content of the submission. K. Johnson, L.S. Robinson, and L. Mays Disclosures: they proclaim they have no conflict of interest.

References

[1] Rosenberg HJ, Rosenberg SD, Wolford GL 2nd, et al. The relationship between trauma, PTSD, and medical utilization in three high risk medical populations. Int J Psychiatry Med 2000;30(3):247–59.

[2] Bilbao Bourke J, Dobrovolny J, Eaton M, et al. Complex trauma care pathway: results of a 12-month pilot. Perm J 2021;25; https://doi.org/10.7812/tpp/20.147.

[3] Sandström L, Engström Å, Nilsson C, et al. Experiences of suffering multiple trauma: a qualitative study. Intensive Crit Care Nurs 2019;54:1–6.

[4] MacNeill LA, Krogh-Jespersen S, Zhang Y, et al. Lability of prenatal stress during the COVID-19 pandemic links to negative affect in infancy. Infancy 2022;28(1):136–57.

[5] McEwen BS. Allostasis and the epigenetics of brain and body health over the life course: the brain on stress. JAMA Psychiatr 2017;74(6):551–2.

[6] McEwen BS, Gray JD, Nasca C. 60 years of neuroendocrinology - redefining neuroendocrinology: stress, sex and cognitive and emotional regulation. J Endocrinol 2015;226(2): T67–83.

[7] Picard M, McEwen BS. Psychological stress and mitochondria: a conceptual Framework. Psychosom Med 2018;80(2):126–40.

[8] Lee SY, Park CL, Pescatello LS. How trauma influences cardiovascular responses to stress: contributions of posttraumatic stress and cognitive appraisals. J Behav Med 2020;43(1): 131–42.

[9] NeSmith EG, Medeiros RS, Holsten SB Jr, et al. Accelerated biologic aging, chronic stress, and risk for sepsis and organ failure following trauma. J Trauma Nurs 2020;27(3):131–40.

[10] Landes SD, Ardelt M, Vaillant GE, et al. Childhood adversity, midlife generativity, and later life well-being. J Gerontol B Psychol Sci Soc Sci 2014;69(6):942–52.

[11] Skiendzielewski K, Forke CM, Sarwer DB, et al. The intersection of adverse childhood experiences and neighborhood determinants of health: an exploratory spatial analysis. Psychol Trauma 2022; https://doi.org/10.1037/tra0001320.

[12] Substance Abuse and Mental Health Services Administration. SAMHSA's concept of trauma and guidance for a trauma-informed approach. Substance Abuse and Mental Health Services Administration. Available at: https://scholarworks.boisestate.edu/cgi/viewcontent.cgi?article=1006&context=covid.

[13] Shinebourne P. Trauma and culture: on Freud's writing about trauma and resonances in contemporary cultural discourse. Br J Psychother 2006;22(3):335–45.

[14] Hallett CE. Portrayals of suffering: perceptions of trauma in the writings of First World War nurses and volunteers. Can Bull Med Hist 2010;27(1):65–84.

[15] Zaki J, Wager TD, Singer T, et al. The anatomy of suffering: understanding the relationship between nociceptive and empathic pain. Trends Cogn Sci 2016;20(4):249–59.

[16] McCleary J, Figley C. Resilience and trauma: expanding definitions, uses, and contexts. Traumatology 2017;23:1–3.

[17] Robinson AM. Let's talk about stress: history of stress research. Rev Gen Psychol 2018;22(3):334–42.

[18] Fanselow MS. Fear and anxiety take a double hit from vagal nerve stimulation. Biol Psychiatry 2013;73(11):1043–4.

[19] McEwen BS. Neurobiological and systemic effects of chronic stress. Chronic Stress 2017;1; https://doi.org/10.1177/2470547017692328:247054701769232.

[20] Szabo S, Tache Y, Somogyi A. The legacy of Hans Selye and the origins of stress research: a retrospective 75 years after his landmark brief "letter" to the editor# of nature. Stress 2012;15(5):472–8.

[21] Selye H. The stress of life. New York: McGraw-Hill; 1956. p. 554.

[22] Fink G. Stress: concepts, definition and history. Neuroscience and biobehavioral psychology, . Reference Module. New York: Elsevier; 2017.

[23] McCarty R. Chapter 2 - The alarm phase and the general adaptation syndrome: two aspects of Selye's inconsistent legacy. In: Fink G, editor. Stress: concepts, cognition, emotion, and behavior. New York: Academic Press; 2016. p. 13–9.

[24] Miller-Karas E. Building resilience to trauma: the trauma and community resiliency models. New York: Routledge; 2015.

[25] Duncan AR, Jaini PA, Hellman CM. Positive psychology and hope as lifestyle medicine modalities in the therapeutic encounter: a narrative review. Am J Lifestyle Med 2021;15(1):6–13.

[26] LeBlanc NJ, Toner ER, O'Day EB, et al. Shame, guilt, and pride after loss: exploring the relationship between moral emotions and psychopathology in bereaved adults. J Affect Disord 2020;263:405–12.

[27] Felitti VJ, Anda RF, Nordenberg D, et al. Relationship of childhood abuse and household dysfunction to many of the leading causes of death in adults. The Adverse Childhood Experiences (ACE) Study. Am J Prev Med 1998;14(4):245–58.

[28] Tan SY, Yip A. Hans Selye (1907-1982): founder of the stress theory. Singapore Med J 2018;59(4):170–1.

[29] D'Amico D, Amestoy ME, Fiocco AJ. The mediating role of allostatic load in the relationship between early life adversity and cognitive function across the adult lifespan. Psychoneuroendocrinology 2022;141:105761.

[30] Fava GA, McEwen BS, Guidi J, et al. Clinical characterization of allostatic overload. Psychoneuroendocrinology 2019;108:94–101.

[31] Juster RP, McEwen BS, Lupien SJ. Allostatic load biomarkers of chronic stress and impact on health and cognition. Neurosci Biobehav Rev 2010;35(1):2–16.

[32] McEwen B. Sex, stress and the hippocampus: allostasis, allostatic load and the aging process. Neurobiol Aging 2002;23(5):921–39.

[33] Anda RF, Croft JB, Felitti VJ, et al. Adverse childhood experiences and smoking during adolescence and adulthood. JAMA 1999;282(17):1652–8.

[34] McPeters SL, Bryant PH, Speck PM. The quagmire of social determinants of health for the legal nursing consultant: evaluating failure to thrive. J Leg Nurse Consult 2021;32(3):10–25.

[35] Speck PM, Connor DP, Small E, et al. Never-served populations: addiction, risk, and health in drug court clients in Memphis TN. Washington, DC: American Public Health Association; 2007 presented at.

[36] Speck PM, Connor PD, Hartig MT, et al. Vulnerable populations: drug court program clients. Nurs Clin North Am 2008;43(3):477–89, x-xi.

[37] Mann FD, Cuevas AG, Krueger RF. Cumulative stress: a general "s" factor in the structure of stress. Soc Sci Med 2021;289:114405.

[38] Kredlow MA, Fenster RJ, Laurent ES, et al. Prefrontal cortex, amygdala, and threat processing: implications for PTSD. Neuropsychopharmacology 2022;47(1):247–59.

[39] Bremner JD. Traumatic stress: effects on the brain. Dialogues Clin Neurosci 2006;8(4):445–61.

[40] Shonkoff JP, Boyce WT, McEwen BS. Neuroscience, molecular biology, and the childhood roots of health disparities: building a new framework for health promotion and disease prevention. JAMA 2009;301(21):2252–9.

[41] Freed S, D'Andrea W. autonomic arousal and emotion in victims of interpersonal violence: shame proneness but not anxiety predicts vagal tone. J Trauma & Dissociation 2015;16(4):367–83.

[42] Aubert G, Lansdorp PM. Telomeres and aging. Physiol Rev 2008;88(2):557–79.

[43] Chan SR, Blackburn EH. Telomeres and telomerase. Philos Trans R Soc Lond B Biol Sci 2004;359(1441):109–21.

[44] Heijmans BT, Tobi EW, Stein AD, et al. Persistent epigenetic differences associated with prenatal exposure to famine in humans. Proc Natl Acad Sci U S A 2008;105(44):17046–9.

[45] Champagne FA. Epigenetic influence of social experiences across the lifespan. Dev Psychobiol 2010;52(4):299–311.

[46] Gudsnuk K, Champagne FA. Epigenetic influence of stress and the social environment. ILAR J 2012;53(3–4):279–88.

[47] Palma-Gudiel H, Fañanás L, Horvath S, et al. Psychosocial stress and epigenetic aging. Int Rev Neurobiol 2020;150:107–28.

[48] Skinner MK. Environmental stress and epigenetic transgenerational inheritance. BMC Med 2014;12:153.

[49] Shammas MA. Telomeres, lifestyle, cancer, and aging. Curr Opin Clin Nutr Metab Care 2011;14(1):28–34.

[50] McCarthy MM, Nugent BM. At the frontier of epigenetics of brain sex differences. Front Behav Neurosci 2015;9:221.

[51] Argentieri MA, Nagarajan S, Seddighzadeh B, et al. Epigenetic pathways in human disease: the impact of DNA methylation on stress-related pathogenesis and current challenges in biomarker development. EBioMedicine 2017;18:327–50.

[52] Jones CW, Esteves KC, Gray SAO, et al. The transgenerational transmission of maternal adverse childhood experiences (ACEs): insights from placental aging and infant autonomic nervous system reactivity. Psychoneuroendocrinology 2019;106:20–7.

[53] Slade M, Rennick-Egglestone S, Blackie L, et al. Post-traumatic growth in mental health recovery: qualitative study of narratives. BMJ Open 2019;9(6):e029342.

[54] Linley PA, Joseph S. Positive change following trauma and adversity: a review. J Trauma Stress 2004;17(1):11–21.

[55] Parker VJ, Douglas AJ. Stress in early pregnancy: maternal neuro-endocrine-immune responses and effects. J Reprod Immunol 2010;85(1):86–92.

[56] Lieberman AF. Traumatic stress and quality of attachment: reality and internalization in disorders of infant mental health. Infant Ment Health J 2004;25(4):336–51.

[57] Speck PM, Johnson K, Robinson LS, et al. Caring for women with past trauma using trauma informed care strategies. Adv Family Pract Nurs 1:1 February, 2023 (in press).

Advances in Family Practice Nursing 5 (2023) 151–168

ADVANCES IN FAMILY PRACTICE NURSING

Cannabis Use in Pregnancy and Postpartum: Understanding the Complicated History and Current Recommendations to Facilitate Client-Centered Discussions

Elizabeth Muñoz, DNP, CNM, FACNM[a,*],
Ellen Solis, DNP, CNM, FACNM[b,c],
Stephanie Mitchell, DNP, CNM, CPM[d]

[a]Nurse-Midwifery Pathway, University of Alabama at Birmingham, 1701 University Boulevard, Birmingham, AL 35294, USA; [b]University of Washington, School of Nursing Health Sciences Building, Box 357262, 1959 NE Pacific Street Seattle, WA 98195, USA; [c]Quilted Health, 4300 Talbot Road South Suite 403, Renton, WA 98055, USA; [d]Birth Sanctuary Gainesville, PO Box 40, Gainesville, AL 35464, USA

Keywords

- Cannabis • Pregnancy • Postpartum • Substance-use • CBD • Harm reduction
- Therapeutic communication

Key points

- There is a long history of cannabis as a healing modality across multiple cultures; only recently did the substance become legal in some US states.
- Cannabis is often considered a "safe" substance by the public because of the recent legalization of cannabis products in many states.
- Pregnant people commonly report using cannabis for nausea and vomiting in pregnancy, and many report using the substance in the first trimester during the time of embryogenesis.
- Health care professionals should inform pregnant clients that using cannabis in pregnancy is not recommended due to an increase in poor pregnancy outcomes.
- Health care professionals can apply client-centered to interactions where the use of cannabis in pregnancy is being discussed.

*Corresponding author. Carle Foundation Hospital, 601 W Park Street, Urbana, IL 61801
E-mail address: elizabethgmunoz@gmail.com

https://doi.org/10.1016/j.yfpn.2022.12.002
2589-420X/23/© 2022 Elsevier Inc. All rights reserved.

C annabis has long been used as a form of "natural medicine." More recently, it has been used as a method of evidence-based treatment in westernized medicine, and the use of this substance in pregnancy is not a new trend. Once considered an illicit substance, cannabis is now the most frequently used drug in pregnancy and its use has been increasing annually [1]. More than 14.2 million Americans (5.1% of the population) met criteria for cannabis use disorder, a term used to describe those who cannot stop using cannabis even when it is causing health concerns or problems [2].

Much like its use in nonpregnant individuals, the reasons for cannabis use in pregnancy are varied and include easing symptoms of nausea and vomiting in early pregnancy, stimulating hunger for those struggling to eat while pregnant and for mental health purposes, such as anxiety, depression, and insomnia [3]. Pregnant patients may turn to cannabis under the assumption that it is safer than some medications used for the common complaint of nausea and vomiting. Recent legalization of cannabis products in many states may mean that pregnant people could be likely to review their use of this product with their health care professionals. Health care professionals should be aware of the common uses of products containing cannabis in pregnancy and should be educated on how to talk with clients about their use of these products in a way that is bias-informed and evidence-based [3]. A sample script demonstrating respectful, patient-centered language in three scenarios is provided below. This article provides the reader with background information regarding the history of cannabis as medicine, legal trends, and troubles clients face with cannabis use in pregnancy and postpartum, including potential dangers of cannabis that goes unregulated and a brief review of the available evidence on cannabis use in pregnancy.

HISTORY OF CANNABIS

The mention and use of cannabis throughout the earliest civilizations have been well-documented. So much so that common historical and global uses of cannabis for pain control have continued to be pervasive in both Eastern and Western medicine, increasingly so as documentation of cultures continues to become more readily available [4,5]. *Cannabis Sativa* is the Latin botanic genus and epithet of the Marijuana plant, indigenous to the Indian subcontinent and Central Asia. Globally, it is seen as commercially useful, with a mature cultivated plant yielding essentially all parts of the plant useable, from the dried leaves and edible seeds to a drug resin, and an industrial fiber. Its agricultural versatility for uses in both medicinal and therapeutic has made this plant controversial and highly sought, based on which components of the dioecious flowering plant are desired and which of the three species, namely *sativa, indica,* and *ruderalis* are used [6].

Components of the plant

The military research of the 1930s and 1940s identified the first cannabinoid properties, whereas the 1960s brought about an increased understanding of how cannabinoids acted on the human brain. In addition, the chemical structure of delta-9-tetrahydrocannabinol (THC) was identified and first studied in 1964 [7]. During the 1970s, scientists identified other related compounds collectively called phytocannabinoids, and by the 1980s, scientists were beginning to understand the mechanism of action of these cannabinoids on the central nervous system (CNS). Specifically, there was a better understanding of the psychoactive elements of the plant that refer to the cannabinoid (Cannabinoid Receptor 1 [CB1]) receptors in humans and its ability to produce biological and behavioral responses and changes in perception. These effects became desired elements and have contributed to the exploitation of the substance, making cannabis the most used illicit drug in the world.

Cannabidiol (CBD) is the nonpsychologically altering component within the plant that is used for a variety of therapeutic uses and is used both topically and internally. The biodiversity and varied bioavailability from the related cannabinoid compounds are what makes the pharmacology of cannabis unique as it is considered an anxiolytic, sedative, psychedelic, and an analgesic [8]. Many products containing CBD have entered the public sphere in the last decade, and they often remain unregulated and untested for safety in pregnancy.

Medicinal timeline
The historic use of cannabis as medicine ranges from ancient pharmacopeias to Phase III trials of pharmaceutical grade cannabis. The richly documented history seeped into medical practice paints the picture for the utility of this plant as medicine. The ingestion, inhalation, and application of cannabis were common treatments for a variety of ailments. In 2600 BC, the use of cannabis was documented as pain relief for a Chinese Emperor, whereas in ancient Egyptian societies, cannabis was a treatment for infections and vaginal contractions [9]. From ancient manuscripts to current literature, common medicinal use of cannabis has always seemed to improve the occurrence of convulsions [10]. The 1800s continued to document cannabis and its ability to elicit positive neurologic effects in those with epilepsy, whereas the nineteenth century brought a new wave of usage for rheumatism, tetanus, cholera, and infant seizures.

COMMON MEDICINAL USES OF CANNABIS
Although cannabis has been used across cultures as medicine for generations, the exploration of cannabis as a component of western medicine in the United States came only in recent history. In the mid to late 1900s, modern western medicine began to lean in favor of synthetic pharmacotherapy and cannabis began to decrease in popularity as a medical treatment, leading to increases in the criminalization and outlawing of the use of cannabinoids as medicine. The illegal recreational and social use of cannabis in the United States in the 1960s and 1970s allowed scientists to observe the effects of cannabis on modern humans. What was discovered over the next several decades was the beginning of a well-documented trail of literature, which reported the impact of

cannabis as medicine for several common diagnoses. For example, with regard to the diagnosis of epilepsy, cannabinoids compete for the nerve synapses that exhibit overexcitability as well as decrease the hyperexcitability of CNS. The effects of cannabinoids and the CNS suggested that cannabis may exert an anticonvulsant effect. Today, further scholarship has confirmed what the earlier studies from the 1970s hypothesized, the use of cannabinoids as an independent or adjunct treatment in both children and adults has proven anti-seizure and antiepileptic actions due to the decreasing the availability of the presynaptic neurotransmitter glutamate [11,12]. By the beginning of the twenty-first century, cannabis was relegitimized as a medical modality in the United States, treating diagnoses from anxiety to cancer. Table 1 lists some of the most common medicinal uses of cannabis in the United States.

LEGALITY OF CANNABIS

Cannabis has a history fraught with legal issues, and the earliest noted public bans on cannabis were recorded in the 1300s. History demonstrates a legacy of restriction, persecution, criminalization, banning, and outlawing of cannabis in a variety of ways, including laws created in the twentieth and twenty-first centuries. It was not until the turn of the twenty-first century when the global majority began to shift ideas surrounding the legality of cannabis.

In the United States, federal drug laws classify cannabis in the highest classification as a Schedule I drug, based on the US federal Controlled Substances Act. Proposition 215 made California the first state to legalize cannabis in 1996. Since then, 39 states and the District of Columbia have legalized medical use of marijuana as of 2022, and 19 states and the District of Columbia have also legalized the adult recreational use of marijuana. In states with no legality for distribution, use, or possession, some of the lesser penalties may include fines starting at $100.00. Although some of the harsher penalties may include between 60 days to 30 years in prison, fines of up to $1,000,000.00, or both for large quantities of cannabis. In October of 2022 President Joe Biden pardoned all those who "committed the offense of simple possession of marijuana in violation of the Controlled Substances Act" which was expected to positively affect the criminal records of over 6,500 citizens [13,14]. This policy change may shift the future of drug laws in the United States, including those negatively affecting pregnant people and their families.

Table 1
Common medicinal uses of cannabis

Nausea/vomiting	Chronic pain control	Cachexia
Cancer	Degenerative neurologic conditions	Traumatic brain injury
Epilepsy	PTSD	HIV/AIDS
Spasticity	IBS	Parkinson's
Glaucoma	Schizophrenia	Psychosis

THE DANGERS OF UNREGULATED CANNABIS

The large amount of illicit cannabis seized by the Drug Enforcement Administration (DEA) over the last 10 years in the United States demonstrates that the increased potency, a variety of commercial agricultural growth environments, and individualized breeding practices are several reasons the illegal cannabis market continues to thrive, even in states with legal medical and recreational use [15]. The dangers as highlighted by the DEA have shown an increased incidence in the rise of THC-containing products that are mixed with synthetic but molecularly similar psychoactive compounds. In worse case scenarios, these unregulated cannabis products mixed with unregulated synthetic materials are known to be dangerous and life-threatening. Although similar to agricultural THC, the chemical compounds of these synthetic additives affect the brain more powerfully, at times resulting in psychoactive effects [16].

With the legalization and regulation of cannabis becoming the rule and no longer the exception in the United States, research is now being done on the safety of regulated cannabis products and cannabis products procured from an unregulated source, such as "street" weed [17]. There are risks with unregulated cannabis, ranging from mild, such as mixing of inactive substances such as dried garden herbs to severe, such as the combining of opioids in the cannabis product to increase the sensation and addictive quality of the product. Largely due to the infiltration of lesser cheaper products as additives used to increase the quantities of illicit drug products opens the opportunity and concern for free-market and nonregulated availability of cannabis. Recent evidence shows that the manufacturing of illegal drugs for illicit nonprescriptive recreational use include more powerful, cheaper, dangerous, and often variability of drug concentrations and additives.

Fentanyl

Fentanyl is an opioid that is 100 times the strength of morphine and can be easily overdosed when combined with cannabis due to uneven mixing of the substances [18]. This is a dangerous, common, and purposeful additive to some street drugs, namely cannabis, heroin, and cocaine, largely due to the goal to increase revenue for manufacturers for a decreased volume of product [19]. This concern has been linked to inadvertent drug exposure along with the potential for overdose and death. The dangers of not regulating the cultivation, harvesting, and distribution of cannabis is well-documented, allowing an entry point for those seeking to take advantage of an unregulated industry. With the increased use of recreational cannabis, including e-cigarettes, vaping of cannabis oils, and hookahs, comes to the risk of exposure to additives and variations in production. Irregularities in additives are what make unregulated cannabis consumption particularly dangerous.

It is known that regulating cannabis has increased safety for the general population and one potentially deadly concern is the addition of fentanyl into cannabis products that remain unregulated. As mentioned before, the person purchasing cannabis illegally may be exposed to fentanyl without their knowledge, leading to a dependence on a substance they potentially never intended to use. This unknown exposure to such an addictive opioid can lead to unexpected withdrawal symptoms for the patient and even lifelong substance use disorders [18]. In the case of a pregnant person, exposure to opioids in pregnancy, whether known or not, can lead to neonatal withdrawal and complications for the infant after birth. When counseling pregnant and postpartum patients on the use of unregulated cannabis products, health care professionals should discuss the risk of polysubstance exposure due to the actions of the seller of the product and specifically mention Fentanyl and its risks. Although health care professionals may not agree with their client's substance use in pregnancy, strongly advising the client to use only regulated cannabis is a form of harm reduction which should be practiced by all prenatal care professionals.

CONSIDERATIONS FROM US HISTORY AND POLICY

Although the history of the criminalization of drug use can be traced back to the 1870s, the modern day "War on Drugs" in the United States began in the 1960s with the increase in popularity of psychedelic substances and was made an official federal initiative in 1971 by President Richard Nixon [20]. The new laws, created as a deterrent to drug use, led to the incarceration of 400,000 people in America by 1997 and disproportionately affected black communities [21]. By the early 2000s, the annual arrests for illegal cannabis use peaked in the United States at 900,000 and then began declining, most likely due to the changing political landscape in the country [22]. Current policies on substance use in the general population are trending toward compassion and harm reduction, such as providing clean needles to people with opioid use disorders, though critics of these policies say they are being loosened to keep white Americans out of prisons and do little to address the racist history of incarceration of drug offenses [20].

Policies surrounding pregnancy

The policies mentioned above demonstrate leniency toward cannabis use in the general population, though this cannot be said about laws surrounding drug use in pregnancy. Twenty-four states have current child welfare laws that make drug use in pregnancy a crime because they consider it child abuse, though these offenses often go unprosecuted [23]. In both Alabama and South Carolina, the states' supreme courts upheld that drug use, including the use of cannabis, during pregnancy can be considered child abuse, making it more likely that a pregnant person would be tried and convicted under these laws [23].

Substance use in pregnancy is considered such a problem in America that there are 25 states that require drug use in pregnancy to be reported to the state by the health care professional and 19 states that offer fully funded treatment programs, prioritizing the admission of pregnant people [23]. Clearly, the physical and political landscape of one's surroundings means that location of the pregnant person may drive the outcomes for the use of cannabis during pregnancy. Although location of practice is a factor in the incidence of reporting substance use, screening specifically for cannabis use in pregnancy may be guided by individual clinical practice guidelines. Recent literature reviews have found that health care professionals are not sure how to approach screenings or their recommendations for clients in states where cannabis use is legalized [24]. Even then, provider feelings and biases on the use of cannabis in pregnancy can lead to discriminatory drug screening during pregnancy, and therefore an inequitable sequela of events if those tests are positive for substance use [25]. Table 2 reviews the common methods of cannabis use and their potential adverse fetal effects.

CANNABIS USE IN PREGNANCY AND POSTPARTUM

The reasons a pregnant person may use cannabis in pregnancy center around common discomforts in pregnancy, such as nausea and vomiting, sleep disturbances, and mood disorders. Although many pregnant people avoid substance use, the public perception of the safety of cannabis is one reason that clients may not understand the risks of use in pregnancy. The following paragraphs discuss the most common reasons for use of cannabis in pregnancy.

Nausea and vomiting

The first trimester of pregnancy is known to be the time with the greatest potential use of cannabis, most likely due to its positive effects on the symptoms of nausea and vomiting in early pregnancy [1]. As many as 85% of pregnant people experience nausea and vomiting, which can have a significant impact on their lives, affecting their ability to work or attend school and care for themselves or family members [26]. A pregnant person is more likely to use cannabis if their nausea and vomiting symptoms are severe and negatively impact their quality of life [1]. Of those that report nausea and vomiting during pregnancy, 18% report needing to take medication or supplements to mitigate their symptoms [27]. Unfortunately, frequently prescribed and over the counter medications and supplements have varied success rates, with many pregnant people reporting incomplete or no relief [26,27]. Some people will therefore turn to self-medication with cannabis. In addition to this, 3% to 14% of pregnant individuals may experience hyperemesis gravidarum, defined as "a debilitating and potentially life-threatening pregnancy disease marked by weight loss, malnutrition, and dehydration attributed to unrelenting nausea and/or vomiting," which requires significant intervention, sometimes including hospitalization [26,27]. In the case of hyperemesis, the hunger induction from cannabis may be appealing to the client because of the belief that it can assist with weight gain. Furthermore, there can be a paradoxic response to cannabis use in pregnancy where the person becomes more nauseated instead of experiencing a decrease of symptoms. Although cannabis is considered a legal and evidence-based treatment for severe or persistent nausea for nonpregnant people in the states that legalize the use of the substance as a medical treatment, this is not the case in pregnancy [1].

Table 2
Methods of cannabis use and potential adverse effects in pregnancy

Method	Mechanism of action	Potential adverse effects in pregnancy
Smoking Vaping Hashish resin Hashish oil	Inhaled into the lungs and absorbed into the bloodstream	• Cough and exacerbation of asthma symptoms • Systemic effects, such as tachycardia, postural hypotension, and reddening of the conjunctivae as a result of vasodilation • Risk for bronchitis and emphysema • Crosses the placental barrier to fetus leading to the known risks of cannabis use in pregnancy • Tar from the smoke is considered carcinogenic.
Ingesting	Absorbed by mucous membranes of the mouth and absorbed in the stomach as it is digested.	Crosses the placental barrier to fetus, leading to the known risks of cannabis use in pregnancy
Topical transdermal (CBD)	Transdermal products deliver CBD in a manner that penetrates through the upper barriers of the skin and into the bloodstream.	Crosses the placental barrier to fetus, leading to the known risks of cannabis use in pregnancy
Topical (CBD)	Interacts with cannabinoid receptors. However, it does not penetrate the bloodstream.	Is not known to cross the placental barrier but risks are not fully understood.
Synthetic cannabinoids	Can be smoked, vaped, ingested, and applied topically.	Exposure to synthetic cannabinoids has been shown to potentially have teratogenic effects on the fetus

Data from Fischer B, Russell C, Sabioni P, et al. Lower-Risk Cannabis Use Guidelines: A Comprehensive Update of Evidence and Recommendations [published correction appears in Am J Public Health. 2018 May;108(5):e2]. Am J Public Health. 2017;107(8):e1-e12; and Compton WM, Volkow ND, Lopez MF. Medical Marijuana Laws and cannabis Use: Intersections of Health and Policy. JAMA Psychiatry. 2017;74(6):559–560. https://doi.org/10.1001/jamapsychiatry.2017.0723

The exact reason that cannabis is effective in relieving nausea is not completely understood; however, it is clear that nausea and vomiting is largely regulated through the endogenous endocannabinoid system (ECS) in the brain. The CB1 is an essential component of the ECS [28] that helps to regulate the release of neurotransmitters, such as serotonin, dopamine, and glutamate [29]. CB1 is activated by a class of compounds called cannabinoids, some of which are produced endogenously (endocannabinoids), whereas others can come from plants (phytocannabinoids) or be produced synthetically. THC, one of the active ingredients in the cannabis plant, is a phytocannabinoids that can bind strongly to CB1, thereby triggering a release of the neurotransmitters responsible for nausea regulation, euphoria or feelings of well-being, pain relief, motor impairment, sedation, appetite enhancement, tachycardia, and sedation [30]. Thus, when a person uses a product-containing cannabis to fight nausea, it is possible that it is the stimulation of the CB1 that provides the sought-after relief.

Sleep

Another reason a pregnant person may turn to (or continue) cannabis use in pregnancy is for help with sleep disturbances. It is reported that 66% to 97% of people struggle with changes in their sleep patterns during pregnancy with nocturnal waking becoming more common in the third trimester [31]. The most common sleep disturbances in pregnancy are caused by obstructive sleep apnea, restless leg syndrome, nocturnal leg cramps, snoring, and waking to urinate. The causes of these are multifactorial and happen due to the hormonal and physical changes associated with normal pregnancy. Health care professionals often recommend stress reduction, good sleep hygiene, adequate exercise, and medications to address sleep problems [32]. However, despite this advice, pregnant clients may continue to report inadequate sleep and ask about using cannabis products to help with their symptoms. Cannabis affects sleep by acting on CB1 and stimulating the release of adenosine and suppressing the brain's arousal centers [33]. In many situations, this combination promotes sleep; however, due to the inherent differences in an individual's physiology and the varied chemical compounds in cannabis, sedative effects can vary, and cannabis has not been found to be reliable or consistent sleep aid during pregnancy [34]. Health care professionals need to be prepared to have compassionate, evidence-based discussions about cannabis use and effective remedies for sleep disturbances in pregnancy.

Mood disorders

In addition to using cannabis for help with nausea, vomiting, and sleep, pregnant people may also use it to help manage mood disorders. Depression, anxiety, and other mood disorders are common in pregnancy and the first year after birth, with approximately 10% to 15% of people affected. Several recent studies have reported an increase in cannabis use in pregnancy to manage stress and mood [35] with the most prevalent use among people with a prepregnancy history of trauma, depression, and anxiety. Although the effects of cannabis on mood remain incompletely understood, it is likely that it is the activation of the CB1 causing a release of dopamine and other neurotransmitters and feelings of euphoria and well-being that individuals are seeking to ameliorate their symptoms of depression and anxiety [36]. However, studies have shown little evidence to support the efficacy of cannabis to help with mood disorders, in fact, some studies have indicated worsening feelings of depression and anxiety [35]. As with the efficacy for sleep disturbance, this could be linked to the differences in individual people's reactions to the active ingredients in cannabis (specifically THC and CBD) and the variations in these substances from formulation to formulation. In addition to this, some studies have reported pregnant people feeling guilty or internally conflicted about using cannabis which could exacerbate their depression and anxiety [36].

EVIDENCE REVIEW

The current research gives some insight into the timing of use, reasons for use, and the risks of use for both the pregnant person and the fetus. For example, when cannabis is used in pregnancy, it is more commonly used in the first trimester, and the initial use of the substance decreases with each subsequent trimester [1]. However, if someone begins to use cannabis in pregnancy in the first trimester, they are more likely to continue using throughout the remainder of the pregnancy. This is important to know due to the embryogenesis occurring in the first trimester of pregnancy and the potential risks of disrupting embryogenesis and establishment of the placental bed (placentation). It is also known that exposure during pregnancy could lead to dysregulation of innate and adaptive immune system responses of the developing fetus [37,38]. In addition, some studies demonstrate that epigenetic changes may lead to weakening of immune defenses against infections and cancer later in life. Although the evidence struggles to define the level of risks to a pregnant person and fetus if cannabis is used in pregnancy, there are several risks that are better understood. Table 3 addresses both maternal and fetal risks increased by the use of cannabis in pregnancy.

Limitations to the evidence

It is difficult to distinguish if the potential risks assessed by the current evidence were from cannabis use because multi-substance use is common in pregnancy [1]. In addition, current cannabis strains are known to be stronger than those of previous decades, with approximately 8% increase in strength from strains

Table 3
Risks of cannabis use in pregnancy

Affects the Pregnant person	Risk	Affects the fetus
✔	Cannabinoid induced hyperemesis	
✔	Placenta previa	✔
✔	Prolonged premature rupture of membranes	✔
✔	Prolonged hospital stay	✔
✔	Anemia	✔
✔	Intrauterine growth restriction	✔
	Low birth weight	✔
	Neonatal Intensive Care Unit (NICU) Admission	✔

Key:
Affect only pregnant person
Affect both pregnant person and fetus
Affect only fetus

Table 4	
Care considerations for pregnant patients using cannabis [39]	
Topic	Recommendation
Substance use screening	Screen all pregnant people for substance use early in pregnancy. Preconception screening is also recommended.
Counseling	Pregnant people should be counseled on negative outcomes when cannabis is used in pregnancy.
	Stop using cannabis when you become pregnant. Preconception discontinuance is also encouraged.
	Breastfeeding while using cannabis is discouraged due to the lack of evidence to support it [40].
	Discuss legal ramifications with pregnant people using cannabis during prenatal care so that they are aware of the legal reporting requirements that the health care professional may face.
Considerations	Risk of stillbirth may be "slightly increased" in pregnant patients using cannabis. Consider fetal testing at term if indicated.

used in 1995 [1]. This is important to note because many of the studies with limited evidence regarding safety in pregnancy were performed with weaker strains of cannabis [1]. Another limitation to the evidence regarding cannabis use in pregnancy is that substance use in pregnancy has a predisposed negative public bias. Because of this, many of the articles that are considered foundational for this topic contain the bias of the era in which they were written.

CONSIDERATIONS FOR CARE

Health care professionals must recommend that pregnant people avoid using cannabis in pregnancy but should do so knowing that the use of cannabis in pregnancy shows no signs of diminishing. Therefore, it becomes paramount for health care professionals to understand the care recommendations from the leading national sources. Table 4 consolidates the current recommendations from the American College of Obstetricians and Gynecologists and The Society for Maternal Fetal Medicine [41,42].

SCRIPTING FOR HEALTH CARE PROFESSIONALS TO HAVE BIAS-INFORMED DISCUSSIONS

Client-centered language, also known as person-centered language, places the person before their health care choices and diagnoses [43]. Client-centered language aligns with the nursing model of care and can be used in any clinical situation, including substance use in pregnancy. Table 5 contains several

Table 5
Examples of client-centered language options for healthcare professionals

Case study	Biased clinician language	Client-centered language	General counseling questions on safety and cannabis use
A 22-year old G1P0 presents with a severe case of nausea and vomiting after eating. She has a body mass index (BMI) of 21.0 and is losing weight in early pregnancy. She wants to be able to eat but cannot keep food down, and family members are worried and beginning to voice their concern. She asks if it is ok for her to continue eating edibles to stimulate hunger and suppress	*Of course it is not ok for you to continue using drugs while you're pregnant. You are harming your baby, your family, and yourself. It is very selfish of you to treat your symptoms with something harmful to your child.*	*Thank you for sharing this with me. I am glad you brought this up today and I want to work with you to address your symptoms. If it is ok with you, I would also like to talk about some options for medications approved for use in pregnancy. While I cannot recommend that you continue using cannabis while you are pregnant, it does not mean you will have to suffer with your symptoms. Let's*	*Thank you for sharing your questions about cannabis use in pregnancy with me. I understand that you've been uncomfortable during this pregnancy and I want you to find relief from that discomfort. I must share that I cannot recommend you use cannabis while you are pregnant. There is not enough research to say what an OK amount of exposure would be for your baby. What I can recommend if you*

nausea and vomiting.

A pregnant client with a history of chronic pain presents for a prenatal visit with a new onset of lower back pain and symphysis pubis pain and asks if vaping cannabis is ok in pregnancy as a means of pain relief.

find a solution together.

I hear the pain you are experiencing is becoming intolerable for you. At your last visit, we reviewed the concerns with cannabis use but I do not think we talked about vaping. Thanks for clarifying with me. Vaping is not considered safe in pregnancy, so I do not recommend that for your symptoms. I have a few more questions about when you experience this pain and if it is ok with you, we can discuss the options for treatment that address your specific needs.

continue to use cannabis is that you'll need some extra ultrasounds as you get closer to your due date to check on your baby's growth. Also, I want to let you know that we would like to do a drug screen every trimester and one on admission to the labor and delivery unit. Would this be ok with you?

I told you at your last appointment that you should not be using illicit substances while pregnant. Use the pelvic support band I gave you and tough it out like everyone else.

A client with postpartum anxiety is smoking marijuana daily and reports this on their intake forms when they arrive for a postpartum visit.

I am sorry to hear about the anxiety you are

What do you mean you are smoking weed? Why are you doing that? I have known you for a long time and you have never been a drug user. This is not going to help you be less worried.

(continued on next page)

Table 5
(continued)

Case study	Biased clinician language	Client-centered language	General counseling questions on safety and cannabis use
	experiencing postpartum. Are you open to discussing this today? [client says yes] Please tell me about your symptoms and how often they are occurring. I'm here for you if you want to talk about this in the future. If you are open to discussing medications to treat anxiety, I have recommendations when you are ready.		

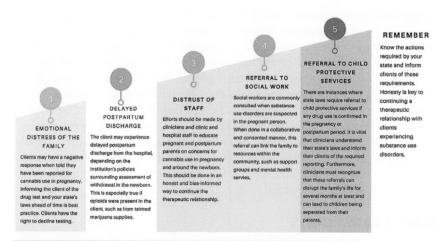

Fig. 1. Potential sequelae of reporting cannabis use in pregnancy.

scenarios with and offers different approaches to discussions about cannabis use in pregnancy and postpartum.

COUNSELING ON LEGAL CONSEQUENCES

When counseling pregnant people on cannabis use in pregnancy, provider attention should focus on the reasons for the use and if there are evidence-based options that can be recommended for the client's specific complaints. Reasons for the use of cannabis vary widely, and patients should not be stigmatized by their health care professional. It is very important to note that counseling should include education regarding the potential legal sequelae for cannabis use in pregnancy. Clients should be informed on the legal requirements in their state and whether or not there is potential for involvement from the Department of Child Protective Services. Because of the growing public acceptance of cannabis use in the United States, clients may not know they could face legal problems in some states that could lead to separation from their newborns. Health care professionals should alert clients to any danger of incarceration for cannabis use in pregnancy in states with the most restrictive laws. The goal of the discussion should be to inform the client and support their best health, not to intimidate them. Fig. 1 depicts a range of potential sequelae for clients who use cannabis in pregnancy and can be used by health care professionals as a starting point for this discussion.

SUMMARY

The history of cannabis use as medicine is long and multicultural, and discussing cannabis use with pregnant clients can be challenging for health care professionals who may struggle to discuss the substance in a bias-informed manner. Although approved as a medicinal product in nonpregnant people to improve nausea in states that have legalized the substance, cannabis is not approved for use in pregnancy and may exacerbate nausea and vomiting in this population. Other known risks of cannabis use in pregnancy exist, such as an increased chance of premature rupture of membranes, placenta previa, prolonged hospital stay, and intrauterine growth restriction. In addition, there could be an even greater risk to using cannabis while pregnant because products on the market today are known to be stronger than those used before the turn of the century and unregulated cannabis can contain other stronger substances, such a fentanyl, which can be life-threatening in small amounts. Health care professionals should educate clients who begin or continue to use cannabis in pregnancy that there is no known safety threshold for cannabis use in pregnancy and it should be avoided.

CLINICS CARE POINTS

- Pregnant clients may prefer "natural" remedies, such as cannabis products, over pharmaceutical methods to ease the discomforts of pregnancy
- Cannabis is the most commonly used illicit substance in pregnancy, and all pregnant clients should be screened for substance use at the first prenatal visit.
- Clients may not understand the dangers associated with cannabis use in pregnancy due to the growing acceptance of cannabis as a non-illicit drug.
- The risks of cannabis use in pregnancy include risks for the fetus and the pregnant client, and the use of cannabis in pregnancy can affect multiple systems of the body.
- Health care professionals can apply therapeutic communication techniques when discussing cannabis use in pregnancy to build a better health care professional–client relationship.

DISCLOSURE

The Authors have nothing to disclose.

References

[1] Volkow ND, Compton WM, Wargo EM. The Risks of Marijuana Use During Pregnancy. JAMA 2017;317(2):129–30.

[2] Substance Abuse and Mental Health Services Administration, Key substance use and mental health indicators in the United States: results from the 2020 national survey on drug use and health (HHS publication No. PEP21-07-01-003, NSDUH series H-56), Center for Behavioral Health Statistics and Quality, Substance Abuse and Mental Health Services Administration, Rockville, MD, 2021 Available at: https://www.samhsa.gov/data/. Accessed August 12, 2022.

[3] Vanstone M, Panday J, Popoola A, et al. Pregnant People's Perspectives On cannabis Use During Pregnancy: A Systematic Review and Integrative Mixed-Methods Research Synthesis. J Midwifery women's Health 2022;67(3):354–72.

[4] Narconon, History of Marijuana Use Available at: 2022. https://www.narconon.org/drug-information/marijuana-history.html. Accessed August 12, 2022.

[5] Britannica ProCon, Historical Timeline: History of Marijuana Available at: 2022. https://medicalmarijuana.procon.org/historical-timeline/. Accessed August 12, 2022.

[6] Behere AP, Behere PB, Rao TS. cannabis: Does it have a medicinal value? Indian J Psychiatry 2017;59(3):262.

[7] Compton WM, Volkow ND, Lopez MF. Medical Marijuana Laws and cannabis Use: Intersections of Health and Policy. JAMA Psychiatry 2017;74(6):559–60.

[8] Ashton C. Pharmacology and effects of cannabis: A brief review. Br J Psychiatry 2001;178(2):101–6.

[9] Mechoulam R. Marihuana chemistry. Science 1970;168(3936):1159–66.

[10] Friedman D, Sirven JI. Historical perspective on the medical use of cannabis for epilepsy: ancient times to the 1980s. Epilepsy Behav 2017;70:298–301.

[11] Capasso A. Do cannabinoids confer neuroprotection against epilepsy? An overview. Open Neurol J 2017;11:61.

[12] Consroe PF, Wood GC, Buchsbaum H. Anticonvulsant nature of marihuana smoking. JAMA 1975;234(3):306–7.

[13] J.R. Biden Jr., A Proclamation on Granting Pardon for the Offense of Simple Marijuana Possession. The White House Briefing Room Available at: 2022. https://www.npr.org/2022/10/10/1127708285/marijuana-pardon-biden-black-people-war-on-drugs-harm. Accessed August 12, 2022.

[14] A. Wise, Bident pot pardon to help reverse war on drugs harm to Black people, advocates say, National Public Radio, 2022 Available at: https://www.npr.org/2022/10/10/1127708285/marijuana-pardon-biden-black-people-war-on-drugs-harm. Accessed August 12, 2022.

[15] ElSohly MA, Chandra S, Radwan M, et al. A Comprehensive Review of Cannabis Potency in the United States in the Last Decade. Biol Psychiatry Cogn Neurosci Neuroimaging 2021;6(6):603–6.

[16] NIDA, February 5. Synthetic Cannabinoids (K2/Spice) DrugFacts Available at: 2018. https://nida.nih.gov/publications/drugfacts/synthetic-cannabinoids-k2spice. Accessed August 12, 2022.

[17] DISA, Marijuana Legality by State Available at: 2022. https://disa.com/maps/marijuana-legality-by-state. Accessed August 12, 2022.

[18] DEA, Drug Fact Sheet: Fentanyl Available at: 2020. https://www.dea.gov/factsheets/fentanyl#:~:text=Fentanyl%20is%20a%20synthetic%20opioid,100%20times%20stronger%20than%20morphine. Accessed August 12, 2022.

[19] Boddiger D. Fentanyl-laced street drugs "kill hundreds". Lancet 2006;368(9535):569–70.

[20] Beckett K, Brydolf-Horwitz M. A kinder, gentler drug war? Race, drugs, and punishment in 21st century America. Punishment Soc 2020;22(4):509–33.

[21] Drug Policy Alliance, A History of the Drug War Available at: 2022. https://drugpolicy.org/issues/brief-history-drug-war. Accessed August 12, 2022.

[22] NORML Foundation, Marijuana Arrests Fall Precipitously Nationwide in 2020 Available at: 2022. https://norml.org/blog/2021/09/27/marijuana-arrests-fall-precipitously-nationwide-in-2020/. Accessed August 12, 2022.

[23] Guttmacher Institute, Substance Use During Pregnancy Available at: 2022. https://www.guttmacher.org/state-policy/explore/substance-use-during-pregnancy. Accessed August 12, 2022.

[24] Panday J, Taneja S, Popoola A, et al. Clinician responses to cannabis use during pregnancy and lactation: a systematic review and integrative mixed-methods research synthesis. Fam Pract 2022;39(3):504–14.

[25] Emily L, Ilina DP, Deanna W, et al. The impact of state legalization on rates of marijuana use in pregnancy in a universal drug screening population. J Maternal-Fetal Neonatal Med 2022;35(9):1660–7.

[26] McParlin C, O'Donnell A, Robson SC, et al. Treatments for Hyperemesis Gravidarum and Nausea and Vomiting in Pregnancy: A Systematic Review. JAMA 2016;316(13): 1392–401.

[27] MacGibbon KW. Hyperemesis Gravidarum: Strategies to Improve Outcomes. J Infus Nurs 2020;43(2):78–96.

[28] Parker LA, Rock EM, Limebeer CL. Regulation of nausea and vomiting by cannabinoids. Br J Pharmacol 2011;163(7):1411–22.

[29] Matsuda LA, Lolait SJ, Brownstein MJ, et al. Structure of a cannabinoid receptor and functional expression of the cloned cDNA. Nature 1990;346(6284):561–4.

[30] Stith SS, Li X, Orozco J, et al. The effectiveness of common cannabis products for treatment of nausea. J Clin Gastroenterol 2022;56(4):331–8.

[31] Kryger MH, Roth T, Dement WC. Principles and practice of sleep medicine. Philadelphia, PA: Elsevier; 2017.

[32] Bacaro V, Benz F, Pappaccogli A, et al. Interventions for sleep problems during pregnancy: a systematic review. Sleep Med Rev 2020;50:101234.

[33] Conroy DA, Kurth ME, Strong DR, et al. Marijuana use patterns and sleep among community-based young adults. J Addict Dis 2016;35(2):135–43.

[34] Murnan AW, Keim SA, Li R, et al. Marijuana use and sleep quality during pregnancy. J Maternal-Fetal Neonatal Med 2021;35(25):7857–64.

[35] Young-Wolff KC, Sarovar V, Tucker L, et al. Association of Depression, Anxiety, and Trauma With Cannabis Use During Pregnancy. JAMA Netw Open 2020;3(2):e1921333.

[36] Chang JC, Tarr JA, Holland CL, et al. Beliefs and attitudes regarding prenatal marijuana use: perspectives of pregnant women who report use. Drug Alcohol Depend 2019;196:14–20.

[37] Grant KS, Petroff R, Isoherranen N, et al. cannabis use during pregnancy: pharmacokinetics and effects on child development. Pharmacol Ther 2018;182:133–51.

[38] Corsi DJ, Donelle J, Sucha E, et al. Maternal cannabis use in pregnancy and child neurodevelopmental outcomes. Nat Med 2020;26(10):1536–40.

[39] Committee Opinion No. 722. Marijuana use during pregnancy and lactation. Obstet Gynecol 2017;130:e205–9, American College of Obstetricians and Gynecologists.

[40] Bertrand KA, Hanan NJ, Honerkamp-Smith G, et al. Marijuana Use by Breastfeeding Mothers and Cannabinoid Concentrations in Breast Milk. Pediatrics 2018;142(3): e20181076.

[41] American College of Obstetricians and Gynecologists (ACOG), Marijuana and Pregnancy Available at: https://www.acog.org/-/media/project/acog/acogorg/womens-health/files/infographics/marijuana-and-pregnancy.pdf?la=en&hash=8A0BAAF57A1AF22F663045414C977ECB. Accessed August 12, 2022.

[42] J. Ecker, A. Abuhamad, W. Hill, et al., Substance use disorders in pregnancy: clinical, ethical, and research imperatives of the opioid epidemic: a report of a joint workshop of the Society for Maternal-Fetal Medicine, American College of Obstetricians and Gynecologists, and American Society of Addiction Medicine, Am J Obstet Gynecol 221 (1) (2019) B5–B28 Available at: https://www.smfm.org/publications/275-smfm-special-report-substance-use-disorders-in-pregnancy-clinical-ethical-and-research-imperatives-of-the-opioid-epidemic. Accessed August 12, 2022.

[43] K. Hyams, N. Prater, J. Rohovit, et al., Person-centered language. Clinical Tip No, 8 Available at: 2018. https://www.mhanational.org/person-centered-language. Accessed August 12, 2022.

Advances in Family Practice Nursing 5 (2023) 169–182

ADVANCES IN FAMILY PRACTICE NURSING

Gaps in Social Determinants of Health History Taking, Clinical Documentation, and Billing/Coding Errors During Women's Health Patient Encounters

Melissa LeBrun, DNP, MPH, APRN, FNP-C*,
Kim Brannagan, PhD, RN, MSN, MBA, BS Ed,
Antiqua N. Smart, DNP, APRN, FNP-BC, PHNA-BC, COI

Loyola University New Orleans, 6363 Street Charles Avenue, New Orleans, LA 70118, USA

Keywords
- Social determinants of health • Screening tools • Health history
- Clinical documentation • Billing • Coding • Advanced practice registered nurses

Key points
- Despite the widespread acknowledgment of the relationship between social determinants of health (SDOH) and health outcomes, SDOH are not routinely screened among health-care professionals and organizations.
- The 5 key areas of SDOH include economic stability, education, social and community context, health and health care, and neighborhood and built environment. Each area is described below including examples of how each factor might affect the health of women.
- Health inequalities related to gender have a long history in the United States. Women also have a history of discrimination and violence related to gender.

INTRODUCTION

Population health initiatives address the health of populations and individuals from a holistic perspective. At the foundation of these initiatives are social determinants of health (SDOH). Despite the widespread acknowledgment of the

*Corresponding author. 6363 Street Charles Avenue, New Orleans, LA 70118. *E-mail address:* mplebrun@loyno.edu

https://doi.org/10.1016/j.yfpn.2022.11.009
2589-420X/23/

relationship between SDOH and health outcomes, SDOH are not routinely screened among health-care professionals and organizations [1]. Specifically, gaps in assessing SDOH during the health history exist, particularly in women's health. Assessing and purposefully identifying the SDOH that affects an individual's health allows providers to have a complete or holistic picture of the person's health needs. Often these issues are "hidden" within patient data and documentation. Because one's health is significantly affected by the determinants of health outside of access to health care, it is critical for health-care organizations to be mindful and purposeful about capturing and documenting these factors. Systematic screenings for SDOH will permit providers to determine unmet health-related social needs, including the effectiveness of referrals and the availability and accessibility of community services.

SDOH screenings are also not clearly defined or fully reimbursed by payers. An overview of SDOH, related billing codes, SDOH screening tools, and recommendations for health assessment and history are presented.

SOCIAL DETERMINANTS OF HEALTH DEFINED

The World Health Organization (WHO) Commission defines SDOH as "the conditions in which people are born, grow, live, work, and age, including the health system shaping the conditions of daily life. These forces and systems include economic policies and systems, development agendas, social norms, social policies, and political systems." [2,3].

The 5 key areas of SDOH include economic stability, education, social, and community context, health and health care, and neighborhood and built environment. Each area is described in Table 1 including examples of how each factor might affect the health of women.

The SDOH that are not specific to health-care access have not traditionally been considered part of the health-care provider's responsibility. Because health behaviors account for 30% of an individual's health status, there has been more focus placed on behavior change initiatives with the goal of improving health outcomes. Despite efforts to address behavioral factors such as smoking, diet, exercise, and stress through behavior change programs and marketing, these efforts have not proven to be effective [2]. The rates of smoking, obesity, physical inactivity, and stress-related mental health disorders continue to increase in the United States. A major factor is that individuals do not always have control over the things that make them sick or prevent them from being able to practice health-seeking behaviors, particularly those who are of low economic status [4]. Thus, without addressing the reasons that individuals may not have control over these factors, health improvement is hindered.

Assessing for individual SDOH needs to be integrated into primary and secondary prevention and the treatment of diseases [5]. In America where access to health care is often more limited for certain portions of the population such as women, individuals who live in situations of lower economic and inadequate social environments, the impact is tremendous. Therefore, beyond behavior change counseling, initiatives such as improving the public transportation

Table 1
Social determinants of health

SDOH key area	Contribution to healthy outcomes	Description	Impact on Women's health
Economic stability	40%	Economic status, employment status, food security, and housing stability affect health	Women often received lower wages than men in the same jobs. Employment status is influenced by the added responsibilities of caregiver
Education		Higher levels of education are correlated with better health and longevity. Low performing early childhood education programs and K-12 schools have a negative impact on health. Language and literacy also affect health	College-educated women are living longer. Racial disparities exist in education
Social and community context		Positive relationships, sense of social cohesion, and civic participation all have a positive impact on health. Discrimination, unsafe neighborhoods, and incarceration all have negative impacts on health	Women experience relationship violence at higher levels than men. The rate of death for women in the United States is four times the rate of other developed countries
Health and health care	20%	Access to health care, including primary care, access to health insurance, preventative screenings, and health literacy impact an individual's health	From medical research to women's life expectancy, women are less likely to have access to health-care services
Neighborhood and built environment	10%	Housing quality, crime, violence, environmental conditions, and access to healthy food make up an individual's environment	As caregivers, women are more likely to have limited housing options and have to provide food for entire families
Health behaviors	30%	Tobacco use, diet and exercise, alcohol and drug use, and sexual activity	Often women

system, urban planning to improve access to parks, bicycle and walking paths, and other recreational activities, and the promotion of community gardens are necessary to address the barriers faced by many. Other issues, such as socioeconomic inequalities, discrimination, poor housing, poor educational systems, violence, abuse, and more are also community issues that must be addressed. Although no one entity can take on every social issue, when communities band together, including health care, to address poor social conditions, an impact can be made. Models to develop coordinated systems to integrate and transform the health of populations are currently being created to assist communities in developing a shared mission [6].

Social determinants and health equity in Women's health

Health inequalities related to gender have a long history in the United States. Women also have a history of discrimination and violence related to gender. For example, medical research often purposefully excluded women [7]. It was not until the 1970s and 1980s that change occurred in this area. Still today, the health of women in United States is poorer than the health of women in other high-income countries. Currently, women in the United States have a life expectancy of 81 years, with a three-year difference between White and Black women. The last 16 years of life for women are often spent with at least two chronic health conditions. Based on data from the National Health and Aging Trends Study, only 23.7% of women aged 65 years and older are able to conduct "basic self-care and mobility activities, compared with 36.6% of men." [7].

In addition to the economic inequality between White and Black women, the disproportionate health status related to education level is significant [7]. College-educated women have a longer life expectancy than those who have not completed high school. Mood and anxiety disorders also have a major impact on women's health. Although the rate of depression among adult men is 5.5%, the rate among women is 10.4%. Autoimmune diseases are also disproportionately higher among women (6.4%) than men (2.7%) [7]. Interestingly, women are also most often misdiagnosed at rates higher than men.

Not surprisingly, menstruation, menopause, and pregnancy have been much of the focus for women's health. Compared with research and advances in men's health, women's health advances are limited [7]. For example, research and treatment advances related to menopause are minimal, often rationalized by the belief that menopause and its related symptoms are natural occurrences related to aging. In similar issues that naturally occur in men, significant advances have been made.

Birth rates among women have declined on average, reaching a record low in 2020 of 1.64 children per woman and the average age of first birth has increased from 24.9 to 27.0 [7]. Even today, many women in the United States have limited access to contraception, especially among marginalized individuals who reside in states where Medicaid funds are regulated for contraception products. Maternal mortality is also poor in the United States as compared with other high-income countries, and pregnancy-related mortality rates are about three times higher among Black women (40.8) compared with White women (12.7) . Cervical cancer rates also disproportionately affect Black women. Endometriosis is a condition that many women (10%–15%) endure but there has been very little advancement in diagnosis and treatment [7]. Finally, violence is a tremendous issue for women in the United States. The leading cause of death for girls and young women and for pregnant or post-partum women is homicide [7]. Partner violence is also a significant issue with estimates of 30.6% of women experiencing physical violence. Moreover, 43.6% of women in the United States have experienced some form of sexual violence in her lifetime [7].

SCREENING TOOLS FOR ASSESSING SOCIAL DETERMINANTS OF HEALTH

Assessing and purposefully identifying the SDOH that impacts an individual's health allows providers to have a complete or holistic picture of the person's health needs. Often these issues are "hidden" within patient data and documentation. Because one's health is significantly affected by the determinants of health outside of access to health care, it is critical for health-care organizations to be mindful and purposeful about capturing and documenting these factors. Systematic screenings for SDOH will permit providers to determine unmet health-related social needs, including the effectiveness of referrals and the availability and accessibility of community services.

Although most clinicians realize that addressing the underlying causes of health issues is critical to healing, it is often challenging to address social issues in which providers feel they have no control [2]. Clinicians on the front lines of health care are faced with the realization of the impact that social factors have on their patients' health. Asking patients about social factors may also be avoided due to time constraints, lack of personnel to follow up on the issues presented, or even the belief that the discussion is outside of the clinician's role. However, "failure to identify hidden social challenges can lead to misdiagnosis and a path of inappropriate investigations," such as issues related to violence or abuse [2]. Additionally, inappropriate plans of care can be recommended such as prescribing a heart healthy diet to someone who struggles with providing food for their family.

It is imperative that clinicians view each encounter as an opportunity to address the factors that have the largest impact on their patients' health. Clinicians can assess patients in a variety of ways. For example, asking individuals about their social history may help to uncover issues that can be addressed through local support services [2]. Speaking to patients about social issues that are typically considered off-limits in a sympathetic, concerned, and nonjudgmental manner can help to build trust and create a safe place for opening up. The difficult conversations may be the first step to getting the individual help. Further, incorporating community services navigation, health outcomes tracking, and having a community-wide mindset to address continuity of care will contribute to the improvement of health outcomes for individuals and the community [8].

In addition to engaging in conversation about social issues, a standardized screening process with clear guidelines and procedures may provide more efficiency and consistency in addressing the SDOH. According to Moen and colleagues, approximately 50% of patients who have SDOH needs are being missed due to failure to conduct routine screenings [9]. A screening process can also assist in contributing to the SDOH data needed to address gaps in care associated morbidity and mortality, resource needs, social inequities, and health outcomes. Unfortunately, existing SDOH screening tools lack standardization creating inconsistencies in measurements. Social needs data are being used to support value-based payment reform and to determine how to "integrate and finance nonmedical services as part of health insurance benefit design." [9].

Since the World Health Organization released its report on the SDOH in 2008, several tools that screen for health-related social conditions have been developed [9]. Many of the screening tools can be uploaded into the organization's electronic health record (EHR). Several are offered in multiple languages and can be either self-administered or administered by clinical or nonclinical staff. Examples of screening tools include the following:

- The National Association of Community Health Centers' Protocol for Responding to and Assessing Patients' Assets, Risks, and Experiences tool (PRAPARE) [10].
- The American Academy of Family Physicians Social Needs Screening Tool through the EveryOne Project [11].
- Centers for Medicare and Medicaid Services Accountable Health Communities' Health-Related Social Needs Screening Tool [12].

Common documentation pearls for social determinants of health and coding in Women's health

The EHR has been integral in providing clear, consistent charting in clinical practice as well as providing standardization essential for coding processes. Documentation is key to interoperability and functionality of patient care. Coding from proper documentation aids in reimbursement measures that sustains health-care organizations. The Subjective, Objective, Assessment and Plan (SOAP) note format is most commonly used by health-care providers and is typically integrated into the EHR system [13]. The National Committee on Quality Assurance (NCQA) reports guidelines for medical record documentation and notes 21 essential elements in completing a chart [14]. A gap in knowledge and practice exists in reference to assessing and documenting SDOH and the related coding principles. For example, providers will often not address SDOH in the subjective history taking sections of documentation, thus potentially reducing the likelihood that the patient will receive the care and services needed to achieve optimal health outcomes. Alternatively, providers may address related SDOH during history taking but fail to document the information thereby foregoing the opportunity to capture the associated reimbursement for the service. Being familiar with best practices related to assessing and screening for SDOH and the associated billable services and codes will allow the practitioner to provide care that improves continuity of care and access to appropriate services. To assist practitioners in providing complete and consistent documentation, the NCQA has provided guidelines for medical record documentation in Table 2.

Clinical documentation components for Women's health and social determinants of health screening

History of presenting illness

Subjective documentation encompasses the client's chief complaint, history of presenting illness (HPI), review of symptoms and current medications and allergies. An acronym most commonly used when completing the HPI is OLD-CARTS—onset, location, duration, characterization, alleviating and aggravating factors, radiation, temporal factors, and severity [13]. The HPI is the most common component of the assessment where missed SDOH information occurs. The HPI involves the collection of subjective history that depends on the client answering questions accurately. The review of systems (ROS) is a component of the documentation that elicits client subjective symptoms that would otherwise be missed. The ROS is designed as systematic questions based on each body system. The past medical and surgical history is a component of charting that both helps with the plan of care (POC) as well as provides the provider and client a reference source for care management. Past family history is a pertinent part of charting because this may trigger certain preventative screenings based on familial components. The social history component of a client chart details information such as smoking, alcohol use, and sexual orientation. Social history can also guide preventative measures. Objective findings include the physical assessment findings. Documentation mistakes commonly occur when trying to distinguish between signs and symptoms. Signs consist of objective findings and symptoms are the patient's description [13]. Under the assessment section, there are elements that must be listed. First, the problem list is important and the differential diagnosis list [13]. The POC is a significant part of the chart documentation. A detailed plan helps disseminate client information for continuity of care as well as provides a framework for future client visits.

As previously noted, underlying causes of health issues are often hidden within various SDOH, such as financial barriers, access to affordable healthy food options, living in an area that is unsafe for outdoor activities, lack of transportation, poor performing educational programs, history of abuse, and more. When providers and patients are not accustomed to discussing these issues during medical encounters, it is the provider's responsibility to create a safe space for patients to share information that might affect their ability to carry out the POC as prescribed. Helping patients to understand the rationale behind asking

Table 2
The National Committee on Quality Assurance essential guidelines and the 21 essential charting elements

Element I	Each page in the record contains the ID number or the patient's name [14]
Element II	Including personal biographic data such as the address, employer, home and work telephone numbers, and marital status [14]
Element III	Includes all entries in the medical record contain identification of the author which can be electronic signatures or a handwritten signature [14]
Element IV	All entries are dated [14]
Element V	Record is legible [14]. The fifth element is that significant illnesses and medical conditions are listed as part of the problem list [14]
Element VI	Medication allergies and any adverse reactions are noted in the clinical documentation [14]
Element VII	Clinical notation of the past medical history is easily identified and includes traumas, surgical operations, and illnesses [14]. It is important to note that for children and adolescents, past medical history relates to prenatal care, birth, operations, and childhood illnesses [14]
Element VIII	Patients 12 years of age and older, there is clinical documentation detailing the use of cigarettes, alcohol, and illicit substance use [14]
Element IX	Comprises the history and physical examination that identifies subjective and objective information pertinent to the patient's presenting complaints [14]
Element X	Includes laboratory and other studies are documented when ordered [14]
Element XI	All diagnoses are consistent with the clinician's findings [14]
Element XII	Requires that the client's treatment plans are consistent with diagnoses given [14]
Element XIII	Details that the client encounter forms or notes have a notation, regarding follow-up care, calls or visits, if needed [14]
Element XIV	Should include the specific time of return is noted in weeks, months, or as needed in the chart documentation [14]
Element XV	Must identify unresolved problems from previous office visits and make sure those are addressed in subsequent visits [14]
Element XVI	Includes the review for underutilization or overutilization of consultants [14]
Element XVII	Requires that any consultation, imaging, or laboratory reports filed in the chart are initialed by the practitioner who ordered them [14]
Element XVIII	Requires that a consultation, abnormal laboratory, or imaging results have a notation in the record of follow-up plans [14]
Element XIX	

(continued on next page)

Table 2 (continued)	
Element I	Each page in the record contains the ID number or the patient's name [14]
Element XX	Must meet the requirement that there is no evidence that the client is placed at inappropriate risk by a procedure, both diagnostic and therapeutic [14]
	Must include an immunization record is up to date for children or an appropriate history has been made in the medical record for adults [14]
Element XXI	Requires that there is evidence that preventive screening and services are offered in accordance with the organization's practice guidelines [14]

Data from The National Committee for Quality Assurance (NCQA). Guidelines for Medical Record Documentation. Available at https://www.ncqa.org/wp-content/uploads/2018/07/20180110_Guidelines_Medical_Record_Documentation.pdf

what may seem to be personal questions may be the first step in creating an open dialog for potentially sensitive topics. For example, sharing that the information may assist the provider/health-care organization in identifying available resources in the patient's local area that are needed for achieving optimal health outcomes may reduce the barriers to capturing that information.

In addition to gathering SDOH information during the face-to-face HPI, providers should be aware of situations that may result in an unintended unsafe space for patients, inhibiting the sharing of information. Examples include power differentials, gender concerns, external fears (e.g., partner learning that abuse is reported), embarrassment, age differences, personal relationship with facility employees, and previous experience with breaches of privacy. A standardized screening process offers an excellent supplement to face-to-face dialog. Screening tools allow organizations to collect consistent data and to track changes in the patient's social needs. Keep in mind that when patients share critical information in the screening process, the issues should be acknowledged during the face-to-face visit. Otherwise, trust may be diminished, prohibiting future sharing of information. Without exception, current and complete documentation is critical for continuity of care and proper reimbursement.

INSUFFICIENT DOCUMENTATION

Insufficient documentation is a major barrier to reimbursement and continuity of care. For example, unsigned charts or lack of date of service on documentation can prolong the reimbursement process [15]. Evaluation and management (E/M) services have some of the most documentation errors according to the Centers for Medicare and Medicaid. Insufficient or no documentation and incorrect coding are lacking many times to support the billing of E/M services [15].

PREVENTATIVE MEDICINE SERVICE CODING FOR WOMEN'S HEALTH

Counseling Risk Factor for Reduction and Behavioral Change. The codes for counseling risk factors include the current procedural terminology (CPT) codes: (99401–99412) [15]. The counseling for this intervention must be completed at a separate encounter from the preventative service [15]. The codes should not be reported when a client is seen for an established condition [15]. Conditions that qualify are behaviors such as substance abuse or tobacco abuse [15].

Preventative Medicine E/M Services. The CPT codes for preventative medicine E/M are (99381–99387) [15]. These specific codes are used in reporting annual well-woman examinations [15].

Emergency Contraception Coding. There are codes used for Levonorgestrel and Ulipristal contraceptive pills (Plan B contraception) [15]. The ICD-10 diagnosis code used is Z30.012 for emergency contraception prescription. J3490 is the CPT code for unclassified drugs (supply) and S4993 for contraception pills for birth control [15]. There is also coding associated with natural family planning. For initial counseling and surveillance, the ICD-10 code is Z30.02, which codes for counseling and education on natural family planning to avoid pregnancy.

Procedure Codes for Preventative Services. Screening for interpersonal and domestic violence during the annual well-woman examination is critical to identifying these issues and creating an action plan to address them. Some example diagnosis codes are as follows: T74.0 Neglect or abandonment; T74.1 Physical abuse, confirmed; T74.2 Sexual abuse, confirmed; Psychological abuse, confirmed; T74.9 Unspecified maltreatment, confirmed [15].

BILLING AND CODING SOCIAL DETERMINANTS OF HEALTH

Because health-care providers and systems strive to find methods of identifying and addressing the social needs of patients and communities, the challenging task of identifying how to fund these initiatives has been underway. Further, determining standard definitions and measures for social needs is ongoing. Tracking social needs is the first step to being able to integrate the data into payment models. Integrating SDOH data into EHRs will provide information for risk adjustment [16]. Using Z Codes (Z55-Z65) hospitals can capture the social needs of their patients. Current Z codes address information related to "education and literacy, employment, housing, lack of adequate food or water, or occupational exposure to risk factors such as dust, radiation, or toxic agents." [16] Self-reported data by the patient can also be incorporated into the medical record once the providers sign off on the information. Then the information can be used to select appropriate Z codes. A description of the SDOH Z codes is illustrated below (Table 3).

E/M codes are a category of CPT codes used for outpatient and ambulatory services [17]. In January 2021, revisions to the medical decision making (MDM) grid and new E/M codes were developed to capture specific areas of risk related to the SDOH. MDM refers to the complexity of establishing a diagnosis and selecting a POC. The levels of MDM are affected by the number of

Table 3
Social determinants of health Z codes

ICD-10-CM Code Category	Problems/Risk Factors
Z55 Problems related to education and literacy	Illiteracy, less than high school diploma
Z56 Problems related to employment and unemployment	Unemployment, change of job, threat of job loss, stressful work schedule, military deployment
Z57 Occupational exposure to risk factors	Occupational exposure to noise, radiation, toxic agents, noise
Z58 Problems related to physical environment	Inadequate drinking-water supply
Z59 Problems related to housing and economic circumstances	Sheltered and unsheltered homelessness, inadequate housing, housing instability, lack of adequate food, food insecurity, poverty
Z60 Problems related to social environment	Adjustment to life-cycle transitions, social exclusion and rejection, target of adverse discrimination and persecution
Z62 Problems related to upbringing	Inadequate parental supervision and control, parental overprotection, institutional upbringing, personal history of child abuse in childhood
Z63 Other problems related to primary support group, including family circumstances	Absence of family member, disruption of family by separation and divorce, stressful life events affecting family and household, alcoholism and drug addiction in family
Z64 Problems related to certain psychosocial circumstances	Unwanted pregnancy, multiparity
Z65 Problems related to other psychosocial circumstances	Imprisonment and other incarceration, release from prison, other legal circumstances, victim of crime and terrorism, exposure to disaster, ware and other hostilities

(Adapted from American Hospital Association (AHA). (2022). ICD-10-CM coding for social determinants of health. Available at https://www.aha.org/system/files/2018-04/value-initiative-icd-10-code-social-determinants-of-health.pdf; with permission)

possible diagnoses, the complexity of medical records, and the risks associated with the presenting problem [18]. Patient complexity ranges from minimal to high. SDOH are captured under the risks category related to establishing a diagnosis and selecting care management options. Thus, accurate documentation and screening are critical to representing the social elements that influence the treatment.

COMMON CLINICAL DOCUMENTATION ERRORS RELATED TO SOCIAL DETERMINANTS OF HEALTH
Advanced practice registered nurses (APRNs) should obtain SDOH components during the health history interview of the women's comprehensive

wellness examination. More specifically, the family history and social history sections of the SOAP Note contain identifiable information that should prompt SDOH screening and documentation. Kepper and colleagues state that methodical SDOH screening and correct documentation of SDOH findings is necessary for social needs-informed care that can create health-care delivery systems resulting in cost-effective, early interventions which prevent hospitalizations, reduce repeated hospitalizations and outpatient care visits, curtail missed moments for diagnoses during visits, increase patient treatment plan adherence, and ease patient's accessibility to affordable prescriptions [19].

SOLUTIONS TO REDUCE SOCIAL DETERMINANTS OF HEALTH CLINICAL DOCUMENTATION ERRORS

Solutions for reducing SDOH clinical documentation errors are different for board-certified, licensed APRNs and matriculating APRN students providing women's health care. Board-certified, licensed APRNs require on the job training or formal continuing education programs to become proficient in their SDOH clinical documentation skills. Keeper and colleagues list the following SDOH clinical documentation error solutions suggested by board-certified, licensed APRNs: (1) utilization of clinical documentation improvement specialists to increase SDOH screening and documentation; (2) collaboration with the billing department, compliance department, and clinical documentation team to create a Z-code guidebook; and (3) incorporation of a provider-specific SDOH documentation and billing course [19].

Conversely, APRN students need more intense education that incorporates SDOH clinical documentation concepts and skills throughout their APRN specialty courses. The American Association Colleges of Nursing provided a call to action for both undergraduate and graduate nursing education programs to integrate SDOH content into their curricula [20]. For example, Davis and colleagues incorporated the use of a virtual unfolding case study in which APRN students are assigned a simulated family that has limited financial and social support services [21]. Each semester, the case study scenario changed but the simulated family remained the same as students matriculated in the program [21]. Reflection and discussion board assignments were also used as teaching-learning activities to ensure students had a basic understanding of SDOH and were competent in SDOH clinical documentation and billing before graduation [21].

Due to the major impact that SDOH have on an individual's health providers, health providers would be remiss if these issues are not assessed and considered in the development of a POC for their patients. Health-care organizations and schools of nursing that prepare APRNs must ensure that practitioners are well versed in SDOH concepts. These entities also must be aware of the effect SDOH have on the patient's health outcomes.

SUMMARY

SDOH are important elements of holistic care often overlooked by APRNs responsible for the management and treatment of common diseases diagnosed among the female patient population. During every patient–provider encounter, APRNs should assess each of the five key SDOH areas that include economic stability, education, social and community context, health and health care, and neighborhood and built environment. APRNs providing women's health care can no longer focus on medical diagnoses in isolation but must learn to identify how SDOH attributes to the exacerbation of episodic and chronic disease processes. The assessment, screening, clinical documentation, and billing and coding associated with SDOH requires a different set of competencies and skills not often taught in APRN education programs. More discussion and research articles are needed to assist board-certified, licensed APRNs develop a better foundational knowledge of SDOH concepts and to properly translate that knowledge into clinical practice. Quality improvement projects related to SDOH care can also aid in the creation of clinical practice guidelines that allow APRNs to implement the best SDOH interventions needed to reduce health disparities and inequities among women.

CLINICS CARE POINTS

- Insufficient documentation is a major barrier to reimbursement and continuity of care.
- Because health-care providers and systems strive to find methods of identifying and addressing the social needs of patients and communities, the challenging task of identifying how to fund these initiatives has been underway.
- APRN students need more intense education that incorporates SDOH clinical documentation concepts and skills throughout their APRN specialty courses.

DISCLOSURE

The authors have nothing to disclose.

References

[1] Bradywood A, Leming-Lee T, Watters R, et al. (2021). Implementing screening for social determinants of health using the Core 5 screening tool. Br J Med (Bjm) Open Qual 2021; https://doi.org/10.1136/bmjoq-2021-001362.
[2] Andermann A. Taking action on the social determinants of health in clinical practice: A framework for health professionals. Can Med Assoc J (Cmaj) 2016;188:17–8.
[3] Nash DB, Skoufalos A, Fabius RJ, et al. Population health: creating a culture of wellness. Burlington, MA: Jones & Bartlett; 2021.
[4] Wang J, Geng L. Effects of socioeconomic status on physical and psychological health: Lifestyle as a mediator. Int J Environ Res Public Health 2019;6(2):281.
[5] National Academies of Sciences, Engineering, and Medicine, (2019). Integrating social care into the delivery of health care: moving upstream to improve the nation's health, U.S. National Academies of Sciences, Engineering, and Medicine, United States, 2019

Available at: http://nap.nationalacademies.org/25467, Accessed October 3, 2022. doi:10.17226/25467.

[6] Madhavan P, Rouse & Rappuoli. Vision for a systems architecture to integrate and transform population health. Proc Natl Acad Sci (Pnas) 2018;9:2018.

[7] Short SE, Zacher M. Women's health: Population patterns and social determinants. Annu Rev 2022;48:277–98.

[8] Centers for Disease Control and Prevention (CDC). Social determinants of health: Know what affects health. 2021. Available at: https://www.cdc.gov/socialdeterminants/index.htm.

[9] Moen M, Storr C, German D, et al. A review of tools to screen for social determinants of health in the United States: A practice brief. Popul Health Management 2020;23(6); https://doi.org/10.1089/pop.2019.0518.

[10] National Association of Community Health Centers, Protocol for responding to and assessing patients' assets, risks, and experiences tool (PRAPARE) Available at: 2019. https://prapare.org/. Accessed August 30, 2022.

[11] American Academy of Family Physicians (AAFP), Social determinants of health guide to social needs screening, The EveryOne Project, 2018 Available at: https://www.aafp.org/dam/AAFP/documents/patient_care/everyone_project/hops19-physician-guide-sdoh.pdf. Accessed August 30, 2022.

[12] Centers for Medicare & Medicaid Services (CMS), Accountable health communities' health-related social needs screening tool (AHC-HRSN) Available at 2017. https://innovation.cms.gov/files/worksheets/ahcm-screeningtool.pdf. Accessed September 16, 2022.

[13] Podder V, Lew V, Ghassemzadeh S. SOAP notes. [Updated 2021 sep 2]. In: StatPearls [internet]. Treasure Island (FL): StatPearls Publishing; 2022. Available at: https://www.ncbi.nlm.nih.gov/books/NBK482263/.

[14] NCQA.org. MCQA Guidelines. Available at: https://www.ncqa.org/wpcontent/uploads/2018/07/20180110_Guidelines_Medical_Record_Documentation.pdf. Accessed August 12, 2022.

[15] Women's Preventative Health. Coding Guide. Available at: https://www.womenspreventivehealth.org/wpcontent/uploads/2020_WPSI_CodingGuide.pdf. Accessed August 12, 2022.

[16] American Hospital Association (AHA), ICD-10-CM coding for social determinants of health Available at: 2022. Available at: https://www.aha.org/system/files/2018-04/value-initiative-icd-10-code-social-determinants-of-health.pdf. Accessed August 31, 2022.

[17] American Academy of Professional Coders (AAPC). (2021). 99202-99215: Office/outpatient E/M coding in 2021 Available at: https://www.aapc.com/evaluation-management/em-codes-changes-2021.aspx. Accessed August 31, 2022.

[18] Centers for Disease Control and Prevention (CDC), Evaluation and management services guide: MLN booklet, MLN00674 January 2022 Available at: 2022. https://www.cms.gov/outreach- and-education/medicare-learning-network-mln/mlnproducts/downloads/eval-mgmt-serv- guide-icn006764.pdf. Accessed August 31, 2022.

[19] Kepper MM, Walsh-Bailey C, Prusaczyk B, et al. The adoption of social determinants of health documentation in clinical settings. Health Services Research; 2022. p. 1–11; https://doi.org/10.1111/1475-6773.14039.

[20] American Association of Colleges of Nursing. The essentials: Core competencies for professional nursing education. 2021. Available at: https://www.aacnnursing.org/Portals/42/AcademicNursing/pdf/Essentials-2021.pdf.

[21] Davis VH, Murillo C, Chappell KK, et al. Tipping point: Integrating social determinants of health concepts in a college of nursing. J Nurs Educ 2021;60(12):703–6.

Advances in Family Practice Nursing 5 (2023) 183–192

ADVANCES IN FAMILY PRACTICE NURSING

Sexual Dysfunction in Biologic Females for Family Practice Providers

Assessment, Diagnosis, and Treatment

Christina M. Wilson, PhD, CRNP, WHNP-BC

School of Nursing, Division of Gynecologic Oncology, Department of Obstetrics & Gynecology, University of Alabama at Birmingham and Heersink School of Medicine, NB 573E 1720 2nd Avenue South, Birmingham, AL 35294-1210, USA

Keywords

• Sexual dysfunction • Female • Assessment • Treatment

Key points

• Female sexual function has multiple domains; therefore, dysfunction can occur in any of those aspects.

• A thorough history and physical examination are needed to determine the root cause of sexual dysfunction.

• Clinicians should be aware of other diagnoses, medications, and treatments that can cause secondary sexual dysfunction.

• Adequate management of sexual dysfunction can encompass both non-pharmacologic and pharmacologic therapies, as deemed necessary by the treating clinician.

INTRODUCTION

Sexual health is an important component of most individuals' lives and encompasses a broad range of aspects including sexuality, sexual function, and sexual relationships. Optimal sexual health is defined as "a state of physical, emotional, mental, and social well-being in relation to sexuality, not merely the absence of disease, dysfunction, or infirmity, [and] a positive and respective approach to sexuality, sexual relationships, as well as the possibility of having pleasurable and safe sexual experiences ..." [1] Although sexual health is a broad term, sexual function refers to the specific aspects of engaging in sexual

E-mail address: wilsoncm@uab.edu

https://doi.org/10.1016/j.yfpn.2023.01.005
2589-420X/23/© 2023 Elsevier Inc. All rights reserved.

activity. For purposes of this article, the specific focus was on female sexual dysfunction. Therefore, when the word "female" was used, it is being used to describe the biologic sex of an individual, not gender or one's gender identity. If an individual is transgender and/or undergoing transition, certain considerations related to hormone usage, or surgical treatment could affect their sexual function.

Female sexual function has been described in many models and has advanced in knowledge from the linear models, similar to male sexual function, of the 1960s and 1970s. Current models, describe female sexual function in nonlinear paths, recognize that there are the components of desire, arousal, orgasm but also that there may be additional aspects that factor into the female sexual response cycle [2,3]. For example, Basson's model recognizes that desire may be responsive, and not spontaneous, leading to a simultaneous experience of desire and arousal [2]. Additionally, Janssen and Bancroft's model expands even further to explain the interaction between sexual excitement and inhibition in female sexual response [3]. To clarify, excitement is defined as interest or things that lead one to want to engage (eg, partner's touch), whereas inhibition, in this context, means things that prohibit or impair one from wanting to engage (eg, pain, stress) [3,4]. Excitement and inhibition are physiologic processes occurring within the brain and are not always easy for one to distinguish [3,4].

Female sexual dysfunction occurs when there is difficulty with one or more of the domains of sexual function: desire, arousal, lubrication, orgasm (satisfaction/pleasure), or when pain occurs [5]. These difficulties can occur in relation to a disease, illness, with the cessation of menstruation, or may present idiopathic. Sexual dysfunction occurs in approximately 41% of premenopausal females, and studies report it can occur around 60% in postmenopausal females [6–9].

Because sexual dysfunction is common among females, both premenopausal and postmenopausal, it is crucial for all clinicians, who encounter these issues, to be privy to the assessment, diagnosis, and treatment of female sexual dysfunction. This is especially important for family practice providers, who may be the first clinician that the patient speaks to about their sexual health or dysfunction issues. Therefore, the purpose of the article is to detail the initial approach to care for females presenting with sexual dysfunction. Specifically, the assessment, along with subsequent diagnosis (for dysfunction), as well as treatment recommendations for sexual health issues and dysfunction will be discussed.

APPROACH TO CARE

Assessment

A complete history and physical examination are pertinent to accurate diagnosis and management of sexual function. Sexual dysfunction can occur for many reasons and all areas should be examined. It is important to gain both subjective and objective data before making a definitive diagnosis.

History

A thorough history is one of the first steps in determining if or why the patient may be experiencing sexual dysfunction. First, having the patient provide a chief complaint, or reason for why they are presenting is important. If the patient states "sexual problems" or something similar, an investigation into what dimension of sexual function is affected (desire, arousal, orgasm, lubrication, or if pain is present) is required. The type of sexual activity that the issue is present in should also be documented, whether it is intercourse, oral sex, masturbation, or other type of sexual activity. These domains have been developed and assessed through, a reliable and valid instrument, the Female Sexual Function Index [5], which could also be used to help quantify dimensions of the history of present illness (HPI). After obtaining a chief complaint and detailed HPI related to the patient's sexual dysfunction, a thorough review of systems should be obtained. A complete review of systems, not just sexual symptoms, should be reviewed. Subjective report of symptoms in other areas can provide important clues to the diagnosis and management of sexual dysfunction.

After obtaining a complete review of systems, a detailed history, including but not limited to social, family, medical, surgical, sexual, gynecologic (eg, pregnancies, deliveries, sexually transmitted infections), and medications, is also important. Not only recognizing that medical and surgical history can play a role but also noting the types of medical history or surgical history is important. Medical issues, including psychological issues affect sexual function. Moreover, various surgical procedures, not limited to those in the genitalia, can lead to sexual problems. For example, brain surgeries that affect the hypothalamus or pituitary gland can not only affect sexual function from the hypothalamus-pituitary-ovary axis but also breast surgeries such as mastectomies can affect arousal from sensation changes. Pay particular attention to both physical and mental health concerns, along with medications that have known impacts on sexual function. In assessing social history substance use (eg, opiates, other drugs), alcohol, and tobacco use should also be noted because they can contribute to sexual dysfunction [10]. Specifics in the history can alert one to illnesses, treatments, or medications that predispose one to sexual dysfunction. When obtaining a sexual history, the provider should not only include the traditional aspects of a sexual history but also detail the engagement in sexual activity, types of sexual activity, and if dysfunction occurs with each one is important. In addition to documenting these aspects, noting partner status, and if the partner has sexual issues can be helpful in determining the cause of sexual dysfunction. An additional aspect of the sexual history in past or current trauma because physical, emotional, and sexual trauma have been shown to affect sexual function [11,12].

Psychological and physical assessment

A thorough psychological assessment and physical assessment are important to determining a cause for sexual dysfunction. First, obtaining information and screening for depression, anxiety, and stress are important to consider when assessing for sexual dysfunction. Depression, anxiety, and stress have all been found to be associated or related to sexual dysfunction [13–15]. Additionally, body image changes, or mental health issues specifically associated with them, such as eating disorders, can impact sexual function [16,17].

A physical assessment should not be limited to a gynecologic examination. Assessment of all systems should be conducted because various medical conditions have been shown to cause sexual dysfunction. Although, not a complete overview of assessments for sexual dysfunction, the following areas are recommended and should be used in conjunction with the clinician's clinical judgement and expertise. First, pain should be assessed as well as any medications prescribed to treat it (eg, opiates, selective serotonin reuptake inhibitors, neuropathic agents) should be noted. Pain, anywhere in the body, and specifically in the genito-pelvic area can cause sexual dysfunction. A detailed endocrine evaluation should be conducted, as multiple endocrine conditions have been associated with changes in sexual function. Thyroid disorders, hyperprolactemina, diabetes, and obesity have all been shown to have an influence on overall sexual function. More specifically, difficulties with desire, arousal, orgasm, and lubrication have been shown in patients with these disorders [18–22]. Immunologic or autoimmune assessment should be completed. Autoimmune conditions, such has Sjogren syndrome and scleroderma, can lead to lubrication difficulties, which can lead to dyspareunia [23–25]. Genitourinary and gastrointestinal assessments should also be considered because urinary incontinence, urinary tract infections (UTIs) and inflammatory bowel disease can affect sexual function [26,27]. Neuromuscular conditions should be assessed. Parkinson, seizures, spinal cord injuries, and fractures of the pelvis and/or lower extremities can all impact sexual function in various ways [28–32]. In addition to these assessments, other conditions that affect multiple systems including cancer can affect sexual function [33]. Furthermore, the actual medical condition leading to sexual dysfunction, the clinician should also determine if related medications, procedures, or treatments to the condition are causing or if they are related to the sexual dysfunction.

In conducting a gynecologic/pelvic examination, specific assessment findings should be noted. First, in assessing the external genitalia, look for any anatomical abnormalities, female circumcision, fistulas, lacerations, or lesions that may be present. Note the color and moisture of the vulva, labia, clitoris, introitus, and perineum. Before inserting a speculum, permission from the patient should be obtained, to ensure the patient is aware and comfortable with the procedure. This uses the trauma informed care approach allowing for patient autonomy. If permission is not obtained, the examination should be stopped, and the patient should be informed about the next steps. When doing a speculum examination, be sure to use adequate lubrication to reduce friction, and note any pain on insertion or on opening the device. Again, take note of any abnormalities, as well as color and moisture within the vagina and on the cervix. Note any discharge that may be in the vaginal canal because certain infections (eg, sexually transmitted infections, bacterial vaginosis) can affect sexual function [34,35]. In conducting the bimanual examination, it may be helpful to insert one finger before both and note any pain response. If pain occurs with one finger, do not proceed to two. Although conducting the bimanual examination, note tenderness above the mons pubis and in the adnexa. Additionally, generally assess the depth and width of the vaginal canal. Throughout the examination, note for tensing or contraction of pelvic muscles, tenderness and/or pain. Specifically, determine where the pain occurs and if pain occurs on the vulva, or introitus.

Testing
As part of a thorough physical examination, certain laboratory testing may be needed to rule in or out certain causes of sexual dysfunction. Medical causes previously discussed, such as Sjogren syndrome, thyroid disease, diabetes, sexually transmitted infections, and UTIs can cause sexual dysfunction. Therefore, the appropriate blood work or urine testing should be obtained. Additionally, progression of life changes can lead to sexual dysfunction or changes. Both pregnancy, postpartum, breastfeeding and menopause have been shown to affect sexual function and should be assessed through appropriate testing [8,9,36–38].

Diagnosis
Determining whether there is a pathophysiologic cause (eg, underlying illness, medication) or physiologic (ie, lack of knowledge about the female sexual response cycle) is crucial to adequate and accurate treatment. A complete review of the history, physical examination, and testing will provide insight into the diagnosis.

Physiologic
If after conducting a thorough assessment, the clinician determines that key information in the history demonstrate a lack of knowledge related to female sexual function, and the findings seem within normal limits, the root cause of the sexual dysfunction may be physiologic. Physiologic sexual dysfunction may not be sexual dysfunction at all but a lack of knowledge regarding the differentiation and distinguishing differences between male and female sexual response cycles and patterns. For this, the diagnosis would be sexual health counseling, and a comprehensive overview should be provided to the patient. For example, if the patient's chief complaint is decreased desire, and per the HPI, the clinician elicits that the patient lacks spontaneous desire, but that instead desire occurs in response to a stimulus, then a sexual health counseling diagnosis should be made, and the patient provided education. Responsive desire in females is not a pathophysiologic issue but commonly occurs in many females. Additionally, arousal and desire can occur close together or concurrently in women [2].

Pathophysiologic
If an underlying cause was identified during the assessment, be it a medical issue, medication, substance use, procedure or treatment, the diagnosis should be "sexual dysfunction" due to the related cause (eg, medical condition, substance use). The medical condition should be treated, and the sexual dysfunction should also be treated based on the domains (eg, desire, lubrication) it

interferes with. A diagnosis of sexual dysfunction or the medical illness can be documented, in conjunction with a diagnosis of the root cause (eg, vaginal dryness, dyspareunia). If the sexual dysfunction is related to a medication that the patient must be on, or a condition and/or treatment that cannot be reversed (eg, a cancer treatment), treating the sexual dysfunction long-term is important.

In the absence of a secondary sexual dysfunction because of another medical cause, sexual dysfunction can be a primary diagnosis based on the history and physical examination findings. Although sexual dysfunction itself can be the diagnosis, tapering down to the exact cause of the sexual dysfunction makes it easier to treat. Sexual function has many domains, and therefore, dysfunction does as well. Adequate lubrication can be a significant issue for many patients, whether it is related to another condition, an adverse effect of treatment, or a natural progression in life (eg, menopause), which can lead to vaginal dryness. Vaginal dryness may present with tissue that is pale, thin, shiny, erythematous, and without noticeable moisture [39]. In this case, the diagnosis would be vulvovaginal atrophy or atrophic vaginitis. A female desire or arousal disorder, in the absence of other causes, is defined as meeting 3 of the 6 criteria in the American Psychiatric Association's Diagnostic and Statistical Manual V (DSM-V) relating to lack of interest or arousal [40]. Desire whether impaired by other causes or not can be diagnosed as decreased libido, decreased desire, or female sexual interest disorder. Similar to desire and arousal, orgasm difficulties, in the absence of another reason (eg, medication, cancer treatment), are diagnosed according to the DSM-V, which defines it as lack of or change in the timing or frequency of orgasm sensations between 75% and 100% of sexual encounters [40]. Either by organic causes or by the absence thereof, orgasm difficulties are typically diagnosed as either anorgasmia or female orgasmic disorder. Pain disorders come in various forms. Similar to all of the sexual dysfunction disorders, they can be a symptom of a primary illness, its treatment, a medication, or they can occur in the absence of those things. Dyspareunia is painful intercourse, whereas vagismus is the tensing/or constant tension of pelvic floor muscles during intercourse, which can even occur during pelvic examinations. In the absence of other causes, these together are diagnosed as a genito-pelvic pain and penetration disorder, per the DSM-V criteria [40]. Other types of pain conditions can affect sexual function but do not have to occur with sexual dysfunction. Two common pain conditions, vulvodynia (pain in the vulva) and vestibulodynia (pain in and around the opening of the vagina) can not only affect sexual function but also commonly occur outside in women outside of engagement in sexual activities [41].

Treatment Options
Nonpharmacologic
Nonpharmacologic treatments range in type: counseling, physical therapy, and devices. Sexual health counseling, or sex therapy, has been shown to benefit women with sexual dysfunction [42]. If a sex therapist is not available, counseling in itself may be beneficial to patients with sexual dysfunction. Cognitive behavioral therapy has been shown to be effective at improving desire, arousal,

and orgasm disorders [43]. Pelvic physical or physiotherapy has been shown to have significant benefit in those with sexual dysfunction, especially related to pelvic muscle tension and tightness [44,45]. Additionally, medical devices like dilators can help improve dyspareunia and/or vagismus. The purpose of a dilator (or a dilator kit) is to gradually help the patient become comfortable with larger diameter of sizes being inserted into the vagina. In certain populations, it can help to prevent or stretch the vaginal tissues. Vibrators can have a similar effect but can also help those with arousal, or orgasm difficulties.

Pharmacologic
Although nonpharmacologic treatments can help improve sexual dysfunction in some patients, they may not improve it in all patients. Vaginal moisturizers and lubricants, although over the counter, play an important role in treating vaginal atrophy, and some have been shown to be equivalent to vaginal estrogen use in menopause [46–48]. If the patient has vaginal atrophy, besides other conditions that require the use of a dilator, the use of lubricants and moisturizers need to be emphasized to the patient. There are some approved medications for desire disorders but most are off label, as are those for arousal and orgasm. Pain conditions should be treated based on the root cause and location of the pain, which may vary in the type of pain medication that can be prescribed (eg, neuropathic drugs, topical lidocaine).

SUMMARY
Sexual dysfunction is a common occurrence among both premenopausal and postmenopausal females. A thorough history and physical examination are crucial to the accurate diagnosis and adequate treatment of the dysfunction. It is important not to rule out underlying medical conditions, medications, and other treatments that could be contributing to the sexual dysfunction. If they are the root cause and can be treated or managed, then they should be addressed first, and sexual dysfunction managed concurrently if appropriate. In the case that the cause is unable to be addressed, then the sexual dysfunction should be treated. Both nonpharmacologic and pharmacologic based treatments should be considered, and the patient should be treated based on symptoms, diagnosis, and other pertinent factors.

CLINICS CARE POINTS

- Sexual dysfunction commonly occurs in women, therefore clinicians should routinely assess for it.
- Knowledge of medications and illnessses that can cause secondary sexual dysfunction can expedite the root cause of sexual dysfunction.
- Adequate diagnosis and management of sexual dysfunction can improve quality of life in individuals.

DECLARATION OF INTERESTS

The author has no funding related to this article. The author has no conflicts of interest to disclose.

References

[1] World Health Organization. Sexual Health and Its Linkages to Reproductive Health: an operational approach. Geneva 2017. Available at: https://apps.who.int/iris/handle/10665/258738. Accessed July 20, 2022.

[2] Basson R. The female sexual response: a different model. J Sex Marital Ther 2000;26(1):51–65.

[3] Janssen E, Bancroft J. The dual control model: The role of sexual inhibition and excitation in sexual arousal and behavior. In: Janssen E, Bancroft J, editors. The psychophysiology of sex. Bloomington, IN: Indiana University Press; 2007. p. 197–222.

[4] Bancroft J, Graham CA, Janssen E, et al. The dual control model: current status and future directions. J Sex Res 2009;46(2–3):121–42.

[5] Rosen R, Rosen R, Brown C, et al. Th e Female Sexual Function Index (FSFI): a multidimensional self-report instrument for the assessment of female sexual function. J Sex Marital Ther 2000;26:191–208. Available at: http://www.fsfiquestionnaire.com/Published Format.pdf. Accessed September 6, 2017.

[6] McCool ME, Zuelke A, Theurich MA, et al. Prevalence of female sexual dysfunction among premenopausal women: a systematic review and meta-analysis of observational studies. Sex Med Rev 2016;4(3):197–212.

[7] Yoldemir T, Garibova N, Atasayan K. The association between sexual dysfunction and metabolic syndrome among Turkish postmenopausal women. Climacteric 2019;22(5):472–7.

[8] Trento SRSS, Madeiro A, Rufino AC. Sexual function and associated factors in postmenopausal women. Rev Bras Ginecol Obstet 2021;43(7):522–9.

[9] Nazarpour S, Simbar M, Ramezani Tehrani F, et al. Quality of life and sexual function in postmenopausal women. J Women Aging 2018;30(4):299–309.

[10] Ghadigaonkar DS, Murthy P. Sexual dysfunction in persons with substance use disorders. J Psychosexual Health 2019;1(2):117–21.

[11] Van Berlo W, Ensink B. Problems with sexuality after sexual assault. Annu Rev Sex Res 2000;11:235–57. Available at: https://pubmed.ncbi.nlm.nih.gov/11351833/. Accessed August 4, 2022.

[12] Kelley EL, Gidycz CA. Posttraumatic stress and sexual functioning difficulties in college women with a history of sexual assault victimization. Psychol Violence 2019;9(1):98–107.

[13] Yazdanpanahi Z, Nikkholgh M, Akbarzadeh M, et al. Stress, anxiety, depression, and sexual dysfunction among postmenopausal women in Shiraz, Iran, 2015. J Family Community Med 2018;25(2):82.

[14] Basson R, Gilks T. Women's sexual dysfunction associated with psychiatric disorders and their treatment. Womens Health (Lond Engl). 2018;14; https://doi.org/10.1177/1745506518762664.

[15] Tutino JS, Ouimet AJ, Shaughnessy K. How do psychological risk factors predict sexual outcomes? A comparison of four models of young women's sexual outcomes. J Sex Med 2017;14(10):1232–40.

[16] Castellini G, Lelli L, Ricca V, et al. Sexuality in eating disorders patentis: etiological factors, sexual dysfunction and identity issues. A systematic review. Horm Mol Biol Clin Investig 2016;25(2):71–90.

[17] Castellini G, Rossi E, Ricca V. The relationship between eating disorder psychopathology and sexuality: etiological factors and implications for treatment. Curr Opin Psychiatry 2020;33(6):554–61.

[18] Krysiak R, Drosdzol-Cop A, Skrzypulec-Plinta V, et al. Sexual function and depressive symptoms in young women with elevated macroprolactin content: a pilot study. Endocrine 2016;53(1):291.

[19] Gabrielson AT, Sartor RA, Hellstrom WJG. The impact of thyroid disease on sexual dysfunction in men and women. Sex Med Rev 2019;7(1):57–70.

[20] Esposito K, Ciotola M, Marfella R, et al. The metabolic syndrome: a cause of sexual dysfunction in women. Int J Impot Res 2005;17(3):224–6.

[21] Esposito K, Giugliano D, Ciotola M, et al. Obesity and sexual dysfunction, male and female. Int J Impot Res 2008;20(4):358–65.

[22] Elyasi F, Kashi Z, Tasfieh B, et al. Sexual dysfunction in women with type 2 diabetes mellitus. Iran J Med Sci 2015;40(3):206. Accessed August 4, 2022.

[23] Chris Saad S, Pietrzykowski JE, Lewis SS, et al. Vaginal lubrication in women with scleroderma and sjogren's syndrome. Sex Disabil 1999;17(2):103–13.

[24] Isik H, Isik M, Aynioglu O, et al. Are the women with Sjögren's Syndrome satisfied with their sexual activity? Rev Bras Reumatol 2017;57(3):210–6.

[25] Al-Ezzi M, Tappuni AR, Khan KS. The impact of Sjögren's syndrome on the quality of sexual life of female patients in the UK: a controlled analysis. Rheumatol Int 2022;42(8); https://doi.org/10.1007/S00296-021-04830-6.

[26] Salonia A, Zanni G, Nappi RE, et al. Sexual dysfunction is common in women with lower urinary tract symptoms and urinary incontinence: results of a cross-sectional study. Eur Urol 2004;45(5):642–8.

[27] Zhang J, Wei S, Zeng Q, et al. Prevalence and risk factors of sexual dysfunction in patients with inflammatory bowel disease: systematic review and meta-analysis. Int J Colorectal Dis 2021;36(9):2027–38.

[28] Varanda S, Ribeiro da Silva J, Costa AS, et al. Sexual dysfunction in women with Parkinson's disease. Mov Disord 2016;31(11):1685–93.

[29] Bhattacharyya KB, Rosa-Grilo M. Sexual dysfunctions in parkinson's disease: an underrated problem in a much discussed disorder. Int Rev Neurobiol 2017;134:859–76.

[30] Merghati-Khoei E, Emami-Razavi SH, Bakhtiyari M, et al. Spinal cord injury and women's sexual life: case-control study. Spinal Cord 2017;55(3):269–73.

[31] Rathore C, Henning OJ, Luef G, et al. Sexual dysfunction in people with epilepsy. Epilepsy Behav 2019;100(Pt A); https://doi.org/10.1016/J.YEBEH.2019.106495.

[32] Duramaz A, Ilter MH, Yıldız Ş, et al. The relationship between injury mechanism and sexual dysfunction in surgically treated pelvic fractures. Eur J Trauma Emerg Surg 2020;46(4):807–16.

[33] Zhou ES, Frederick NN, Bober SL. Hormonal changes and sexual dysfunction. Med Clin North Am 2017;101(6):1135–50.

[34] Şimşir C, Coşkun B, Coşkun B, et al. Effects of bacterial vaginosis and its treatment on sexual functions: A cross-sectional questionnaire study. Arch Clin Exp Med 2019;4(2):99–102.

[35] Cai T, Mondaini N, Migno S, et al. Genital Chlamydia trachomatis infection is related to poor sexual quality of life in young sexually active women. J Sex Med 2011;8(4):1131–7.

[36] Ninivaggio C, Rogers RG, Leeman L, et al. Sexual function changes during pregnancy. Int Urogynecol J 2017;28(6):923–9.

[37] Aydin M, Cayonu N, Kadihasanoglu M, et al. Comparison of Sexual Functions in Pregnant and Non-Pregnant Women. Urol J 2015;12(5):2339–44. Available at: https://pubmed.ncbi.nlm.nih.gov/26571317/. Accessed August 5, 2022.

[38] Fuentealba-Torres M, Cartagena-Ramos D, Fronteira I, et al. What are the prevalence and factors associated with sexual dysfunction in breastfeeding women? A Brazilian cross-sectional analytical study. BMJ Open 2019;9(4); https://doi.org/10.1136/BMJOPEN-2018-025833.

[39] Bleibel B, Nguyen H. Vaginal Atrophy - StatPearls - NCBI Bookshelf 2022. Available at: https://www.ncbi.nlm.nih.gov/books/NBK559297/. Accessed August 5, 2022.

[40] American Psychiatric Association. Diagnostic and Statistical Manual of Mental Disorders. 5th edition. Washington, D.C: American Psychiatric Association Publishing; 2013. https://doi.org/10.1176/appi.books.9780890425596.

[41] Stenson AL. Vulvodynia: diagnosis and management. Obstet Gynecol Clin North Am 2017;44(3):493–508.

[42] Karakas S, Aslan E. Sexual Counseling in Women With Primary Infertility and Sexual Dysfunction: Use of the BETTER Model. J Sex Marital Ther 2019;45(1):21–30.

[43] Mirzaee F, Ahmadi A, Zangiabadi Z, et al. The effectiveness of psycho-educational and cognitive-behavioral counseling on female sexual dysfunction. Rev Bras Ginecol Obstet 2020;42(6):333–9.

[44] Berghmans B. Physiotherapy for pelvic pain and female sexual dysfunction: an untapped resource. Int Urogynecol J 2018;29(5):631–8.

[45] Wallace SL, Miller LD, Mishra K. Pelvic floor physical therapy in the treatment of pelvic floor dysfunction in women. Curr Opin Obstet Gynecol 2019;31(6):485–93.

[46] Mitchell CM, Reed SD, Diem S, et al. Efficacy of vaginal estradiol or vaginal moisturizer vs placebo for treating postmenopausal vulvovaginal symptoms: a randomized clinical trial. JAMA Intern Med 2018;178(5):681–90.

[47] Jokar A, Davari T, Asadi N, et al. Comparison of the hyaluronic acid vaginal cream and conjugated estrogen used in treatment of vaginal atrophy of menopause women: a randomized controlled clinical trial. Int J Community Based Nurs Midwifery 2016;4(1):69. Accessed August 5, 2022.

[48] Nachtigall LE. Comparative study: Replens versus local estrogen in menopausal women. Fertil Steril 1994;61(1):178–80.

Pediatrics

Advances in Family Practice Nursing 5 (2023) 193–205

ADVANCES IN FAMILY PRACTICE NURSING

The Importance of Sleep for Normal Growth and Development

Ann Sheehan, DNP, CPNP

Michigan State University, College of Nursing, 1355 Bogue Street A124, East Lansing, MI 48824, USA

Keywords

- Sleep • Growth and development • Sleep hygiene • Sleep architecture
- Emotional regulation • Sleep quality

Key points

- Adequate sleep is necessary for growth and development to occur normally.
- Advance practice registered nurses need to understand what is normal and what constitutes abnormal sleep to prevent long-term health consequences.
- Quality sleep is crucial to all physiologic, psychological, and social functioning.
- Brain plasticity of infants and toddlers suggests that this is the right time to introduce sleep routines.
- Culture plays a big part in how sleep issues are defined as problems.

INTRODUCTION

Sleep is a necessity for human life and daily functioning. Sleep is the primary activity of the developing brain. Without sleep, humans are not able to maintain adequate growth, regulate emotions, or have adequate memory recall. Many physiologic processes take place during sleep, including neurologic, metabolic, and endocrine [1]. Healthy sleep habits develop over time and need to be part of children's daily routines from birth. Poor sleep quality puts children at high risk for developing chronic illness and decreased quality of life. In addition, inadequate sleep has been associated with poor academic performance, difficulty regulating emotions, poor attention span, obesity, and an increase in risk-taking behaviors [2].

While conducting a literature review for this article, it was discovered that very little has been written on the topic of pediatric sleep in the last 5 years.

E-mail address: sheeha49@msu.edu

https://doi.org/10.1016/j.yfpn.2022.11.012

Sleep and sleep issues are a common topic of discussion during well-child examinations. It has been reported in the literature that 25% to 30% of all children experience some type of sleep difficulty [2–4]. The prevalence of sleep issues goes up as children age [2]. It is imperative that primary care providers have a firm grasp on the pathophysiology of sleep, developmental issues that impact sleep and have confidence in coaching parents and children on appropriate sleep habits.

The purpose of this article was to review how sleep–wake cycles develop, why sleep is important for children, and the way developmental milestone achievement affects sleep. In addition, this article provides the advance practice registered nurse (APRN) with anticipatory guidance for parents to promote better sleep quality and quantity for children. It is not the intention of this article to do a deep dive into the pathophysiology of sleep. The reader is referred to a pathophysiology textbook to review this process.

SLEEP BASICS
In general, the state of sleep is a period of decreased responsiveness to the environment when the mind and body recuperate. However, there is significant neurologic and physiologic activity during sleep [5]. The sleep–wake cycle is governed by three processes: circadian rhythm, homeostasis, and ultradian rhythm. These systems interact independently and interdependently to influence the amount, timing, and depth of sleep [5,6]. A regular routine for sleep and awake activities creates strong internal clock functioning and promotes sleep quality [6]. Alternatively, when there is no routine to the sleep–wake cycle the quality of sleep is reduced [6]. The ability or inability to sleep is impacted by several factors: psychological, physiologic, cultural, and environmental. The developing brain is highly susceptible to environmental influences [7].

Circadian rhythm process
The circadian rhythm process is the internal clock that regulates wakefulness and sleep. The circadian cycle matures over the first 6 months of life and is influenced by brain and nervous system development, social cues, and environmental cues [1]. One of the most influential environmental cues is light and darkness. Studies show that early morning light exposure sets the internal clock for the day [5]. Similarly, light exposure just before bedtime can interrupt sleep onset. This light exposure comes from a multitude of sources: television, bright bedroom or bathroom lighting, sunlight, or personal electronic devices (screens). Alternatively, light exposure can be helpful to accelerate waking [5]. There are a variety of other cues that can affect the circadian rhythm, including hunger, room temperature, medications, and bedtime routines [5]. Therefore, the circadian rhythm process regulates the timing of an individual's sleep.

Homeostasis process
The sleep homeostasis process is individual self-regulation of sleep. Homeostasis drives the brain to sleep. The literature describes the drive to sleep as

pressure on the brain to sleep. This pressure to sleep builds up during waking h [6]. This pressure is relieved by sleeping. The pressure to sleep gets stronger the longer individuals are awake. Given this process, the longer the brain has been awake, the longer and deeper an individual tends to sleep [6]. Sleep pressure is the lowest after individuals have sufficient quantity and quality of sleep. This process can be interrupted by medications, alterations in or no bedtime routine, and sleeping too little or too much [6]. Therefore, the homeostasis process regulates an individual's length and depth of sleep to restore alertness.

Ultradian rhythm process

Although homeostasis and circadian rhythm process dictate when an individual sleeps and how restorative that sleep is, the ultradian rhythm process determines the timing and duration of sleep [4,6]. This process is commonly referred to as sleep architecture. These states are known as nonrapid eye movement (NREM) and rapid eye movement (REM) sleep. These sleep states are associated with differing levels of arousal, brain activity, autonomic response, and muscle tone [8].

NREM sleep is a period of sleep with relatively low brain activity where regulatory activity of the brain is ongoing [8]. This type of sleep can be divided into four stages starting at approximately 6 months of age. Stage 1 is a transitional state of sleep between wakefulness and sleep. Children can be easily aroused from this stage of sleep. This stage of sleep represents less than 5% of the children's total time sleeping. Stage 2 is where children spend about half of their total sleep time. In this stage, there is a decrease in eye movement, muscle tone and respiratory rate. Children are more difficult to arouse from this state but will be alert shortly after awaking from this stage. Stages 3 and 4 are similar and occur when the body is the most relaxed [8]. About 20% of children's total sleep time is spent in these two stages [8]. During these stages, it is difficult to arouse children and they may be confused and disoriented on awaking from these stages.

REM sleep is when dreaming occurs [5,8]. Children experience muscle paralysis during this stage of sleep. Dreams seem real to children, and they may remember vivid detail about their dreams. Dreams during this stage are generally about things that children experience during the day and are a way for them to process the events of the day [5]. REM sleep time decreases as children age. By the time children are 5 years of age, they spend only 20% to 25% of their time in REM sleep, compared with infants who spend roughly 55% of their time in REM sleep [5].

SLEEP AND DEVELOPMENT

Sleep architecture changes significantly as children grow and mature from newborn through adolescence. In addition, sleep behaviors change with external and internal influences. External influences include parenting practices, environmental factors, and cultural practices. Internally, sleep architecture is affected by the normal developmental process. Infants need to achieve two sleep milestones: sleep consolidation and sleep regulation. Sleep consolidation is the ability to sleep for a prolonged, continuous period, allowing infants to sleep through the night. In addition, infants must learn to regulate their sleep. Sleep regulation is the ability to control internal states of arousal that allow infants to self-soothe and initiate sleep without parent involvement. These two developmental milestones are normally achieved in the first 6 months of life. The ability for infants to achieve sleep consolidation and sleep regulation predicts their ability to achieve quality sleep in the future [8]. In addition, as children achieve various developmental milestones, their ability to achieve quality and quantity of sleep can be affected. Table 1 provides the reader with a summary of sleep recommendations by age group.

NEWBORNS (0 TO 2 MONTHS)
Newborns' average 14 h of sleep per 24 h. There is no nocturnal or diurnal sleep pattern established in this age group. Newborns' sleep wake cycles are dependent upon their hunger. Bottle-fed newborns tend to sleep for longer stretches of time than breastfed infants. This age group does not have an established circadian rhythm, so predictability of their sleep pattern is not possible [5]. When talking with parents of newborns it is important to teach them how to recognize signs of drowsiness so their newborn can be put down to sleep. This is important to help set or establish the circadian rhythm and support the homeostasis process.

INFANTS (2 TO 12 MONTHS)
Infants average 13 h of sleep per 24 h. Achievement of gross motor milestones, such as rolling over and crawling, cause infants to begin to fight sleep. Infants' attachment and level of social engagement affect the quality and quantity of their sleep. These milestones are accompanied by infants' ability to begin to regulate their sleep through self-soothing behaviors. These behaviors allow infants to consolidate their sleep patterns and space out their naps. The decrease in napping and the ability to self-soothe makes it possible for infants to sleep

Table 1
24-h pediatric sleep recommendations

Age	Range	Average	Night waking	Number of naps	Nap length
Newborn (0 to 2 months)	12 to 18 h	14 h	Varies widely	Varies widely	1 to 3 h
Infant (2 to 12 months)	12 to 16 h	13 h	1 to 3	2 to 4	1 to 3 h
Toddler (12 to 36 months)	11 to 14 h	13 h	0 to 1	1	1 to 3 h
Preschool (3 to 5 years)	10 to 13 h	12 h	0	0	—
School age (6 to 12 years)	9 to 12 h	10 h	0	0	—
Adolescent (12 to 18 years)	8 to 10 h	9 h	0	0	—

through the night between 6 and 12 months of age [5]. At this stage, infants begin to associate a routine of activities with the onset of sleep. Transitional objects, such as a pacifier, blanket or toy, are important to support self-soothing. This is the emergence of the ultradian rhythm process.

Teaching parents the importance of developing a consistent sleep schedule for nighttime sleep and for napping by 3 months of age supports the circadian rhythm and homeostasis processes for sleep [5]. Infants should be taught to put themselves to sleep. This is accomplished by putting them down to sleep while they are drowsy but still awake with a transitional object. Parents should also understand that it is common for infants to have transient sleep problems. It is important to support infants' self-soothing to transition back to sleep as opposed to getting them out of bed each time they awaken. This process helps protect infants from developing a chronic sleep problem.

TODDLERS (12 TO 36 MONTHS)

Toddlers' average 13 h of sleep in 24 h. The amount of napping that is required in this age group decreases as they get older. By 18 months of age, most toddlers are napping only once per day. The toddlers' circadian rhythm process is beginning to mimic the adult rhythm with distinct consolidation of sleep at night and being awake most of the daylight h [2].

This age group has a rapid achievement of developmental milestones across all domains. Toddlers are easily mobile and enjoy autonomous play and interactions, making it difficult to settle down to sleep [4]. Toddlers' naturally curious minds lead them to get out of bed frequently and test the limits which overrides the homeostasis process [4]. Toddlers are reliant on transitional objects and are developing an imagination. The imagination can lead to frequent nighttime fears. However, they have limited language to express these fears. Therefore, toddlers may be awake and getting out of bed or crying frequently in the night.

The achievement of mobility and independence makes it difficult for toddlers to get adequate sleep. When toddlers are tired, they have difficulty regulating their emotions [2]. Therefore, it is common for toddlers to have temper tantrums frequently throughout the day when they are not getting sufficient sleep. It is important for parents to understand the value of maintaining a consistent bedtime and nap routine. The frequent nighttime waking, and bedtime resistance is generally transient in toddlers. Like the infant, encouraging a transitional object and self-soothing enables the toddler to regulate their sleep so the sleep issues do not become chronic.

PRESCHOOL (3 TO 5 YEARS)

Preschool children average about 12 h of sleep per 24 h. Over the course of these years, preschool children stop taking naps and consolidate their sleep to the nighttime h. Most preschoolers have stopped napping by 5 years of age [2]. Unfortunately, preschool children's sleep can be interrupted be almost any stimuli, including temperature, bedding, light, hunger, family/cultural practices, illness, medications, temperament, and attachment issues [4]. Pre-school children experience further development of their imagination and develop fantasy thinking. This can be the cause of frequent nightmares or nighttime fears [2].

Consistent bedtime routine remains important in this age group. If sleep issues arise, they should be addressed as soon as possible to prevent them from becoming a chronic problem. When preschool children do not get enough sleep, they tend to have behavioral issues. Like toddlers, these behavior issues can include temper tantrums, but can also include hitting, kicking, biting, and head banging. Screens, such as television, tablets, and cell phones, tend to become a common part of life during the preschool years. The American Academy of Pediatrics (AAP) recommends no screens in the bedroom or as part of the bedtime routine throughout childhood and adolescence [9]. It has been well established in the literature that sleep duration for preschool children is decreased with the use of screens [2]. Rather, the AAP recommend reading as part of the regular bedtime routine. Reading helps support the natural language development of this age group and supports a longer duration of sleep and a decreased incidence of sleep disturbances [2].

Screens have been shown to decrease the natural surge of melatonin in the evening that supports sleep [2]. When preschoolers use screens, they can get a "second wind" which causes difficulty in settling down for nighttime sleep or for napping [4], thus overriding the natural circadian rhythm and homeostasis processes that support quality sleep.

SCHOOL AGE (6 TO 12 YEARS)

School-age children should average 10 h of sleep per night. Children in this age group are eager to please and easily develop healthy habits. Sleep habits of this age group are affected by a wide variety of stimuli including school activities and sporting events. School-age children are concrete thinkers so nighttime fears are grounded in reality. For instance, if they hear about a burglar in the neighborhood, they may be awake at night worrying when the burglar will enter their house. This age group may also lose sleep due to worry about keeping up academically and socially. As they age, school-age children become increasingly busy interacting with their peers, participating in sports, and extracurricular activities at school. Along with these activities comes an increase in screen use, which reduces sleep quality and quantity [2].

In this age group, individual circadian rhythm patterns begin to emerge that favors evening sleepiness or alertness that can affect sleep onset [2]. Sleepiness affects children's ability to pay attention which can adversely affect school performance. Insufficient sleep causes issues with mood dysregulation that manifests as symptoms of depression and/or anxiety. Along with a consistent sleep schedule, the AAP recommends a wind-down period for school-age children to support the homeostasis process for sleep [9]. Consistent daytime drowsiness and decreased alertness is a red flag. School-age children with these complaints need to have their sleep quality and quantity evaluated, by a pediatric health care provider.

Adolescents (12 to 18 years)

Adolescents should average 9 h of sleep each night. Like school-age children, adolescents are engaged in a multitude of activities that impinge upon their ability to get this amount of sleep each night. These activities include sporting events, school functions, work obligations, and socializing with peers, both virtually and in person. These commitments cause an alteration in the circadian rhythm process and adolescents override their drive to sleep (homeostasis). Alternations in both processes negatively affect the quality and quantity of sleep for adolescents. Therefore, adolescents have the desire to sleep long h on the weekends or days off from school. Unfortunately, this does not change their sleep deficit or feeling of fatigue because they still do not get the quality sleep that is restorative. It is not uncommon for adolescents to always complain of feeling tired.

The adolescent circadian rhythm pattern naturally develops a 2-h delay from what it was for school-age children [2]. This means that adolescents are programmed to go to bed about 2 h later and awaken at least 2 h later in the day. It is not unusual for adolescents to suddenly feel wide awake around 2200 and not be able to settle down to sleep until 0200 to 0300. This shift in adolescents' circadian rhythm pattern makes early school start times and early h for work very difficult.

For these reasons, it is important for adolescents to have a routine sleep wake cycle, even on weekends or days off from school. This helps reset their circadian rhythm and supports the homeostasis process. The pediatric provider needs to engage the parents and the adolescent in this type of discussion. Developmentally, it is normal for adolescents to gain more independence in setting their own schedules. However, the natural adolescent changes make it difficult for them to maintain a good sleep–wake pattern on their own. One way to help reset adolescents' circadian rhythm is to get light exposure upon waking [5]. In addition, adolescents should not use any screens at least 2 h before bedtime [9]. As previously noted in this article, screen use suppresses the surge of melatonin that naturally occurs at nighttime [9]. When the melatonin surge does not occur, it becomes easier to override homeostasis and fight the drive to sleep.

HEALTHY SLEEP PROMOTION

It is estimated that 34.9% of children do not regularly get the recommended amount of sleep for their age [10]. The human body's need for restorative sleep is evident; however, there are a multitude of stimuli that can impact children's ability to achieve adequate quality and quantity of sleep. Evidence supports several interventions that should be implemented early in the life of children and maintained throughout life to support sleep. Maintaining children's circadian rhythm and homeostasis processes are imperative to achieving adequate quantity and quality sleep. Parents and children may need coaching to achieve restorative sleep.

A multitude of learned organizations have developed normative values for sleep duration based on age. These organizations are identified with websites in Box 1. Although these values are quantitative yardsticks for parents and pediatric providers, it is important to realize that not all children will fall into these normative ranges. Table 1 provides the reader with a summary of normative sleep and wake values.

Cultural and family practices

Cultural and family practices and beliefs can affect children's ability to achieve adequate sleep quantity and quality. While talking with families about sleep practices, the pediatric provider needs to keep in mind that what constitutes an issue with sleep varies based on the family and cultural practices. The current evidence-based practices focus on changing the individual child or parent's behavior rather than assessing for specific cultural and family practices. Thus, identifying the cultural norms that determine the boundaries of normal and problematic sleep issues for an individual child are lost [11].

There are many sleep practices that vary across cultures. Sleep duration and sleep need are perceived differently. Although it seems that all children get the same amount of sleep across a 24-h time period, they get this sleep in different ways [11]. These differences are even present in the United States and are dependent on socioeconomic status (SES). For instance, the literature suggests that American minority children tend to go to bed later and wake up later than their White counterparts [7].

Bedtime routines seem to be specific to Americans. Many cultures, other than America, have no formal bedtime and allow children to fall asleep when they are tired and where they want to sleep [11]. In addition, many cultural beliefs support co-sleeping with parents and/or siblings [11]. The AAP evidence does not support this practice [9]. Outside of the American culture, putting children to sleep alone and in their own bed is looked upon as neglectful or unkind [3,7,11]. Many cultures believe sleeping alone leaves the person vulnerable to spiritual risks (at any age) [7]. Americans value independence and therefore, encourage children to learn to sleep alone, at an early age [5].

Using transitional sleep objects tends to be common in industrialized cultures but not common in nonindustrialized cultures [7]. This author believes there is a correlation between co-sleeping and a decreased need for a transitional object to promote sleep. The use of a transitional object to support sleep through self-soothing is necessary developmentally. The transitional object supports independents and helps children work through Piaget's stage industry versus initiative [12].

Napping is a practice that is not consistent between cultures. Melatonin naturally dips in the late afternoon to early evening [2]. Some cultures encourage

Box 1: Resources for patient education materials

American Academy of Pediatrics: www.healthychildren.org

American Academy of Sleep Medicine: https://aasm.org/clinical-resources/practice-standards/practice-guidelines/

National Foundation of Sleep: https://www.thensf.org/

late afternoon napping because of this melatonin dip. In these cultures, children nap after school and are awakened in the later evening, given dinner, and then left to do their homework late into the night, after the parents have gone to bed. Many cultures have siestas during the heat of the day. This is a time when most family members nap. This alters the bedtime to a much later time and children are socialized into the adult routine of eating late at night and going to bed late at night. In American culture, the literature reports that lower SES families tend to nap later in the day and stay up later at night [3]. This is compared with higher SES families that nap earlier in the day to support an early bedtime so the parents can have time alone [3].

Sleep hygiene

Taking all of this information into consideration, the pediatric provider should review sleep hygiene at every well-child visit to ensure children continue to get adequate sleep. Sleep hygiene is the overarching term used to describe best sleep practices. The main principle to establishing good sleep hygiene is the creation of a safe, comfortable sleep environment to support good quality and quantity of sleep. A consistent bedtime routine is important to provide children with the cues that it is time to wind-down and get ready for sleep (homeostasis). The bedtime routine should include fun, quieting or calming activities that help children feel loved and secure. These positive interactions at bedtime may help reduce bedtime struggles because children will look forward to this one-on-one time with parent(s) [2].

The bedtime routine activities should be very structured with a defined duration, so children know there is an endpoint to the interaction with their parent(s). A bath, brushing teeth, reading a book or singing, and then hugs or snuggles while tucking children into their beds is an adequate routine. These activities should occur in the same order at the same time every night, thus promoting sleep onset association (homeostasis). Likewise, children should be awakened at about the same time every morning with the gentle introduction of light into the room [13]. These activities support the circadian rhythm process.

Children's sleep environment should be calm, quiet, dark, and cool. Children should have their own designated sleeping space that is developmentally appropriate. Newborns and infants up to the age of 6 months should sleep in their own bed in the parents' room [9]. After 6 months of age, infants can be moved into their own room into their own crib [9]. Newborns and infants should be placed on their backs to sleep [9]. When toddlers begin to climb out of the crib, they should be transitioned into a bed of their own. All children, including newborns should be put into bed drowsy but awake. This promotes their ability to self-soothe as they fall asleep. This practice has been shown to decrease night waking as infants and toddlers self-soothe to fall back to sleep during the night and do not require parental intervention [13].

Screen and media exposure should be avoided as part of the bedtime routine. These activities have been shown to interfere with the evening surge of melatonin due to light exposure [13]. Televisions and digital screens of all kinds should be removed from children's bedrooms to prevent sleep onset issues. If children have difficulty reaching a relaxed state to fall asleep, a short period of quiet activity (10 to 15 min) in the dimly light bedroom may be beneficial [13]. These activities might include looking at a book, coloring, or writing in a journal, for older children.

Children should not be put to bed hungry. The literature reports that children tend to wake up frequently during the night if they are hungry [7]. Breast-feeding or bottle feeding for newborns and infants is appropriate. For toddlers and older children, a light snack with a protein source is appropriate just before the bath and teeth brushing. These snacks support brain growth by providing proper nutrition. Satiety promotes the feeling of sleepiness thus supporting homeostasis [7].

Bathing as part of a bedtime routine helps promote the feeling of sleepiness. The bedtime bath supports sleep by initially raising the core body temperature and then lowering it, which promotes the feeling of sleepiness [7]. Brushing teeth at bedtime is a positive hygiene practice to prevent dental caries and other diseases. These activities not only support good sleep but also facilitate learning proper self-care.

The AAP encourages reading and singing lullabies at bedtime [9]. This creates a calming environment that supports homeostasis and the circadian rhythm process for sleep. These activities also promote language development [9]. During this time, the parent(s) can cuddle, rock, and/or massage their children. This interaction promotes the feeling of security which can extinguish separation anxiety that may cause bedtime resistance and night waking.

CONSEQUENCES OF POOR SLEEP QUALITY AND QUANTITY

Sleep issues are among the most common concerns expressed during well-child examinations. Bedtime struggles and frequent night waking are experienced by 20% to 25% of the toddler and preschool population [3]. Nightmares and night terrors account for night waking in 11% to 40% of school-age children [3]. If left untreated, these developmentally normal sleep issues will become chronic sleep issues.

Poor sleep quality and quantity can cause permanent developmental deficits in all domains [14]. The literature shows the consequences of poor sleep include behavioral problems, poor school performance and learning deficits, sports injuries, mood, and emotional dysregulation, obesity, and impaired social skills [7]. One author detailed additional consequences for sleep-deprived adolescents, including high-risk behaviors such as substance use, suicidality, drowsy driving, and sexual risk taking [15,16].

IMPLICATIONS FOR ADVANCED PRACTICE REGISTERED NURSES

Pediatric providers need to do a thorough assessment of sleep patterns when parents present a psychological, social, or physiologic concern for their children. The promotion of good sleep habits is essential to good quality and quantity of sleep throughout childhood and adolescence. Intervening early when a sleep issue is identified helps extinguish the behavior to promote good health. This will also facilitate referral to a specialist for accurate diagnosis when appropriate.

Cultural and family traditions can impact children's ability to achieve the requisite amount of daily sleep. The pediatric provider needs to take time to determine how a sleep problem is framed by the parent and family before determining how to help a family deal with a sleep issue. Determining adherence to a previous treatment plan is imperative. Developing a plan to solve sleep issues may not be as simple as this author has laid out in Box 2. Children do suffer from primary and secondary sleep disorders that require further medical evaluation and treatment. However, pediatric providers need to know what is normal for each age group to understand how to appropriately intervene to solve sleep issues.

Box 2: Bedtime routine

Schedule
- Regular bedtime
- Regular morning awakening
- Put infants, toddlers, and preschool children to bed drowsy but awake

Nutrition
- Feeding
- Light snack

Hygiene
- Brush teeth
- Bath

Communication
- Read story
- Sung lullaby

Physical contact
- Massage
- Cuddling
- Rocking
- Kisses

Avoid screen and light exposure
- No screens in the bedroom
- No frightening or stimulating television, videos, or video games
- Use dim lighting during bedtime routine

SUMMARY

Sleep is a period of intense brain growth and restorative activity. Quality sleep is an important part of physiologic, emotional, and cognitive development. Individual variability in sleep need is influenced by behavioral, medical, environmental, and cultural factors. This article provided an overview of the development of the sleep–wake cycle, how achievement of developmental milestones can affect the sleep–wake cycle, and the requirements for creating a bedtime routine to support quality sleep and adequate sleep quantity throughout childhood and adolescence. The consequences of poor sleep quality and insufficient quantity of sleep results in chronic health conditions, mood dysregulation, school failure, obesity, and an increase in risk-taking behaviors. The brain plasticity of infants and toddlers suggests that the introduction and consistency of the bedtime routine in these age groups prevents adverse consequences throughout childhood and adolescence [14]. The next edition of this journal will present an article related to special circumstances/considerations and a discussion on the assessment for sleep disorders and common sleep disorders.

CLINICS CARE POINTS

- It has been estimated that about a third of all children experience some type of sleep difficulty [2,3,4].
- When parents mention concerns or have questions about their child's sleep, the pediatric provider must obtain a detailed history on the child's sleep pattern and routine before being able to offer any guidance.
- The guidance provided to the parent should center around sleep hygiene evidence.
- These elements include promotion of a sleep schedule[9, 13], ensuring that the child is not hungry [7], providing a hygiene routine [7], communicating verbally and physically with the child [2], and avoiding digital screen light exposure [13].
- The reader is referred to Box 2 for more specific detail on these clinical care points.

Disclosure
The author has nothing to disclose.

References

[1] Rodgers B. Sleep. In: Foret Giddens J, editor. Concepts for nursing practice. 2nd ed. St. Louis, MO: Elsevier; 2013. p. 94–103.

[2] Hines S. Sleep. In: Garzon Maaks D, Starr N, Brady M, et al, editors. Burns' pediatric primary care. 7th ed. St. Louis, MO: Saunders; 2020. p. 281–92.

[3] Grover G, Schopathy T. Sleep: normal patterns and common diseases. In: Berkowitz CD, editor. Pediatrics: a primary care approach. 5th ed. Elk Grove Village, IL: American Academy of Pediatrics; 2020. p. 153–9.

[4] Mindell JA, Owens JA. Sleep problems in pediatric practice: clinical issues for the pediatric nurse practitioner. J Pediatr Health Care 2003;17(6):324–31.

[5] Finn Davis K, Parker K, Montgomery G. Sleep in infants and young children: part one: normal sleep. J Pediatr Health Care 2004;18(2):65–71.

[6] Deboer T. Sleep homeostasis and the circadian clock: do the circadian pacemaker and the sleep homeostat influence each other's functioning? Neurobiol Sleep Circadian Rhythms 2018;5:68–77.

[7] Mindell JA, Williamson AA. Benefits of a bedtime routine in young children: sleep, development and beyond. Sleep Med Rev 2018;40:93–108.

[8] Mindell JA, Owens JA. A clinical guide to pediatric sleep: diagnosis and management of sleep problems. 3rd ed. Philadelphia, PA: Wolters Kluwer; 2015.

[9] Hagan JF, Shaw JS, Duncan PM. Bright futures: guidelines for health supervision of infants, children, and adolescents. 4th ed. Elk Grove Village, IL: American Academy of Pediatrics; 2017.

[10] Wheaton A, Claussen A. Short sleep duration among infants, children and adolescents aged 4 months-17 years – United States, 2016-2018. MMWR Morb Mortal Wkly Rep 2021;70(38):1315–21.

[11] Oskar GJ, O'Connor BB. Children's sleep: an interplay between culture and biology. Pediatrics 2005;115(1):204–15.

[12] Piaget J. The theory of stages in cognitive development. New York, NY: McGraw-Hill; 1969.

[13] Jiang F. Sleep and early brain development. Ann Nutr Metab 2019;75:44–53.

[14] Boysan M. Developmental implications of sleep. Sleep Hypnosis 2016;18(2):44–52.

[15] Fernandez S. Adolescent sleep: challenges and solutions for pediatric primary care. Pediatr Ann 2019;48(8):e292–5.

[16] Paruthi S, Brooks L, D'Ambrosio C, et al. Recommended amount of sleep for pediatric populations: a consensus statement of the american academy of sleep medicine. J Clin Sleep Med 2016;12(6):785–6.

Advances in Family Practice Nursing 5 (2023) 207–215

ADVANCES IN FAMILY PRACTICE NURSING

Fever of Unknown Origin in Pediatrics

Emily Davis, MNSc, APRN, CPNP-AC*,
Teresa Whited, DNP, APRN, CPNP-PC

University of Arkansas for Medical Sciences College of Nursing, 4301 West Markham Street, Slot 529, Little Rock, AR 72205, USA

Keywords

• Fever • Neonates • Infants • Children • Pediatrics • Fever of unknown origin
• Pyrexia • Pyrexia of unknown origin

Key points

• The length of time fever occurs before intervention will vary based on age range.
• The potential cause of fever of unknown origin can be broad.
• Guidelines delineate laboratory and radiology workup based on age range.
• High-risk conditions must be considered and presumptively treated especially in infants and younger children.

Fever is a common symptom in pediatric patients and is defined as a rectal temperature of 38°C or greater [1,2]. Most causes of fever are short in duration and commonly caused by viral illnesses [3]. Occasionally, fever is caused by a bacterial infection, which can typically be diagnosed with a history and physical and then treated with an antibiotic. Sometimes, when the source of the fever cannot be identified or when the fever lasts more than 1 week without an identified source, further workup is required because most typical infections should have resolved within this time frame [1,4,5]. Less than 1% of children with fever will present with a serious infection in a primary care office, and this increases to 25% in an emergency department [6].

PATHOPHYSIOLOGY

Fever of unknown origin (FUO) was first defined in 1961 as a temperature greater than 38.3°C that persists for more than 3 weeks with a failure to reach

*Corresponding author. E-mail address: edavis2@uams.edu

https://doi.org/10.1016/j.yfpn.2022.11.013
2589-420X/23/© 2022 Elsevier Inc. All rights reserved.

a diagnosis after 1 week of inpatient investigation [1,7]. Since that time, many definitions have occurred to include outpatient and inpatient workup and varying time durations. Due to no standard definition for FUO in pediatrics, the incidence and prevalence is unclear [4,7]. The accepted definition, at this time, is fever lasting 7 to 21 days with a workup of 1 week or less [6,8]. There are many causes of FUO including infections, connective tissue disorders, and malignancies [9] (Table 1). Current data reveal 90% of cases have an identified cause with 50% as infectious, 10% to 20% as collagen-vascular, and 10% as oncology [4,6] (see Table 1).

EVALUATION

Fever evaluation includes a thorough history and physical examination to investigate potential causes or disease processes [4,6]. Some key findings include confirmation of the duration and pattern of fever as well as the age and underlying risk factors of the patient [4]. The history of the patient provides clues to potential causes and underlying risk of severe illness. For example, children aged younger than 6 years are more likely to have a respiratory infection, genitourinary infection, localized infection, and juvenile rheumatoid arthritis (JRA). Additional data to collect would include potential contacts with an infectious person, exposure to wild animals, travel history, chronic disease history, and medication history [6]. The remainder of the history and physical examination will be guided by potential differential diagnoses.

The FUO diagnostic workup needs to be completed in stages and based off the history and physical examination findings. Each stage of workup will become more invasive as more data are collected and analyzed by the provider. How quickly the provider proceeds through each state of testing will depend on how ill the patient seems to be at presentation [4]. Examination is typically based on the patient presentation, provider experience, geography, symptoms, exposures, and available testing [4]. Physical examination should always include obtaining temperature, heart rate, and respiratory rate as well as a head-to-toe physical examination to identify potential sources for the fever. Following the physical examination, the patient should undergo a laboratory workup in a staged fashion.

The initial laboratory work includes a complete blood count with differential (CBC), C-reactive protein (CRP), and blood culture, at a minimum. Additional laboratory evaluation would be based on the patient's history but could include a CBC, blood culture, CRP, erythrosedimentation rate, procalcitonin, liver enzymes, renal function tests, lactate dehydrogenase, urinalysis (UA), urine culture (UCX), and chest radiograph. Further laboratory and radiology workup include tuberculin skin test, cytomegalovirus (CMV) antibodies, Epstein-Barr virus (EBV) antibodies, *Toxoplasma gondii* Immunoglobulin M (IgM) antibodies, transthoracic echocardiogram, and abdominal-pelvic ultrasound [1]. If any abnormalities are present on the initial workup, some considerations for other laboratory and radiology studies include chest-abdomen-pelvis computed tomography,

Table 1
Common causes of fever of unknown origin

Bacterial Infection	Viral Infection	Other Infections	Oncology	Autoimmune	Noninfections
Abscess	Adenovirus	Blastomycosis	Leukemia	Inflammatory Bowel disease	Diabetes Insipidus
Bartonella	Arbovirus	Cryptosporidium	Lymphoma	Hyperthyroidism	Drug fever
Brucellosis	CMV	Ehrlichiosis	Langerhans cell histiocytosis	JIA	Factitious fever
E coli	Enterovirus	Histoplasmosis	Neuroblastoma	Kawasaki disease	Familial dysautonomia
Mastoiditis	EBV	Malaria		Sarcoidosis	Periodic fever syndromes
Mycoplasma	Hepatitis	Q fever		SLE	Pancreatitis
Osteomyelitis	HSV	Rocky Mountain spotted fever		Subacute thyroiditis	Serum sickness
Pyelonephritis	HIV	Toxoplasmosis			Cyclic neutropenia
GBS					
Salmonellosis					
Tuberculosis					
Nontuberculous Mycobacterium					

(Data from Antoon JW, Potisek NM, Lohr JA. Pediatric Fever of Unknown Origin. Pediatr Rev. 2015;36(9):380-391. https://doi.org/10.1542/pir.36-9-380)

paranasal sinuses radiography or tomography, radionuclide scan, bone marrow aspirate, and transesophageal echocardiography depending on the underlying suspected cause of the fever. Finally, to workup potential rheumatologic, infectious, and other rare causes the provider would consider protein electrophoresis; antinuclear antibodies; anti-dsDNA antibodies; antineutrophil cytoplasmic antibodies; complement C3 and C4; angiotension-converting enzyme; specific bacterial, viral, spirochetes, rickettsia, parasites, and fungi; and thyroid stimulating hormone (TSH) and T4 [1,7]. Empiric treatment of the fever with antibiotics and other therapies should be judicious and based on the provider's judgment in relation to the age of the child, risk factors, and severity of the illness [4]. The workup of neonates is very different than the workup of older children with FUO. Refer to Table 1 for potential differential diagnoses.

Neonates (8–21 Days)

All febrile neonates should be hospitalized with extensive evaluation and empiric antibiotic treatment. Due to prenatal group beta strep (GBS) screening, the incidence of bacteremia with this organism has significantly decreased but GBS remains the leading cause of meningitis in this age group. *Escherichia coli* is the most cause organism leading to bacteremia in neonates [1,7]. Listeria remains a concern worldwide but is less common in the United States secondary to food safety improvements.

With a well-appearing, febrile, without source of infection neonate ages 8 to 21 days old, the provider will need to obtain a UA with UCX, blood culture, and perform a lumbar puncture (LP) at a minimum [10]. The provider can also consider obtaining inflammatory markers. If the provider is suspicious of prenatal or antenatal transmission of herpes simplex virus (HSV), samples need to be sent for HSV studies [10]. Parental antibiotics with or without acyclovir need to be initiated and the neonate needs to be admitted to the hospital for close observation [10]. If all culture results and HSV studies are negative at 24 to 36 hours, antimicrobials can be discontinued and the patient can be discharged to go home [10]. With any positive culture or studies, the infection needs to be treated appropriately based on the culture and sensitivities [10]. With a urinary tract infection (UTI) or no identified focus, an infant should be started on ampicillin IV or intramuscular (IM) 150 mg/kg divided every 8 hours and either ceftazidime IV or IM 150 mg/kg divided every 8 hours or gentamicin IV or IM 4 mg/kg every 24 hours [10]. With bacterial meningitis, the infant should be started on ampicillin IV or IM 150 mg/kg divided every 8 hours and ceftazidime IV or IM 150 mg/kg divided every 8 hours [10] (Fig. 1).

For well-appearing, febrile, 22 to 28-day-old neonates, the provider should obtain an UA, blood culture, and inflammatory markers [10]. If the UA is concerning, the provider should send a UCX. If the inflammatory makers are abnormal, the provider should complete an LP and start on parental antibiotics [10]. If the inflammatory markers are normal, the provider can choose to wait to perform an LP based on the remainder of the workup [10]. Based on the LP

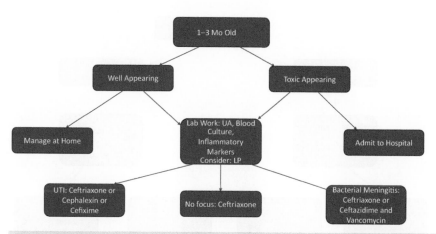

Fig. 1. Management of fever in 1 to 3-month-old infants. (*Data from* Pantell RH, Roberts KB, Adams WG, et al. Evaluation and Management of Well-Appearing Febrile Infants 8 to 60 Days Old [published correction appears in Pediatrics. 2021 Nov;148(5):]. Pediatrics. 2021;148(2):e2021052228.doi:10.1542/peds.2021-052228)

results, the provider can decide rather to admit for parental antibiotics or observe the patient closely at home with frequent follow-up [10]. With a UTI or no identified focus, the infant should be started on ceftriaxone IV or IM 50 mg/kg every 24 hours [10]. With bacterial meningitis, the infant should on ampicillin IV or IM 150 mg/kg divided every 8 hours and ceftazidime IV or IM 150 mg/kg divided every 8 hours [10] (Fig. 2).

Infants 1 to 3 Months old

Most infants in this age group will likely have a viral illness. Ill-appearing infants do need to be admitted and started on empiric antibiotics. Infants in this age group can be managed with IM ceftriaxone with pending blood, urine, and cerebral spinal fluid (CSF) cultures [1,7].

All well-appearing, febrile infants between 29 and 60 days should have a UA, blood culture, and inflammatory markers drawn [10]. With abnormal inflammatory markers, the provider should consider a UA and UCX with consideration of a LP [10]. Infants in this age group can be managed either at home or in the hospital with appropriate antibiotic coverage as needed [10]. With normal inflammatory markers, the infants can be managed at home with close follow-up [10]. With a UTI, the infant should be started on ceftriaxone IV or IM 50 mg/kg every 24 hours or cephalexin PO 50 to 100 mg/kg divided every 6 hours or cefixime PO 8 mg/kg daily [10]. With no identified focus, the infant should be started on ceftriaxone IV or IM 50 mg/kg every 24 hours [10]. With bacterial meningitis, the infant should be started on ceftriaxone IV 100 mg/kg divided every 12 to 24 hours or ceftazidime IV 150 mg/kg divided every 8 hours and vancomycin IV 60 mg/kg divided every 8 hours [10] (Table 2).

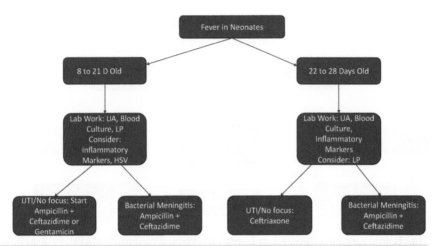

Fig. 2. Management of fever in neonates. (*Data from* Pantell RH, Roberts KB, Adams WG, et al. Evaluation and Management of Well-Appearing Febrile Infants 8 to 60 Days Old [published correction appears in Pediatrics. 2021 Nov;148(5):]. Pediatrics. 2021;148(2):e2021052228. https://doi.org/10.1542/peds.2021-052228)

Infants and toddlers 3 Months to 3 Years of age

Most children in this age group will likely have a viral illness. Nontoxic appearing children can be managed outpatient. Children with a temperature greater than 39°C should have a laboratory investigation performed with the basic workup and then consider additional items based on initial laboratory and radiology findings. Toxic appearing children need to be admitted and started on empiric antibiotics. Children who are well-appearing should have a CBC, BMP, LFT, UA, and radiologic examinations as indicated [4]. Toxic appearing children should have a CBC, BMP, LFTs, UA, cultures, and CSF, CRP, and radiologic examinations as indicated [4]. If this initial workup does identify the source of the fever, further workup can be completed based on suspicion of the provider [4].

Children aged older than 3 Years

Children aged older than 3 years to adulthood often have a more focused workup such as a CBC, BMP, LFTs, and UA with the remainder of laboratory and radiologic examinations based on suspected diagnoses [11]. Infectious causes remain the primary cause in this age group with rheumatologic and malignancy remaining important considerations [12]. Most children can be managed on an outpatient basis with judicious use of antimicrobials based on underlying risk factors and condition of the child. Items such as travel outside the United States, sexually transmitted infections and inflammatory diseases must be considered in older children and adolescents [13,14]. If the child seems toxic or has significant risk factors for bacteremia, the provider may

Table 2
Antibiotics used for fever of unknown origin

Antibiotic	Route	Dose	Susceptible organisms	Cautions	Monitoring
Ampicillin	IV or IM	Neonates: 150 mg/kg/d divided every 8 h; Infants and children: 100–400 mg/kg/d divided every 4–6 h	Group B strep, Staphylococcus, Shigella, Salmonella, Klebsiella	Hypersensitivity to drug or class, renal impairment, asthma, HIV infection, abx-associated colitis	Cr at baseline and then if prolonged therapy: Cr, CBC, LFTs
Ceftazidime	IV or IM	150 mg/kg/d divided every 8 h	Gram-negative organisms: Citrobacter, Enterobacter, Klebsiella, Proteus, Serratia, E coli, Hemophilus influenzae, Neisseria, Pseudomonas, and some gram-positive bacteria	Hypersensitivity, renal impairment, abx-associate colitis	Cr at baseline, If prolonged therapy, Cr, CBC, and LFTs
Gentamycin	IV	Neonates: 2.5–4.5 mg (depending on gestation) IV or IM every 24 h 3mo to 2y: 9.5 mg/kg/dose IV q 24 h 2–8 y: 8.5 mg/kg/dose IV q 24 h 8y and older: 7 mg/kg/dose IV q 24 h	Primarily gram-negative- Pseudomonas, Proteus, E coli, Klebsiella, Enterobacter, Serratia, and some gram-positive Staphylococcus	Nephrotoxicity and ototoxicity	Drug levels (trough and peaks), BUN/Cr, UA, audiometry for high risk/hearing impairment concern
Ceftriaxone	IV or IM	50-100mg/kg/day divided q 12-24 hours (max 4 g/24 h)	Broad spectrum 3rd generation, broader and stronger gram-negative coverage than 1st or 2nd gen. Good coverage against multi-drug resistant Enterobateriaceae	Hypersensitivity to drug class or PCN, renal impairment, hepatic impairment, abx-associated colitis	Cr at baseline, prolonged therapy Cr, CBC, LFTs

(Data from Antoon JW, Potisek NM, Lohr JA. Pediatric Fever of Unknown Origin. Pediatr Rev. 2015;36(9):380-391. https://doi.org/10.1542/pir.36-9-380)

want to consider empiric therapy. All children should have careful history, physical, and evaluation by a provider when presenting with FUO.

Implications for advanced practice registered nurses

FUO remains a challenging diagnosis for providers and patients, which requires a careful workup and often thorough evaluation. Young children and infants with this puzzling fever often have prolonged hospitalizations and high-evaluation costs [7]. Although older children and adolescents can be managed on an outpatient basis, younger children, infants, and neonates often require hospitalization and empiric therapy to avoid the devastating consequences of unidentified meningitis and bacteremia [11]. With careful evaluation and a strong diagnostic process, most FUO can have the source identified by the provider and treated appropriately [11,14].

CLINICS CARE POINTS

- FUO is a challenging diagnosis.
- It takes a thorough history and physical along with laboratory and radiology resources as indicated.
- Your management and treatment depends on age and possible diagnosis.

DISCLOSURES

Teresa Whited gets paid speaker fees for NAPNAP primary care review course.

References

[1] Rigante D, Esposito S. A roadmap for fever of unknown origin in children. Int J Immunopathology Pharmacol 2013;26(2):315–26.

[2] Szymanski AM, Clifford H, Ronis T. Fever of unknown origin: a retrospective review of pediatric patients from an urban, Tertiary Care Center in Washington, DC. World J Pediatr 2019;16(2):177–84.

[3] Hu B, Chen T-M, Liu S-P, et al. Fever of unknown origin (FUO) in children: a single-centre experience from Beijing, China. BMJ Open 2022;12:e049840.

[4] Antoon JW, Potisek NM, Lohr JA. Pediatric fever of unknown origin. Pediatr Rev 2015;36(9):380–91.

[5] Chow A, Robinson JL. Fever of unknown origin in children: a systematic review. World J Pediatr 2010;7(1):5–10.

[6] Barbi E, Marzuillo P, Neri E, et al. Fever in children: pearls and pitfalls. Children 2017;4(81):1–19.

[7] Antoon JW, Peritz DC, Parsons MR, et al. Etiology and resource use of fever of unknown origin in hospitalized children. Hosp Pediatr 2018;8(3):135–40.

[8] Hu L, Shi Q, Shi M, et al. Diagnostic value of PCT and CRP for detecting serious bacterial infections in patients with fever of unknown origin: A systemic review and meta-analysis. Appl Immunohistochem Mo Morhol 2017;25(8):e61–9.

[9] Chusid MJ. Fever of Unknown Origin in Childhood. Pediatr Clin North Am 2016;64(1):205–30.

[10] Pantell RH, Roberts KB, Adams WG, et al. Clinical practice guideline: Evaluation and management of well-appearing febrile infants 8 to 60 days old. Pediatrics 2021;148(2); https://doi.org/10.1542/peds.2021-052228.

[11] Wright W, Auwaerter P. Fever and fever of unknown origin: Review, recent advances, and lingering dogma. Open Forum Infect Dis 2020;1–11; https://doi.org/10.1093/ofid/ofaa132.

[12] M. Ward, Fever in infants and children: Pathophysiology and management. UpToDate Available at: https://www.uptodate.com/contents/fever-in-infants-and-children-pathophysiology-and-management. Accessed August 30, 2022.

[13] D. Palazzi, Fever of unknown origin in children: Evaluation. UpToDate Available at: https://www.uptodate.com/contents/fever-of-unknown-origin-in-children-evaluation?search=fever%20of%20unknown%20origin%20in%20children:%20evaluation&source=search_result&selectedTitle=1~73&usage_type=default&display_rank=1. Accessed August 30, 2022.

[14] Attard L, Tadolini M, DeRose D, et al. Overview of fever of unknown origin in adult and paediatric patients. Clin Exp Rheumatol 2018;36(Suppl.110):S10–24.

Advances in Family Practice Nursing 5 (2023) 217–227

ADVANCES IN FAMILY PRACTICE NURSING

Pediatric Asthma for the Primary Care Provider

Sarah Ann Keil Heinonen, DNP, APRN, CPNP-AC/PC[a],*,
Amanda C. Filippelli, MPH, MSN, APRN, PPCNP-BC, AE-C[b],
Nancy Banasiak, DNP, PPCNP-BC, APRN[c]

[a]Division of Pediatric Pulmonology & Sleep Medicine, Children's Hospital Los Angeles, 4650 Sunset Boulevard, Mailstop #83, Los Angeles, CA 90027, USA; [b]Pulmonary Specialty Clinic, Connecticut Children's Medical Center, Hartford, CT, USA; [c]Yale University School of Nursing, Room 22306, 400 West Campus Drive, Orange, CT 06477, USA

Keywords
- Asthma • Pediatrics • Primary care • SMART therapy • Wheeze

Key points
- Asthma remains a significant, complex, and incurable pediatric chronic disease.
- Primary care providers are key collaborators in the multidisciplinary approach to pediatric asthma diagnosis and management.
- Identification of asthma triggers can be challenging as childhood viral infections are often the most common trigger contributing to acute asthma symptoms and exacerbations.
- Single maintenance and reliever therapy is a good option for persistent asthma as a single inhaler for both daily maintenance and reliever therapies.
- Primary care providers' capacity for identifying key indicators for asthma specialist referral is essential in the care of high-risk patients.

INTRODUCTION

In the United States, asthma is one of the most common pediatric chronic diseases affecting 5.8% (~4.2 million) of children under the age of 18 years [1]. The burden of asthma disproportionally affects non-Hispanic Black and children of Puerto Rican descent in addition to children living in low-income households at higher rates [2]. Asthma is a complex disease characterized by airway hyperresponsiveness, inflammation, and obstruction causing symptoms

*Corresponding author. E-mail address: sheinonen@chla.usc.edu

https://doi.org/10.1016/j.yfpn.2022.11.014
2589-420X/23/© 2022 Elsevier Inc. All rights reserved.

including wheezing, coughing, chest tightness, and shortness of breath [3]. The goals of management are improving asthma control, decreasing exacerbations, improving quality of life, maintaining optimal lung function, and decreasing emergency department visits as well as hospitalizations [4]. Poorly controlled asthma is the leading cause of absenteeism from school and caregiver-missed workdays. The annual cost of asthma care including both direct and indirect costs are estimated at $81.9 billion [5]. In recent years, asthma control improvement has been targeted through published guidelines, education, appropriate medication, referrals to specialists, asthma action plans, and improving access to health care providers [6]. The purpose of this review article is to provide an overview of pediatric asthma, diagnosis, and the most current guideline-based management for the primary care provider.

PATHOPHYSIOLOGY

Asthma is a complex, immune-mediated, inflammatory disease involving the infiltration of inflammatory cells, including neutrophils, eosinophils, and lymphocytes into the airway, with activation of mast cells, and damage to the epithelial cells. These inflammatory responses lead to the classic features of airway swelling, increased mucus production, and bronchial muscle dysfunction (smooth muscle constriction), which produce airway flow limitation (airway narrowing) and subsequent asthma symptoms typically in response to an environmental trigger, often in association with a viral upper airway infection. Numerous inflammatory pathways to airway swelling result in the many clinical phenotypes of pediatric asthma. Airway 'remodeling' is a term that refers to persistent changes in the airway structure, which can occur, ultimately leading to fibrosis, mucus hypersecretion, epithelial cell injury, smooth muscle hypertrophy, and angiogenesis [7–9].

DIAGNOSIS

Diagnosing asthma can be challenging and should be suspected in patients who present with cough, recurring wheezing, shortness of breath, and chest tightness. To diagnosis asthma, a comprehensive medical history, physical examination, spirometry in children 5 and older, and additional studies to exclude alternative diagnoses (Box 1) should be performed [10]. A detailed history should focus on the presence of recurrent cough, wheezing, shortness of breath, and chest tightness which may be triggered by viruses, allergens, exercise, mold, smoke, change in weather, and emotions [6]. Symptoms tend to be worse at night and early mornings, when exposed to triggers and certain medications. Improvement in wheezing and coughing after treatment with a short-acting beta agonist (SABA) or steroids may indicate asthma [5]. A family history of atopy diseases (*Triad: asthma, allergies, and eczema*) is also important to elicit. The physical examination should focus on the respiratory system, especially during an exacerbation that may reveal wheezing, decreased breath sounds, and prolonged expiratory phase [5]. In addition, examination of the nose, throat, eyes, and skin may reveal nasal congestion or clear rhinorrhea, allergic

Box 1: Differential diagnoses for wheezing-children [6]

Common causes

- Allergies (seasonal or otherwise)
- Asthma or reactive airway disease
- Gastroesophageal reflux disease (GER)
- Infections
- Bronchiolitis
- Bronchitis
- Pneumonia
- Upper respiratory infection (URI)
- Obstructive sleep apnea (OSA)

Uncommon causes

- Bronchopulmonary dysplasia (BPD)
- Foreign body aspiration

Rare causes

- Bronchiolitis obliterans
- Congenital vascular abnormalities
- Congestive heart failure
- Cystic fibrosis
- Immunodeficiency diseases
- Mediastinal masses
- Primary ciliary dyskinesia
- Tracheobronchial anomalies
- Tumor or malignancy
- Vocal cord dysfunction

shiners, enlarged turbinate's, and eczema [5]. In children younger than 4 years, a clinical diagnosis is based on a detailed medical history, a full physical examination, and a trial of therapy. In addition, Global Initiative for Asthma recommends confirmation of asthma diagnosis with lung function testing, whenever possible, before commencing long-term treatment; specifically spirometry-based testing if available [11]. Lung function testing is not only used for diagnostic confirmation but for monitoring purposes with spirometry recommended beginning between ages 5 and 7 years. At this age, children have the lung capacity and control to perform the test properly [12]. This testing confirms the presence of airway obstruction and determines the partially reversibility with albuterol (12% improvement in FEV1) [9]. Fractional exhaled nitric oxide (FeNO) which measures nitric oxide may be helpful in determining inflammation in the airways. Other tests to rule out differential diagnoses include chest x-ray, chest, or sinus computerized tomography (CT), allergy testing, sputum for eosinophil levels, evaluation for gastroesophageal reflux, bronchoscopy, sweat test, and provocation tests [13].

DIFFERENTIAL DIAGNOSES

When assessing a pediatric patient for asthma, it is important to be aware of other possible causes for respiratory symptoms. When a respiratory symptom does not respond or only partially responds to asthma therapy, it is vital to work a patient up for other causes that may include other referrals or courses of treatment. The age of the child is an important consideration and influences the differential diagnoses particularly when ruling out congenital airway abnormalities that could be the cause for chronic respiratory symptoms. Table 1 provides differential diagnoses for children with wheezing. In addition, there are differential diagnoses based on signs and symptoms as well as identified diagnostics for asthma as shown in Table 1.

ASTHMA CLASSIFICATIONS

Asthma severity classifications (Box 2) are based on an initial visit for a patient with asthma who is not currently taking long-term medications. Asthma severity can change over time depending on control and the various individual triggers for asthma symptoms [6]. Classification of a patient's disease is understood to be based on the current state of impairment as well as future risk. Future risk is categorized by the frequency of oral systemic corticosteroid use [6]. Impairment is determined by patient symptoms and the objective measurement of lung function. Current guidelines for asthma severity categorization recommend that assessment of daytime symptoms, nighttime awakenings, frequency of SABA use for symptom relief, as well as identified interference with normal daily activities be noted [6]. In addition, spirometry is recommended as a component of the determination of current impairment [6]. Determination of disease-severity category should guide initial treatment.

ASTHMA MANAGEMENT

Asthma management should be approached with a stepwise focus to best support goals of reducing symptom frequency and improve asthma control [5]. Once the asthma disease-severity category has been determined, the next steps for consideration in management should be both identification and avoidance of triggers. Avoiding triggers can be a challenging task given that childhood viral infections are often the most common trigger contributing to acute asthma symptoms and exacerbations [5].

Once the diagnosis of asthma has been determined it is important to estimate the patient's level of severity to determine the intensity of their therapy [5]. The current recommendations from the 2020 Focused Updates to the Asthma Management Guidelines identify scheduled, daily inhaled corticosteroid (ICS) treatment as being the preferred pharmacologic controller therapy for persistent asthma that typically varies in level (mild, moderate, or severe) for individuals

Table 1
Differential diagnosis—characteristics of wheezing [6]

Associated symptoms	Possible diagnosis	Additional testing
Feeding, coughing, or vomiting	Gastroesophageal reflux disease (GER/D)	24-h pH monitoring barium swallow
Position changes	Tracheomalacia; anomalies of the great vessels	Angiography Bronchoscopy CT chest radiography or MRI Echocardiography
Auscultatory crackles, and fever	Pneumonia	Chest radiography
Episodic pattern, cough; patient responds to bronchodilators	Asthma	Allergy testing Pulmonary function testing Trial of albuterol (Proventil)
Exacerbated by neck flexion; relieved by neck hyperextension	Vascular ring	Angiography Barium swallow Bronchoscopy Chest radiography CT or MRI
Heart murmurs or cardiomegaly, cyanosis without respiratory distress	Cardiac disease	Angiography Chest radiography Echocardiography
History of recurrent respiratory illnesses; failure to thrive	Cystic fibrosis, primary ciliary dyskinesia, or immunodeficiency	Ciliary function testing Immunoglobulin levels Sweat chloride testing
Seasonal pattern to occurrence, nasal flaring, intercostal retractions	Bronchiolitis (RSV), croup, and allergies	Chest radiography
Stridor with drooling	Epiglottitis	Neck radiography
Sudden onset of wheezing and choking	Foreign body aspiration	Bronchoscopy

of all ages [14]. Starting with low-dose ICS for mild persistent asthma, although leukotriene modifiers may also be an acceptable option [5]. These recommendations are organized by severity, ages (0 to 4 years/> 12 years), and typically response to treatments with or without a short or long-acting beta2-agonist (SABA/LABA) [14].

Children *ages 0 to 4 years* with recurrent wheezing, using a short (7 to 10 day) course of daily ICS with as-needed inhaled short-acting beta2-agonist (SABA) for quick-relief therapy is recommended starting at the onset of a respiratory tract infection. In mild to moderate persistent asthma (STEP 2) current recommendations are for a daily low-dose ICS and as-needed SABA. Individuals with moderate-to-severe persistent asthma (STEP 3) Daily low-dose ICS-LABA and PRN SABA or Daily low-dose ICS + montelukast,* or daily medium-dose ICS, and PRN SABA with progression to STEP 4 with poor control indicating a

Box 2: Asthma severity classification guidelines [6,17]

Classifications: (1) intermittent, (2) mild persistent, (3) moderate persistent, (4) and severe persistent.

*Asthma Severity is divided into three charts to classify age groups (0 to 4 y, 5 to 11 y, and 12 y and older).

Intermittent asthma is characterized as follows:

- Symptoms of cough, wheezing, chest tightness, or difficulty breathing less than twice a week
- Flare-ups are brief, but intensity may vary
- Nighttime symptoms less than twice a month
- No symptoms between flare-ups
- Lung function test FEV 1 is 80% or more above normal values
- Peak flow has less than 20% variability am-to-am or am-to-pm, day-to-day

Mild persistent asthma is characterized as follows:

- Symptoms of cough, wheezing, chest tightness, or difficulty breathing three to six times a week
- Flare-ups may affect activity level
- Nighttime symptoms three to four times a month
- Lung function test FEV 1 is 80% or more above normal values
- Peak flow has less than 20% to 30% variability

Moderate persistent asthma is characterized as follows:

- Symptoms of cough, wheezing, chest tightness, or difficulty breathing daily
- Flare-ups may affect activity level
- Nighttime symptoms 5 or more times a month
- Lung function test FEV 1 is more than 60% but less than 80% of normal values
- Peak flow has more than 30% variability

Severe persistent asthma is characterized as follows:

- Symptoms of cough, wheezing, chest tightness, or difficulty breathing that are continual
- Frequent nighttime symptoms
- Lung function test FEV 1 is 60% or less of normal values
- Peak flow has more than 30% variability

Daily medium-dose ICS-LABA and PRN SABA with STEP 5; a Daily high-dose ICS-LABA and PRN SABA and for STEP 6 the addition of oral systemic corticosteroids [14].

Ages *5 to 11 years* preferred treatment recommendations include as-needed SABA for intermittent asthma. Similar to other age groups, mild persistent asthma (STEP 2) recommendations are for a daily low-dose ICS with an as-

Box 3: Important components of asthma control

Important components in successful asthma control include

1. Patient/family education regarding disease and disease management
2. Individualized asthma action plans
3. Education on asthma medications use
4. Purpose of controller and reliever medications
5. Appropriate use of their inhaler devices with spacers (demonstrations)
6. Recognition and management of exacerbations.
7. Reinforce education with each visit.

needed SABA [14]. STEP 3 for this age group indicates a daily and prn combination low-dose ICS-LABA with STEP 4 indication increase to a daily and prn combination medium-dose ICS-LABA progressing if uncontrolled to STEP 5, daily high-dose ICS-LABA and PRN SABA with STEP 6 adding the mainstay for all groups of oral systemic corticosteroids [14].

Recommendations for preferred treatment for children *ages 12 years and older* with intermittent Asthma is as needed SABA. Mild persistent asthma (STEP 2) recommendations for a daily low-dose ICS and as-needed SABA or as-needed concomitant ICS and SABA, for quick-relief therapy. Intermittent therapy may be initiated at home with regular follow-up [14]. For individuals with moderate-to-severe persistent asthma already taking low (STEP 3)- or medium (STEP 4) -dose ICS, the preferred treatment is a single inhaler with ICS-formoterol (long-acting beta2-agonist–LABA) (referred to as single maintenance and reliever therapy, or "SMART") used both daily and as needed [14]. STEP 5 in this age group (>12 years) recommends medium- or high-dose ICS-LABA + long-acting muscarinic antagonist (LAMA) and as-needed SABA with STEP 6 adding oral systemic corticosteroids [14].

Therapy is subsequently stepped-up based on symptoms in an effort to reach control (Boxes 3 and 4). Scheduled routine follow-up visits should initially occur every 2 to 9 weeks to reassess asthma control with the option for patients to be seen earlier as needed and extended once control is achieved [5,14]. Step-down therapy is not considered until complete asthma control (see Boxes 3 and

Box 4: Goals of asthma control/treatment

1. Achieve symptoms free days/nights.
2. Unlimited exercise tolerance (as appropriate for age).
3. No school or day care absences due to asthma exacerbations.
4. Sleeping through the night without coughing.
5. Normal chest auscultation.
6. Normal pulmonary function testing, for those old enough to perform the test.

4) has been achieved for >3 months and then is done conversely of the increase [14].

SINGLE MAINTENANCE AND RELIEVER THERAPY

In 2000, the safety and efficacy of ICS for maintenance use in children with mild–moderate persistent asthma was established [15], opening the door for recommended use of *Single Maintenance And Reliever Therapy* (SMART) with the Food and Drug Administration (FDA) approved combination maintenance therapy Advair-Diskus for patients not controlled on ICS alone [16]. However, SMART recommendations do not include fluticasone propionate-salmeterol combination products (Advair, AirDuo and/or generic equivalents) as they have slower onset of action, limited interval increase capacity, and increased risk of prolonged QTc interval [13].

SMART is recommended as a single inhaler for both daily maintenance and reliever therapies [14–16] for ages 4 to 11 years and >12 years related to steps 3+ [16]. There have been some cases for consideration for the long-term use in clinical practice of ICS and formoterol as needed for step 1, with transition to titrated low-to-medium dose SMART for steps 2 to 4 [14]. Important point regarding SMART, formoterol has a rapid onset of action (similar to Albuterol) and an added advantage of a longer duration of action [17,18]. Therefore, use of formoterol provides rapid symptom relief with a longer duration of action than that of an SABA; when coupled with the ICS there is an added benefit of earlier anti-inflammatory exposure leading to symptom relief and reduction in exacerbation events [19].

Exacerbations

Acute viral respiratory infections remain the most common cause of asthma exacerbations [5] in children. Exacerbations are classified as mild, moderate, severe, or life-threatening depending on the degree of the severity of signs and symptoms (wheeze, dyspnea, mental status, respiratory rate, peak expiratory flow (PEF), and response to treatment [6]. The main initial therapies in the outpatient primary care setting for asthma exacerbations include repetitive administration of short-acting inhaled bronchodilators via a metered dose inhaler (MDI) or nebulization, early introduction of systemic corticosteroids and controlled flow oxygen supplementation [3,5,6,14]. Studies suggest that the addition of ipratropium bromide with albuterol as a combination nebulization has decreased hospitalization rates [17]. If symptoms worsen, a referral to the emergency department is indicated.

Severe cases

Severe or poorly controlled asthma in children occurs in approximately 2% to 5% of the pediatric asthma population [5]. A variety of factors play a role in this severity and need to be considered by the provider caring for these patients. Often children with asthma may have social determinants that contribute to poor control from nonadherence, lack of access to care or medications, improper medication delivery techniques, poor understanding of asthma action plans or ongoing environmental triggers (smoking and mold pets) [5]. Additional etiologies for poor control can be comorbidities, incorrect diagnoses, or confounding diagnoses. Confounding diagnoses to consider would be those that impact the respiratory system (airway abnormalities, bacterial infections, and obesity) [5].

WHEN TO REFER

Asthma is a complex disease, influenced by various triggers including seasonal changes and individual social factors. Although there are many guidelines and tools designed to manage pediatric asthma in primary care, there are also times when it may be beneficial for a patient to see a pulmonary specialist.

The Expert Panel of the National Heart, Lung, and Blood Institute (the Panel) have specified various scenarios that would warrant referral to an asthma specialist [6]. For example, if a patient has a life-threatening asthma exacerbation, if a patient has required more than two bursts of oral steroids in the past year or had an exacerbation requiring hospitalization, it would be beneficial to see a specialist to work on a treatment plan that prevents the frequency, severity, and duration of illness [6]. Furthermore, patients who aren't meeting the goals of therapy after 3 to 6 months or if there is suspicion that a patient is not responsive to therapy, they may need a specialist to take a more comprehensive approach to investigating why the plan isn't working. Similarly, there may be patients who need additional education to assist with the challenges associated with therapy and how to improve adherence. If patients < 4 years of age are requiring step 3 or 4 level care, additional assistance on treatment plan management with a specialist may be beneficial [6].

Asthma specialists are particularly helpful if asthma has an atypical presentation or comorbidities are suspected as inhibitors to symptom management. Moreover, if history suggests an occupational or environmental cause is exacerbating symptoms, it may be worth consulting with a specialist to confirm history and assist with overall collaborative management. The Panel recommends referral for immunotherapy or additional testing is required that is not offered in the primary care office. These tests include allergy skin testing, rhinoscopy, complete pulmonary function testing, provocative challenge, and bronchoscopy [6].

Overall, if the asthma diagnosis is complex, there is incomplete resolution of symptoms or the patient is at a higher risk of severe exacerbations, an asthma specialist referral should be considered. Primary care providers are critical in assessing patients at the onset of symptoms and although much of pediatric asthma can be managed effectively in the primary care setting, some patients are good candidates for care from an asthma specialist. This is important to help these children to achieve the best clinical outcomes and quality of life.

SUMMARY

Pediatric asthma remains a complex and challenging problem with considerable effects on quality of life, demands on health resources, and remains an economic burden in spite of improved medical understanding and treatment advances [5]. Although typical asthma is often easily identified, atypical presentations can make it challenging to identify asthma as the cause of the child's symptoms. Identification of disease severity is key to the management approach. SMART is a good option for treating many children ages 4 to 11 years and >12 years with known mild-moderate persistent asthma. Overall prognosis for childhood asthma is good; however, there are subsets of the pediatric asthma population that are difficult to control and would benefit from a pulmonary specialist referral.

IMPLICATIONS FOR ADVANCED PRACTICE PROVIDERS
Asthma remains a statistically significant and complex, chronic disease in pediatrics, which if not controlled can lead to severe respiratory failure and even death. Poor medication adherence and trigger exposure are well-known risk factors for increased morbidity and mortality associated with the diagnosis of asthma. Advanced practice providers (APPs) are well situated and essential to address issues and provide education to patients with a diagnosis of asthma and their caregivers. APPs are key members of the interprofessional team and often provide the continuity of care for pediatric asthma patients educating and engaging patients and caregivers in both understanding the disease and adhering to the appropriate medication regime, avoiding asthma triggers, and using appropriate MDI use to manage symptoms. In these ways, the APP helps the pediatric patient and family achieve asthma control through the use of an asthma action plan and mutual goal setting.

CLINICS CARE POINTS

- Annual influenza vaccinations starting at 6 months of age to reduce respiratory illnesses/triggers should be encouraged.
- Treatment with low-dose inhaled corticosteroid (ICS) for most patients with asthma, even those with infrequent symptoms reduces the risk of serious exacerbations.
- Height should be checked annually as poorly controlled asthma can impact growth velocity (ICS effects on growth are not progressive or cumulative).

DISCLOSURE
The authors have nothing to disclose.

References
[1] Centers for Disease Control and Prevention (CDC). Asthma. Available at: https://www.cdc.gov/asthma/most_recent_national_asthma_data.htm. Accessed June 13, 2022.

[2] Zahran HS, Bailey CM, Damon SA, et al. Vital signs: asthma in children-United States, 2001-2016. MMWR 2018;67(5):149–55.

[3] Abellard A, Pappalardo AA. Overview of severe asthma, with emphasis on pediatric patients: a review for practitioners. J Investig Med 2021;69(7):1297–309.

[4] Rosman Y, Gabay L, Landau T, et al. Childhood asthma - the effect of asthma specialist intervention on asthma control: a retrospective review. J Asthma Allergy 2021;14:1367–73.

[5] Hoch HE, Houin PR, Stillwell PC. Asthma in children: a brief review for primary care providers. Pediatr Ann 2019;48(3):e103–9.

[6] National Heart, Lung, and Blood Institute, National Asthma Education and Prevention Program. Expert Panel Report 3: guidelines for the diagnosis and management of asthma. Full report 2007. Washington, DC: U.S. Dept. of Health and Human Services, National Institutes of Health, National Heart, Lung and Blood Institute; 2007. Available at: http://www.nhlbi.nih.gov/guidelines/asthma/asthgdln.pdf.

[7] Patel SJ, Teach S. J. Asthma. Pediatr Rev 2019;40(11):549–67; https://doi.org/10.1542/pir.2018-0282.

[8] Mims JW. Asthma: definitions and pathophysiology. Int Forum Allergy Rhinol 2015;5(Suppl 1):S2–6.

[9] Maslan J, Mims JW. What is asthma? Pathophysiology, demographics, and health care costs. Otolaryngol Clin North Am 2014 Feb;47(1):13–22.

[10] Fainardi V, Saglani S. An approach to the management of children with problematic severe asthma. Acta Biomed 2020;91(3):e2020055.

[11] Global Initiative for Asthma (GINA 2022). Global Strategy for Asthma Management and Prevention. Available at: https://ginasthma.org/. Accessed October 14, 2022.

[12] Papadopoulos NG, Arakawa H, Carlsen K-H, et al. International consensus on (icon) pediatric asthma. Allergy 2012; https://doi.org/10.1111/j.1398-9995.2012.02865.x.

[13] Ullmann N, Mirra V, Di Marco A, et al. Asthma: Differential Diagnosis and Comorbidities. Front Pediatr 2018;6:276.

[14] Expert Panel Working Group of the National Heart, Lung, and Blood Institute (NHLBI) administered and coordinated National Asthma Education and Prevention Program Coordinating Committee (NAEPPCC), Cloutier MM, Baptist AP, Blake KV, et al. 2020 Focused Updates to the Asthma Management Guidelines: A Report from the National Asthma Education and Prevention Program Coordinating Committee Expert Panel Working Group. J Allergy Clin Immunol 2020;146(6):1217–70.

[15] Chipps BE, Murphy KR, Oppenheimer J. 2020 NAEPP Guidelines Update and GINA 2021-Asthma Care Differences, Overlap, and Challenges. J Allergy Clin Immunol 2022;10(1S):S19–30.

[16] Hendeles L, Blake KV, Galbreath A. A Single Inhaler Combining a Corticosteroid and Long-Acting Beta-2 Agonist for Maintenance with Additional Doses for Reliever Therapy (SMART): Obstacles for Asthma Patients in the USA. Pediatr Allergy Immunol Pulmonology 2021;34(2):73–5.

[17] Barber AT, Loughlin CE. Pediatric Pulmonology 2020 year in review: Asthma. Pediatr Pulmonology 2021;56(8):2455–9.

[18] Abrams EM, Shaker M, Greenhawt M, et al. Treatment of mild-to-moderate asthma in childhood and adolescence in 2021. Lancet Respir Med 2021;9(5):443–5.

[19] Reddel HK, Bateman ED, Schatz M, et al. A Practical Guide to Implementing SMART in Asthma Management. J Allergy Clin Immunol Pract 2022;10(1S):S31–8.

Advances in Family Practice Nursing 5 (2023) 229–240

ADVANCES IN FAMILY PRACTICE NURSING

The Weight of Body Image

Elizabeth R. Silvers, MSN, RN, CPNP-PC, PMHS[a],*,
Kimberly J. Erlich, MSN, RN, MPH, CPNP-PC, PMHS,
CIMHP[b,c,1]

[a]UCSF Benioff Children's Hospital, San Francisco, CA, USA; [b]The Healthy Teen Project, Los Altos, CA, USA; [c]Lifestance Health, Burlingame, CA, USA

Keywords
- Adolescent health • Body image • Eating disorder • Mental health • Pediatrics
- Social media

Key points
- Prevalence and severity of eating disorders (EDs) in the adolescent and young adult population have increased since the start of the COVID-19 pandemic, underscoring the need for further education on this topic.
- Health-care providers (HCPs) must be aware of the signs and symptoms of EDs, the scope of treatment, and when to appropriately refer for higher level of care.
- HCPs should be aware of psychological risk factors for the development of EDs and regularly assess for these in their care of older children and adolescents.
- HCPs should be aware of the role of the medical provider in caring for children/adolescents with EDs.
- A Health At Every Size-informed approach is recommended to promote development of healthy body image in children and adolescents.

INTRODUCTION AND RELEVANCE TO PRIMARY CARE
Untreated eating disorders (EDs) lead to devastating health outcomes including heart failure, osteoporosis, seizures, and suicide. Health-care providers (HCPs) in the primary care setting are responsible for providing developmental surveillance and screening for common physical and mental conditions. As gatekeepers, it is essential that HCPs in primary care can identify early disordered eating behaviors and acknowledge the delicate balance in

[1]Present address: 919 Fremont Avenue #100. Los Altos. CA 94024.

*Corresponding author. 675 18th Street, San Francisco, CA 94107. E-mail address: esilvers14@gmail.com

https://doi.org/10.1016/j.yfpn.2022.11.003
2589-420X/23/

promoting a sustainably healthy lifestyle. Improved primary care participation in psychoeducation about development of a healthy body image and early management of EDs can lead to better medical and psychiatric outcomes [1]. Although this is most relevant in the primary care setting, the recommendations apply more broadly to all HCPs.

Increasing "obesity" rates in the United States has necessitated the development of management guidelines in the primary care setting because obesity affects 17% of children [2]. Higher body mass index (BMI) is a risk factor for developing an ED [3]. However, it is important to consider the impact of well-intentioned messaging to overweight adolescent and young adults (AYA): more than half of adolescent women and one-third of adolescent men engage in unhealthy behaviors to manipulate their weight, including fasting, vomiting, skipping meals, smoking cigarettes, and taking laxatives [4].

IMPACT OF THE COVID-19 PANDEMIC ON EATING DISORDERS IN ADOLESCENTS AND YOUNG ADULTS

The rate of EDs has more than doubled from 2000 to 2006 to 2013 to 2018 [5]. Body image dissatisfaction is associated with higher rates of EDs, and research shows this is a global epidemic: around 50% of young American adolescent women reported feeling unhappy with their body; 12% to 26% of adolescent boys report marked dissatisfaction with their bodies, and 35% of UK teens aged 13 to 19 years reported frequent concern with their body image [6–8]. Several studies have concurred that the intensity of and distress caused by body image dissatisfaction increases throughout adolescence [6,9]. Further, the COVID-19 pandemic has negatively influenced the trajectory of body image and prevalence of EDs in the pediatric population. The overall incidence of EDs across all age groups increased 15.3% in 2020 in the United States compared with earlier years [10]. One study showed a link between body image dissatisfaction in adolescent girls and increased depressive symptoms because of appearance concerns on video-chat and changing routines around managing appearance [11]. Use of social media platforms among AYA increased during the pandemic, and it has been established that social comparison within social networking sites leads to body image and eating concerns [12,13]. Further, a study found that more time spent engaging with Facebook during the pandemic predicted greater concern with body weight and shape [14]. Along these lines, there was an overall increase in adolescents and young adults presenting with EDs who needed inpatient or outpatient care. Compared with those seen in 2019, adolescents assessed for an ED in 2020 showed higher rates of nutritional restriction and functional impairment, medical instability, and required more hospitalizations or urgent consultations [15].

PATHOPHYSIOLOGY: RELATIONSHIP OF BODY IMAGE TO EATING DISORDERS

Body image is a multidimensional construct containing many components: body appreciation, body image flexibility, and functionality appreciation [16–

18]. It is hypothesized that these 3 components protect against body image disturbance and EDs.

Although body image formation begins as young as 3 years old, critical reassessment occurs during early adolescence, a time, which coincides with puberty and drastic changes to an individual's physical appearance [19]. The developmental stage of adolescence creates a susceptibility to external influence, increasing the risk that AYA may develop negative body image, which may contribute to a host of poor health outcomes, including disordered eating behaviors, depression, and use of dietary supplements and steroids without medical indication [20].

Weight bias (negative attitudes directed toward individuals who are perceived to have excess body weight) contributes to body image formation [21]. Internalization of weight bias is associated with negative effects including weight cycling, depressive symptoms, and poor self-esteem [22]. AYA are exposed to weight bias in health-care encounters and steps can be taken to change HCPs practice in a way that decreases weight bias and its negative impact on AYA health.

Several factors influence body image: some positively and some negatively. Factors which negatively influence body image include internalization of the thin ideal (societal norms promote a culture of orthorexia, in which "healthy eating" includes restrictive diets without clear medical indication), weight appearance-related anxiety, pressure from the media, and pressure from peers [4,23]. Protective factors for developing intact body image include body satisfaction, self-compassion, and intuitive eating [4,23]. Studies show that negative body image affects many aspects of adolescent health, underscoring the importance of including anticipatory guidance about body image at annual health maintenance examination visits [22].

Children and adolescents engage with various forms of media at high rates and are on their computers for more than an hour per day [3]. Several studies have demonstrated the relationship between exposure to the thin ideal in mass media and disrupted body image as well as internalization of the thin ideal and disordered eating patterns among young women [3]. In particular, social media platforms reinforce unrealistic expectations of body shape ideals through targeting of images and videos, advertising, and digital enhancement, all of which have been shown to contribute to poor body image and disordered eating behaviors [22,24]. The authors and other experts recommend that HCPs provide guidance around the health consequences of viewing and internalizing unattainable beauty expectations and body type ideals, encouraging patients to critically appraise the images in the media they consume [22].

Perceptual body image constructs, including overvaluation of weight and shape; fear of weight gain; and preoccupation with weight, shape, and size are core features of many EDs [25,26]. In parallel to the increase in rates of EDs during the last few decades and most notably throughout the pandemic, rates of "obesity" have also increased [27]. Although there is a clear overlap between individuals with higher weights and incidence of EDs, the medical treatment approach has largely remained focused on weight reduction, which continues to reinforce body shaming and body mistrust [28]. In contrast, the Health at Every Size (HAES)-informed approach in health care shifts the focus from weight loss to weight-neutral outcomes and empowers the individual to challenge internalized negative messaging regarding body size and worth [29,30].

HISTORY

Research shows that challenging negative body and diet talk can support positive body image [31]. HCPs can model challenging negative body talk for patients while simultaneously obtaining a history of thoughts, beliefs, and behaviors in patients and their families that could presuppose a risk for the development of negative body image, body image dissatisfaction, and EDs. HCPs should ask patients specific questions about the perceptual constructs of body image described above including: (1) how the body is viewed; (2) daily eating patterns including whether 3 meals and 2 snacks per day are consumed; (3) whether meals are skipped; and (4) whether they compare their body to that of peers, celebrities, or other ideals. Additional questions about personal and family "food rules" are appropriate. A family history of EDs, mood and anxiety disorders, obsessive-compulsive disorder, and substance use disorders should also be obtained (Box 1).

Box 1: Assessment of personal and familial risk factors for eating disorders

Body Image
- "How do you view your body?"
- "Do you compare yourself to your peers?"

Eating Patterns
- "Are you eating 3 meals and 2 snacks each day?"
- "Are you skipping meals?"
- "Are there any foods or food groups you avoid?"

Family/Personal "Food Rules"
- No junk food, use of nondairy milk, gluten-free diet without medical indication
- Sudden switch to vegetarian or vegan diet coordinating with weight loss

Relationship with Movement
- "What kind of movement do you enjoy?"
- "Do you ever feel you have to 'earn' meals or 'work off' calories through exercise?"

Family History of Eating Disorders, Anxiety/Depression, OCD

SCREENING

Screening for EDs includes evaluating for early medical complications related to disordered eating behaviors. Medical screening includes the evaluation of the following: growth charts (trending increase or decrease of percentiles over time); vital signs (abnormalities such as orthostasis by either heart rate or blood pressure or both, low resting heart rate, and low body temperature); energy intake; activity level; and substance use (including caffeine, laxatives, stimulants, and insulin if diabetic). Psychological screening evaluates many of the historical components given above, including body image, eating patterns, family and personal meal habits, and relationship with movement. A history of excessive concern with weight, inappropriate dieting, and weight loss may require further evaluation. HCPs may elect to use a patient self-report questionnaire, such as the evidence-based *Eating Attitudes Test-26*, which is validated for use in patients aged 13 years and older [32], or the *SCOFF Questionnaire*, which is validated for use in patients aged 16 years and older [33], to obtain some of this information.

ASSESSMENT

Medical assessment for EDs begins with vital signs (blind weight, heart rate, blood pressure, orthostatic vital signs, temperature) and urinalysis for urine pH and specific gravity, as well as a urine pregnancy test [34]. The blind weight procedure involves not disclosing weight values to patient. This is the most common approach to assessment, largely because the fear of weight gain inspires high levels of anxiety during treatment of EDs, and therefore taking blind weights can support treatment engagement [35]. Detailed evaluation of historical growth chart data includes calculation of BMI, although BMI alone does not always provide an accurate clinical picture. For example, a height plateau, particularly during late childhood through middle adolescence, would be concerning for malnutrition that affects growth. Additionally, a stark shift of weight trend, more than one standard deviation of weight loss, or weight oscillation over time, could be indicative of an ED [34]. Many body systems can be influenced by disordered eating behaviors and malnutrition. Signs and symptoms concerning for ED by body system are shown in Table 1.

DIAGNOSIS

On the surface, common differential diagnoses for a chief concern of rapid weight loss or gain, and decreased appetite include hyperthyroidism, malabsorption, inflammatory causes (Crohn disease, celiac disease, ulcerative colitis), malignancy, depression, substance use disorder, conversion disorder, and delusions (eg, due to schizophrenia) [36,37]. In reality, a comprehensive list of disorders that affect different body systems and can present with these symptoms would be both broad and deep: endocrine disorders (diabetes mellitus, Grave disease, Hashimoto thyroiditis, polycystic ovary syndrome [PCOS]), gastrointestinal disorders (malabsorption, gastroparesis), psychiatric disorders, and

Table 1
Signs and symptoms concerning for eating disorder by body system

General	Gastrointestinal	Cardiovascular
Fatigue	Nausea	Palpitations
Weakness	Vomiting	Chest pain
Activity intolerance	Constipation	Acrocyanosis
Dizziness	Diarrhea	*Endocrine*
Syncope	Early satiety	Cold intolerance
Integumentary	Fullness	Menstrual irregularities
Dry skin	Bloating	*Hematologic*
Lanugo	Burping/reflux	Easy bruising/bleeding
Hair loss	Pain	Pallor

Data from [AED Medical Care Standards Committee. Eating Disorders: A Guide to Medical Care. Published 2021. Accessed September 9, 2022. https://higherlogicdownload.s3.amazonaws.com/AEDWEB/ 27a3b69a-8aae-45b2-a04c-2a078d02145d/UploadedImages/Publications_Slider/2120_AED_Medical_Care_4th_Ed_FINAL.pdf.]

other disorders (eg, tumor, pregnancy, other rheumatologic conditions, and metabolic disorders) [37].

It is necessary to consider more than weight loss as a chief complaint or presenting symptom when evaluating EDs, which is why the psychosocial screening is important. The psychosocial assessment will be described later in the article. The Diagnostic and Statistical Manual for Mental Disorders (DSM-V) defines criteria for various categories of EDs, including anorexia nervosa restricting or binge-purge type, bulimia nervosa, binge eating disorder, avoidant restrictive food intake disorder, and other specified feeding and eating disorder (which includes atypical anorexia) [38]. Other diagnoses that are either not traditionally considered to be EDs or not yet published in the DSM-V include orthorexia and diabulimia. Orthorexia is characterized as an obsession with "healthful" eating, including compulsive checking of nutritional facts labels, overall increased concern about the health of foods or ingredients, such that an increasing number of foods/food groups are cut out of the diet without medical rationale (eg, sugar, carbohydrates, dairy, meat, gluten) [39]. People with orthorexia often display a high degree of distress when foods they consider safe are unavailable [39]. Diabulimia entails purposeful restriction of the insulin dose by a diabetic patient in order to lose weight [40].

MANAGEMENT

As EDs affect both medical and psychiatric health, management targets both domains. Multidisciplinary approach to treatment includes a team consisting of a medical provider, therapist, dietitian, and psychiatric clinician, if there are psychiatric comorbidities [41]. ED treatment is provided within a hierarchy of levels of care: outpatient, intensive outpatient, partial hospitalization, inpatient, and residential treatment [42]. There are established criteria that determine appropriateness for the management of patients at each level of care; those criteria are beyond the scope this article [37,42].

Most HCPs who practice in primary care, whether family practice or pediatric clinicians, provide medical management of EDs at the outpatient level of care. This management includes initial laboratory evaluations (complete blood count; comprehensive metabolic panel including calcium, magnesium, and phosphate; lipid function test [LFT]; thyroid function test including total T3; and erythrocyte sedimentation rate) [34]. If purging is suspected or present, amylase should be included [34]. In women who have been amenorrheic for more than 6 months, follicle-stimulating hormone (FSH), luteinizing hormone (LH), estrogen, and prolactin should be included as well as a urine pregnancy and a dual-energy X-ray absorptiometry scan [37]. In men, a testosterone level may also be considered [34]. An EKG should be performed for all patients with a suspected ED [34]. As EDs impact the entire body, a thorough physical examination should include the assessment of the skin, head, eyes, ears, nose, throat, cardiovascular, musculoskeletal, gastroenterological, and neurologic systems [34]. Follow-up appointments should occur every 1 to 2 weeks to track vital signs, hydration status, urine pH, and progress with treatment.

Psychological care for AYA with EDs at the outpatient level of care should be provided by a qualified mental health professional (MHP) who often subspecializes in the care of AYA with EDs (eg, ED-certified therapist, clinical psychologist, or licensed clinical social worker or registered, supervised trainee) [41]. Initial psychological care includes a thorough psychosocial assessment to evaluate the degree of obsession with food and weight, and the impact on their functioning at home, in school, and with peers [34]. The MHP should assess for the presence of comorbid psychiatric symptoms or diagnoses, including nonsuicidal self-harm or suicidal ideation, as well as assess for a history of trauma [41]. If safety concerns are present, a safety plan should be completed, documented in the chart, and shared with the multidisciplinary team. A key component of psychosocial assessment is the patient's and parent or caregiver's understanding of and reaction to the ED diagnosis, as well as their willingness to receive and participate in treatment. Psychiatric comorbidities should be further evaluated by a psychiatric clinician (eg, psychiatric mental health nurse practitioner, pediatric mental health specialist, or child/adolescent psychiatrist). Key components of the psychiatric evaluation include the temporal relationship of psychiatric symptoms to the development of the ED and associated distress and functional impairment [41,43].

Nutrition support for patients with an ED being managed at the outpatient level of care is provided by a registered dietitian who is trained in EDs [41]. Additional training in the HAES-informed approach to treatment is optimal because it reinforces the notion of working toward body neutrality and intuitive eating in the maintenance phase of treatment [44]. Further, intuitive eating can remain effective at decreasing dieting and disordered weight control behaviors several years after the intervention [45].

When treating EDs at the outpatient level of care, there are several medical and psychiatric indications for referral to a higher level of care [37,42]. When considering whether a patient is appropriate for the current level of care, it is essential to consult with the rest of the outpatient team. This team ideally includes a therapist, dietitian, and a psychiatric clinician, all of whom specialize in or have extensive experience with EDs [34]. Consultation with local ED specialists and programs can be helpful in coordinating transition of care as well as assisting in leveraging available resources in the community. Table 2 shows specific indications for considering referral to a higher level of ED-specialized care.

DISCUSSION

Rising rates of EDs across all age groups, hyperfixation on body image, over-valuation of an ideal body type, and higher acuity of AYA presenting with signs and symptoms of ED underscore the need for HCPs to become proficient in early identification through screening, assessment, and comanagement of EDs. However, the weight-focused standard of care has led to HCPs being more focused on the threat of "obesity" rather than the threat of an ED. In doing so, HCPs risk addressing one chronic illness at the expense of another [46].

The historical model of medical care promotes weight management to further health goals (eg, use of BMI as a measure of health, targeting weight loss in public health policy as a way to address the problem of "obesity" and the overall focus on the threat of "obesity," rather than the risk of development of an ED) [29]. Although current practice guidelines are designed to curb increasing "obesity" rates, they do not acknowledge the impact on body image and potential for body dysmorphia. A HAES-informed approach is recommended to promote the development of healthy body image in children and adolescents [29,30]. A HAES-informed approach shifts the focus to weight neutrality, reducing the focus of weight loss as a health-related goal, and reduction of stigma around weight [29]. HCPs can positively influence the development of healthy body image in AYA through changing the philosophy of care, the messaging they provide during patient education, and modeling healthy attitudes during health-care encounters [37]. This can be pursued by using language that promotes weight neutrality and inclusivity, holistic health enhancement (rather than pursuit of an ideal), eating for well-being (rather than weight reduction), and life-enhancing movement (rather than exercise), which are the principles of the HAES-informed approach [30]. The HAES-informed approach to health and health care can be used both in "obesity" management and in ED management.

Table 2	
Indications for referral to a higher level of care	
Medical indications	**Psychiatric indications**
• Weight loss despite intervention	• Continuous self-harm
• Symptomatic or worsening orthostasis	• Increasing suicidal ideation
• Guidelines for inpatient admission	• Increasing frequency/severity of ED
○ Medical instability (variety of markers)	behaviors
○ Acute food refusal (severe and/or	• Other safety concerns
prolonged)	

IMPLICATION FOR ADVANCED PRACTICE NURSES

The COVID-19 pandemic has been associated with increased rates and severity of EDs [10,15]. A 2021 mixed-methods study of pediatric and family medicine clinicians pointed to early identification of EDs in the pediatric population as an area of need within their practices [1]. Advanced practice nurses (APNs) are well poised to expand access to evidence-based treatment of EDs through early identification and collaborative management. Notably, the same study also cited lack of knowledge about the identification and treatment of EDs as a barrier to implementation [1]. The evidence-based strategies presented here provide APNs the knowledge necessary to improve care for AYA patients, including those with EDs. This can be done effectively through the identification of those at risk through psychological screening, medical assessment, early medical management, and early and continuous psychiatric collaborative management. APNs have an established track record as leaders in implementing collaborative care [47,48]. This is highly relevant to ED specialty care, which requires combining medical, psychological, and psychiatric treatment and leverages the APN as an essential member of this interdisciplinary treatment team.

CLINICS CARE POINTS

- Reinforcement of unrealistic expectations of body shape ideals through social media has been shown to contribute to poor body image and disordered eating behaviors.
- Healthcare providers should challenge negative body and diet talk in medical encounters in order to support positive body image.
- Psychological screeners, such as the SCOFF or Eating Attitudes Test-26, can help to identify excessive concern with weight, inappropriate dieting, and weight loss which may require further evaluation.
- The use of a blind weight is the most common in assessment and management of eating disorders in order to support treatment engagement.
- A stark shift of weight trend, more than one standard deviation of weight loss, or weight oscillation over time, could be indicative of an eating disorder.

DISCLOSURE

The authors have nothing to disclose.

References

[1] Lebow J, Narr C, Mattke A, et al. Engaging primary care providers in managing pediatric eating disorders: a mixed methods study. J Eat Disord 2021;9(1); https://doi.org/10.1186/s40337-020-00363-8.
[2] Grief SN, Waterman M. Approach to obesity management in the primary care setting. J Obes Weight-Loss Medic 2019;5:24.

[3] Argyrides M, Anastasiades E, Alexiou E. Risk and protective factors of disordered eating in adolescents based on gender and body mass index. Int J Environ Res Public Health 2020;17(24):9238.

[4] Statistics & Research on Eating Disorders. National Eating Disorders Association. 2021. Available at: https://www.nationaleatingdisorders.org/statistics-research-eating-disorders. Accessed May 12, 2022.

[5] Galmiche M, Déchelotte P, Lambert G, et al. Prevalence of eating disorders over the 2000–2018 period: a systematic literature review. Am J Clin Nutr 2019;109(5):1402–13.

[6] Kearney-Cooke A, Tiger D. Body image disturbance and the development of eating disorders. In: Smolak L, Levine MP, editors. The wiley handbook of eating disorders. 1st ed. Wiley-Blackwell; 2015. p. 1–10; https://doi.org/10.1002/9781118574089.

[7] Bucchianeri MM, Arikian AJ, Hannan PJ, et al. Body dissatisfaction from adolescence to young adulthood: Findings from a 10-year longitudinal study. Body Image 2013;10(1):1–7.

[8] Millions of teenagers worry about body image and identify social media as a key cause – new survey by the Mental Health Foundation. Mental Health Foundation; 2019. Available at: https://www.mentalhealth.org.uk/news/millions-teenagers-worry-about-body-image-and-identify-social-media-key-cause-new-survey. Accessed May 12, 2022.

[9] Rodgers RF, McLean SA, Marques M, et al. Trajectories of body dissatisfaction and dietary restriction in early adolescent girls: a latent class growth analysis. J Youth Adolesc 2015;45(8):1664–77.

[10] Taquet M, Geddes JR, Luciano S, et al. Incidence and outcomes of eating disorders during the COVID-19 pandemic. Br J Psychiatry 2021;220(5):262–4.

[11] Choukas-Bradley S, Maheux AJ, Roberts SR, et al. Picture perfect during a pandemic? Body image concerns and depressive symptoms in U.S. adolescent girls during the COVID-19 lockdown. J Child Media 2022;1–12; https://doi.org/10.1080/17482798.2022.2039255.

[12] Kerekes N, Bador K, Sfendla A, et al. Changes in adolescents' psychosocial functioning and well-being as a consequence of long-term covid-19 restrictions. Int J Environ Res Public Health 2021;18(16):8755.

[13] Holland G, Tiggemann M. A systematic review of the impact of the use of social networking sites on body image and disordered eating outcomes. Body Image 2016;17:100–10.

[14] Mannino G, Salerno L, Bonfanti RC, et al. The impact of Facebook use on self-reported eating disorders during the COVID-19 lockdown. BMC Psychiatry 2021;21(1); https://doi.org/10.1186/s12888-021-03628-x.

[15] Spettigue W, Obeid N, Erbach M, et al. The impact of covid-19 on adolescents with eating disorders: a cohort study. J Eat Disord 2021;9(1); https://doi.org/10.1186/s40337-021-00419-3.

[16] Tylka TL, Wood-Barcalow NL. The Body Appreciation Scale-2: Item refinement and psychometric evaluation. Body Image 2015;12:53–67.

[17] Sandoz EK, Wilson KG, Merwin RM, et al. Assessment of body image flexibility: the body image-acceptance and action questionnaire. J Contextual Behav Sci 2013;2:39–48.

[18] Alleva JM, Tylka TL, Kroon Van Diest AM. The functionality appreciation scale (FAS): development and psychometric evaluation in US community women and men. Body Image 2017;23:28–44.

[19] Christie D, Viner R. Adolescent development. BMJ 2005;330(7486):301–4.

[20] Golden NH, Schneider M, Wood C. Preventing obesity and eating disorders in adolescents. In: American academy of pediatrics. pediatric clinical practice guidelines & policies. 17th Ed. American Academy of Pediatrics; 2017. p. 1067–76; https://doi.org/10.1542/9781610020862-part04-preventing.

[21] Pearl RL, Puhl RM. Weight bias internalization and health: a systematic review. Obes Rev 2018;19(8):1141–63.

[22] Hartman-Munick SM, Gordon AR, Guss C. Adolescent body image: influencing factors and the clinician's role. Curr Opin Pediatr 2020;32(4):455–60.

[23] Linardon J. Positive body image, intuitive eating, and self compassion protect against the onset of the core symptoms of eating disorders: A prospective study. Int J Eat Disord 2021;54(11):1967–77.

[24] Widdows H, MacCallum F. The demands of beauty: editors' introduction. Health Care Anal 2018;26(3):207–19.

[25] McLean SA, Paxton SJ. Body image in the context of eating disorders. Psychiatr Clin North Am 2019;42(1):145–56.

[26] Neves CM, Cipriani FM, Meireles JF, et al. Imagem corporal na infância: Uma revisão integrativa da literatura. Rev Paul Pediatr 2017;35(3):331–9.

[27] Stierman B, Afful J, Carroll M, et al. National health and nutrition examination survey 2017–march 2020 pre-pandemic data files. Natl Health Stat Rep 2021;158; https://doi.org/10.15620/cdc:106273.

[28] Reel J, Voelker D, Greenleaf C. Weight status and body image perceptions in adolescents: Current perspectives. Adolesc Health Med Ther 2015;149; https://doi.org/10.2147/ahmt.s68344.

[29] Bacon L, Aphramor L. Weight science: Evaluating the evidence for a paradigm shift. Nutr J 2011;10(1); https://doi.org/10.1186/1475-2891-10-9.

[30] The health at every size® (HAES®) principles. ASDAH. 2022. Available at: https://asdah.org/health-at-every-size-haes-approach/. Accessed May 13, 2022.

[31] Mills J, Mort O, Trawley S. The impact of different responses to fat talk on body image and socioemotional outcomes. Body Image 2019;29:149–55.

[32] Garner DM, Garfinkel PE. The eating attitudes test: An index of the symptoms of anorexia nervosa. Psychol Med 1979;9(2):273–9.

[33] Morgan JF, Reid F, Lacey JH. The SCOFF questionnaire: a new screening tool for eating disorders. West J Med 2000;172(3):164–5.

[34] AED Medical Care Standards Committee. Eating disorders: a guide to medical care. 2021. Available at: https://higherlogicdownload.s3.amazonaws.com/AEDWEB/27a3b69a-8aae-45b2-a04c-2a078d02145d/UploadedImages/Publications_Slider/2120_AED_-Medical_Care_4th_Ed_FINAL.pdf. Accessed September 9, 2022.

[35] Froreich FV, Ratcliffe SE, Vartanian LR. Blind versus open weighing from an eating disorder patient perspective. J Eat Disord 2020;8(1); https://doi.org/10.1186/s40337-020-00316-1.

[36] Jey S. Unintended weight loss: what's the diagnosis? Guidelines in Practice. 2020. Available at: https://www.guidelinesinpractice.co.uk/gastrointestinal/unintended-weight-loss-whats-the-diagnosis/455063.article. Accessed September 9, 2022.

[37] Hornberger LL, Lane MA. The Committee on Adolescence, et al. Identification and management of eating disorders in children and adolescents. Pediatrics 2021;147(1); https://doi.org/10.1542/peds.2020-040279.

[38] American Psychiatric Association, Diagnostic and statistical manual of mental disorders, DSM-5. 5th ed., Am Psychiatr Assoc, 2013.

[39] Orthorexia. National Eating Disorders Association. Available at: https://www.nationaleatingdisorders.org/orthorexia. Accessed June 3, 2022.

[40] Diabulimia. National Eating Disorders Association. Available at: https://www.nationaleatingdisorders.org/diabulimia. Accessed June 3, 2022.

[41] The iaedptm Nutrition Health Management Committee. Medical management professionals in eating disorder care. Available at: http://www.iaedp.com/upload/iaedp_Medical_Management_Profess.pdf. Accessed June 3, 2022.

[42] Levels of Care. National Eating Disorders Association. Available at: https://www.nationaleatingdisorders.org/treatment/levels-care. Accessed June 3, 2022.

[43] Society for Adolescent Health and Medicine. Medical management of restrictive eating disorders in adolescents and young adults. J Adolesc Health 2022; https://doi.org/10.1016/j.jadohealth.2022.08.006.

[44] Carbonneau E, Bégin C, Lemieux S, et al. A Health at Every Size intervention improves intuitive eating and diet quality in Canadian women. Clin Nutr 2017;36(3):747–54; https://doi.org/10.1016/j.clnu.2016.06.008.

[45] Christoph M, Järvelä-Reijonen E, Hooper L, et al. Longitudinal associations between intuitive eating and weight-related behaviors in a population-based sample of young adults. Appetite 2021;160:105093.

[46] Gotovac S, LaMarre A, Lafreniere K. Words with weight: The construction of obesity in eating disorders research. Health (London) 2020;24(2):113–31.

[47] Schober M, Lehwaldt D, Rogers M, et al. Guidelines on advanced practice nursing. International Council of Nurses; 2020. Available at: https://www.icn.ch/system/files/documents/2020-04/ICN_APN%20Report_EN_WEB.pdf. Accessed September 12, 2022.

[48] Theccanat SM. Integrating psychiatric nurse practitioners into psychiatric practice settings. Psychiatr Serv 2015;66(9):913–5.

Advances in Family Practice Nursing 5 (2023) 241–253

ELSEVIER
MOSBY

ADVANCES IN FAMILY PRACTICE NURSING

Emerging Mental Health Issues in Children and Adolescents Secondary to the Coronavirus Disease-2019 Pandemic

Kellie Bishop, DNP, APRN, CPNP-PC, PMHS*,
Teresa Whited, DNP, APRN, CPNP-PC[1]

College of Nursing, Univeristy of Arkansas for Medical Sciences, 4301 W Markham Street, Slot 529, RAHN Building Room 5202, Little Rock, AR, 72205, USA

Keywords
- COVID-19 • Coronavirus • Pandemic • Adolescents • Depression • Anxiety
- Suicide • Mental health

Key points
- Determine the prevalence of anxiety, depression, and suicide among adolescents before and during the coronavirus disease-2019 (COVID-19) pandemic.
- Identify evidence-based screening tools to assess for mental illness in adolescents.
- Identify strategies to foster resilience and promote well-being in adolescents.
- Implication strategies for advanced practice nurses, including educating adolescents and families on mental health promotion, and advocating for mental health awareness and resources for adolescents.

Once a highly stigmatized and avoided topic, mental health, particularly among children and adolescents, has become widely recognized societally. Children and adolescents have long experienced depression, anxiety, and devastating rates of suicide. These issues are more widely recognized today due in large part to the drastic increase in mental health issues in children and adolescents during the COVID-19 pandemic. This article

[1]Present address: 3080 Windcrest Drive. Conwav. AR. 72034.

*Corresponding author. PO Box 118, Plumerville, AR 72127. E-mail address: kbishop@uams.edu

https://doi.org/10.1016/j.yfpn.2022.11.011
2589-420X/23/© 2022 Elsevier Inc. All rights reserved.

highlights common mental health issues in children and adolescents and the impact of COVID-19 on their overall mental health. It provides practitioners with the screening tools and opportunities to foster resilience in children and adolescents during this unprecedented time.

BACKGROUND

In April 2022, the American Academy of Pediatrics (AAP), the American Academy of Child and Adolescent Psychiatry (AACAP), and the Children's Hospital Association (CHA) declared a national emergency in children's mental health and called on policymakers to join them in taking action [1]. Between March and October 2020, emergency department visits for mental health issues in children aged 5 to 11 years rose by 24% and 31% in adolescents aged 12 to 17 years [1]. Miller and colleagues [2] explain that current evidence indicates that adolescent mental health symptoms of anxiety, depression, and posttraumatic stress disorder (PTSD) during the pandemic range from 21% to 65% incidence rates. Furthermore, preexisting mental health and behavioral concerns in children and adolescents are exacerbated by stressful events, such as the pandemic and its consequences.

SIGNIFICANCE

Understanding the mental and social development of children and adolescents is critical in attempting to understand the drastic increase in mental health issues during the pandemic. The US Surgeon General's Advisory explains that mental health is shaped by two primary factors: biological and environmental [3]. Biological factors include genes and brain chemistry, which are inherent factors in the person. Environmental factors include life experiences, which can determine whether genetic predisposition to mental health disorder manifests. Environmental factors include prenatal considerations, such as drug and alcohol exposure, birth complications, discrimination, racism, and adverse childhood experiences (ACEs), such as abuse, neglect, exposure to violence, and socioeconomic disparities. These ACEs negatively affect the child's sense of safety, stability, bonding, and well-being [3]. The biologic and environmental factors interact with each other so a child who is genetically predisposed to anxiety may be more affected by an environmental stressor than children without the biologic predisposition. Owing to an increase in environmental stressors, social isolations, and shutdowns, many children and adolescents are experiencing increased rates of mental health disorders.

DISCUSSION

Coronavirus disease-2019

The coronavirus disease-2019 (COVID-19) pandemic has caused upheaval and stress in all aspects of life. Children and adolescents are particularly vulnerable to such stressors as they are still learning how to regulate themselves and overcome stressful situations. Daily life changed quickly resulting in a sudden and drastic change in how our youth attend school, interact with peers, receive health care, and participate in activities. Simultaneously, many parents became unemployed, families became financially unstable and many were left with concerns about food, health care, and housing. Many children and adolescents were affected by contracting COVID-19 themselves, watching loved ones become seriously ill, and experiencing death. The US Surgeon General's Advisory reports that as of June 2021, more than 140,000 American children had lost a parent or grandparent caregiver to COVID-19 [3]. Furthermore, vulnerable populations, such as those with lower socioeconomic status, have contracted and died from COVID-19 at higher rates than less vulnerable populations. Therefore, the children and adolescents in those vulnerable populations have the environmental risk factors of socioeconomic disparities, discrimination, and racism, with the added stresses of losing loved ones at higher rates and living in a pandemic. In understanding the concepts of executive function and resiliency, and how children develop those skills, it is logical that the pandemic has led to an increase in mental health issues among our youth.

Depression

The prevalence of depression among children and adolescents has been increasing for years. However, the rates have drastically increased since the beginning of the pandemic in early 2020. In a poll conducted by the Centers for Disease Control and Prevention (CDC) in 2019, pre-pandemic, 36.7% of American high-school students reported experiencing persistent feelings of sadness and hopelessness [4]. In a similar poll conducted by the CDC in 2021, 1 year into the pandemic, 44% of American high-school students reported persistent feelings of sadness and hopelessness [4]. Contributing factors to this increase include stress at home related to the pandemic and increased rates of child abuse. In the 2021 poll, 55% of students reported experiencing emotional abuse by a parent or other adult in their own home, including swearing at and insulting the child [4]. Furthermore, 11% reported experiencing physical abuse by a parent or other adult in their home, including hitting, kicking, and beating the child [4]. Twenty-nine percent reported that a parent or other adult in the home lost a job due to the pandemic, causing increased stress in the home [4]. Social connectedness with peers through school is of vital importance. Owing to the lack of social interaction and alternate methods of teaching during the pandemic, children and adolescents have lacked the social interaction that promotes mental well-being, leading to an increased prevalence of depression (Box 1 for symptoms). In addition, schools and health care providers are pivotal in detecting and reporting child maltreatment. Many of these incidences have gone undetected during the pandemic due to alternate methods of teaching and an increase in the use of telemedicine.

Anxiety

In addition to the increase in depression, there has also been a marked increase in anxiety among children and adolescents during the pandemic. Racine and colleagues [5] note that 11.6% of children and adolescents experienced

Box 1: Common symptoms of depression, anxiety, and suicide in children and adolescents [12–14]

Depression

    At least 2 weeks of a depressed or irritable mood and/or loss of interest or pleasure in most activities

    Symptoms present most of the day, nearly every day

    Appetite increase or decrease

    Sleeping too much or too little

    Decreased energy

    Decreased activity level

    Impaired concentration

    Thoughts of worthlessness, hopelessness, and guilt

    Mood changes

    Irritability

    Suicidal thoughts or actions

Anxiety

    Generalized and persistent fear and worry

    Weight loss

    Pallor

    Tachycardia

    Tremors

    Muscle cramps

    Paresthesias

    Hyperhidrosis

    Headaches

    Abdominal pain

    Specific fears and worries related to type of anxiety-separation, generalized, social, obsessive-compulsive disorder, panic, phobias

Suicide

    Threatening to hurt or kill oneself or talking about wanting to hurt or kill oneself

    Seeking methods to kill oneself (firearms and pills)

    Talking or writing about death, dying, or suicide (out of the ordinary for the person)

    Feeling hopeless and trapped

    Uncontrolled anger or rage

    Seeking revenge

    Reckless and risky behavior

    Increasing substance use

Withdrawing from family, friends, activities
Inability to sleep or sleeping too much, anxious, agitated
Dramatic mood changes
Seeing no reason for living

symptoms of anxiety before the pandemic. The pandemic has shown to increase the prevalence of anxiety symptoms in children and adolescents to 20.5% [5]. Anxiety and depression are often comorbid conditions and have many of the same contributing factors. Social isolation, the unknown of what will happen, and the fear of illness or death of oneself or loved ones all contribute to the rising anxiety in our youth. Hawes and colleagues [6] examined the incidence of mental health symptoms during the pandemic and noted that there were high rates of clinically elevated symptoms (see Box 1) of anxiety during the pandemic in subjects aged 12 to 22 years who were examined. The increased use of technology in place of social interaction has also contributed to the increase in anxiety among children and adolescents. As Gray and colleagues [7] note, social distancing efforts have resulted in interaction primarily via virtual platforms Adolescents, particularly those with existing anxiety or anxious tendencies, are preoccupied with how others perceive them. The increase in social media and virtual platforms during the pandemic has led to adolescents making social comparisons based on online presentations to attain a desired image. This leads to a conflict between the virtual and real self, increasing anxiety. In addition, online bullying can reach people much faster than face-to-face conflict, forcing those who are bullied to socially isolate even further [7]. Children and adolescents with anxiety require stability to feel secure and the unknown nature of the pandemic has led to more dysregulation in these children.

Suicide

The most devastating consequence of mental illness is suicide. Owing to the increase in mental health disorders, there has also been an increase in the prevalence of suicide. Suicide attempt emergency department visits in adolescents aged 12 to 17 years increased by more than 50% in early 2021 in comparison to the same period in 2019, before the pandemic [1]. The contributing factors to the drastic increase in attempted suicide are similar to those of the increased prevalence of depression and anxiety: increased rates of loneliness and sadness, social isolation, losing loved ones to COVID-19, stress at home, online influences, more time at home with things like medications and guns, and an increase in child abuse and maltreatment. It is vital to recognize the risk factors and symptoms of suicidal children and adolescents (see Box 1). The increased prevalence of suicide among our youth is a staggering statistic that demands attention from health care professionals.

Mental health interventions
It is critical that all health care providers evaluating and treating children and adolescents are aware of the emerging mental health issues among this vulnerable population. Thorough wellness visits should include obtaining past medical history, family medical history, family assessment, medications and supplements used, developmental surveillance, physical examination, and anticipatory guidance. As the pandemic continues, it is especially important to fulfill all portions of the wellness exam. The family history and family assessment can alert the provider to a predisposition or environmental factors that could contribute to the child developing a mental health disorder. The developmental surveillance is crucial to identify any developmental issues in younger children, many of which can be worsened by social isolation and alternative methods of teaching. The private interviews with adolescent patients allow the patient to disclose symptoms of mental health issues, as well as any safety concerns they have, such as abuse in the home. Performing proper surveillance allows the provider to determine if further screening for mental health issues is indicated.

Screening and assessment of mental illness. The drastically increasing prevalence rates of mental health issues in children and adolescents make it vitally important for health care providers to be aware of mental health surveillance and screening. Providers serving the pediatric population should approach children and families with an open, empathetic, and nonjudgmental demeanor. Particularly when discussing sensitive topics, such as mental health, it is important to gain trust. Every wellness visit, and episodic visit if indicated, should include a targeted history focused on the child's behavior and any functional impairment [8]. The provider must be aware of developmentally appropriate behavior at various ages to discern if behavior showed is abnormal. It is important to listen to and address behavioral, mental, and functional concerns of both the caregiver and child. If a patient or caregiver indicates a concern about the child's behavior or mental wellness either directly or through developmental surveillance, an appropriate screening tool should be used to assess for mental illness. Several evidence-based screening tools (Table 1) are available to screen for mental health disorders, including depression and anxiety. If the screening tool used indicates a concern for the disorder examined, that is, depression or anxiety, the provider should further inquire about specific symptoms to determine if a diagnosis is indicated. Providers should use the DSM-V diagnostic criteria in assessing and diagnosing mental health disorders. Through a more extensive discussion of symptoms, the provider will be able to discern if the child meets diagnostic criteria for a specific mental illness and what type of treatment or management is indicated. See Fig. 1 for an assessment algorithm.

Treatment of pediatric mental health concerns. Initiating proper treatment of mental health disorders in children is imperative to prevent worsening symptoms. A

Table 1
Evidence-based screening tools [8]

Instrument	Ages (years)	Reporter	Number of items	Time to complete (Min)
General Mental Health				
Pediatric Symptom Checklist (PSC)	4 to 18	Parent Child	35, 17 (different versions for different ages)	5 to 10
Strengths and Difficulties Questionnaire (SDQ)	4 to 18	Parent Child Teacher	25	5
Anxiety				
Self-Report for Childhood Anxiety-Related Emotional Disorders (SCARED)	8 to 18	Parent Child	41	5
Depression				
Patient Health Questionnaire (PHQ-9)	12+	Child	9	< 5
Center for Epidemiological Studies Depression Scale for Children (CES-DC)	6 to 18	Child	20	5
Beck Depression Inventory	7 to 14	Child	21	5 to 10
	13+	Child	20	5 to 10

child who verbalizes suicidal ideation with or without a plan should be referred immediately to a child behavioral health provider or hospitalized. If the patient denies current suicidal ideation and the screening tool use and patient interview do not indicate a diagnosable mental health condition, the patient and caregiver should be educated about signs and symptoms that would indicate the need for a follow-up appointment. Motivational interviewing can be beneficial in these scenarios for stress management and problem-solving [8]. If the patient requests to see a mental health specialist in the absence of a diagnosed condition, a referral should be initiated to a pediatric mental health specialist. Zhang and colleagues [9] show how research-based psychological counseling reduces the symptoms of depression and anxiety in adolescents.

A child who meets diagnostic criteria for a mental health disorder should be treated with medication, if indicated, and referred to a pediatric behavioral health provider for therapy and advanced management. There are no US Food and Drug Administration (FDA)-approved anxiolytic medications for pediatric patients. Patients presenting with an anxiety disorder should be referred for behavioral therapy. The urgency and determination of inpatient or outpatient treatment will depend on the level of severity (see Fig. 1). *Play Therapy* for preschool-aged children and *cognitive-behavioral therapy* (CBT) for school-aged and older are often effective alone in treating pediatric anxiety [8]. In older children and adolescents, or if CBT alone is ineffective, there are several selective serotonin reuptake inhibitors (SSRI) that are FDA

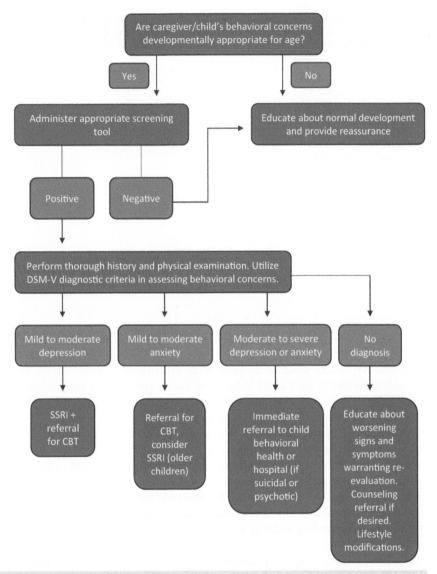

Fig. 1. Assessment and management algorithm [11].

approved for pediatric patients and have proven safe and effective in treating anxiety (Table 2) [8].

The priority intervention in regard to pediatric depression is to determine suicidality. Suicidal risk is greatest within 4 weeks of an initial depressive episode [8]. Patients with acute suicidal ideation and intent with a plan, unstable behavior, psychosis, or risk of abuse should be referred for immediate psychiatric evaluation and treatment at an inpatient pediatric behavioral

Table 2
US Food and Drug Administration-approved medications for depression and anxiety in pediatrics [8]

Drug class and examples	Conditions treated	Primary care drug interactions	Common side effects
Selective Serotonin Reuptake Inhibitors (SSRIs)			
Fluoxetine (prozac, Sarafem) FDA approved 8+	Anxiety Major depressive disorder Obsessive-compulsive disorder Selective mutism	Multiple drug interactions Contraindicated drugs—MAOIs, tryptophan, St. John's wort, thioridazine, TCAs Diet—avoid grapefruit juice and alcohol	Headache, nervousness, insomnia or sedation, fatigue, nausea, diarrhea, dyspepsia, and appetite loss
Escitalopram (lexapro) FDA approved 7+	Depression Anxiety	Same as above but better drug interaction profile	Same as above
Fluvoxamine FDA approved 8+	Major depressive disorder Obsessive-compulsive disorder	Increased risk of bleeding—NSAIDs, aspirin, warfarin	Same as above
Sertraline (zoloft) FDA approved 6+	Major depressive disorder Obsessive-compulsive disorder	Same as above Diet—may interact with grapefruit juice	Same as above
Serotonin Norepinephrine Reuptake Inhibitors (SNRIs)			
Duloxetine (cymbalta, Irenka) FDA approved 7+	Major depressive disorder Generalized anxiety disorder	Multiple drug interactions Risk for toxic levels—SSRIs, amphetamines, guanfacine (potentiates BP effects) Diet—avoid grapefruit juice and alcohol	Nausea, headache, dizziness, diaphoresis, and behavior activation
Venlafaxine (effexor XR) FDA approved 8+	Major depressive disorder Generalized anxiety disorder	Same as above	Same as above

health facility or a hospital. If the patient is at low risk for suicide, the provider can initiate treatment through outpatient modalities. There are several FDA-approved medications for depression in pediatrics (see Table 2). SSRIs are typically first-line treatment. Sertraline and fluoxetine are commonly prescribed as they can be prescribed safely at younger ages (6 years and 8 years, respectively). The evidence indicates that the best treatment responses result from a combination of CBT and SSRIs [8]. Medication maximum response can take 4 to 6 weeks to attain, but doses can be titrated every 2 to 4 weeks if significant side effects are absent [8]. Upon initiating antidepressant therapy, it is important to inform caregivers and patients that activation and mania can occur with antidepressant use. If any concerning symptoms arise, such as decreased impulse control, increased risk-taking behavior, and significantly elevated mood/mania, immediate follow-up is indicated. Providers should make contact with the patient or caregiver within 3 days of initiating pharmacotherapy and follow-up in the clinic weekly through the first 4 weeks of treatment [8]. Once stable, follow-ups should occur every 3 months or as needed for side effects and changes in symptoms [8].

The specialty of pediatrics is unique in that the patient includes the child, but also the family/caregiver and the environment in which the child lives. Therefore, it is crucial to involve the family in the treatment of pediatric mental health conditions. Individual CBT is indicated for children with mental health concerns, but family therapy is also beneficial. A study conducted by Inscoe and colleagues [10] indicated that caregiver involvement in trauma-informed mental health services led to better outcomes for children with co-occurring traumatic stress and suicidal thoughts and behaviors. The COVID-19 pandemic has caused trauma for many children and adolescents, leading to an increased prevalence of mental health issues and suicidal thoughts and behaviors. Therefore, obtaining trauma-informed mental health services for those patients could prove beneficial.

Health care providers may be the only mandated reporters that children and adolescents encounter regularly during the pandemic, so it is crucial to ask important questions and perform thorough physical examinations. Anticipatory guidance of developmental milestones should continue, and providers should also include strategies for fostering resilience in children and adolescents. The concept of resiliency is one that helps many at-risk youth overcome the obstacles that put them at risk for developing mental health problems and is largely determined by executive function and regulation. As Miller and colleagues [2] explain, schools incorporate executive function into their curricula. Executive function involves the processes responsible for regulating emotion, coordinating brain function, and influencing emotional expression to promote healthy social-emotional development and resilience. However, the alternate methods of teaching during the pandemic have limited the ability of the schools to teach those concepts well.

Families can also foster resilience in their children with a variety of positive methods. To promote resilience, it is important to empower children and caregivers to recognize, manage, and learn from their emotions [3]. This includes caregivers addressing their own mental health and substance use problems, modeling positive relationships, and promoting healthy and positive relationships between their children and others, social media, and technology [3]. Caregivers should be educated about the connection between mental health and physical health [2], and that toxic stress affects the long-term health of children and adolescents [3]. Providing thorough education to caregivers allows them to empower and instill resilience in their children.

Implications for advanced practice nurses
Health care providers are patient advocates and trusted professionals. One of the responsibilities of this role is to advocate for policies that promote well-being of the patients served. The evidence indicates a mental health crisis among American children and adolescents, and primary care providers serving this population should be involved in advocating for and promoting access to quality health care and mental health services [1,3]. There are emerging mental health concerns in children and adolescents since the onset of the pandemic. In using the appropriate interviewing strategies, screening tools, and diagnostic and management processes, advanced practice nurses can properly identify and treat the rapidly emerging mental health conditions among America's youth. In addition, the specialty knowledge that advanced practice nurses have regarding mental health and child development equip them to be advocates for enhanced coverage of pediatric mental health services. Many public medical insurances cover mental health services but there remain many private insurance policies that have limited coverage for mental health conditions. Access to care continues to be a barrier for children to obtain mental health services. Unfortunately, there are still many areas in America that lack mental health services for pediatric patients. Advocating for legislation that allows for advanced practice nurses to practice at the full scope of their certification and licensure can create opportunities for advanced practice nurses to serve this underserved population. The role of the advanced practice nurse in providing primary care for pediatric patients spans well beyond the physical health of the child. It is essential for advanced practice nurses to recognize the disparities in pediatric mental health and work diligently to diminish them.

SUMMARY

In conclusion, the literature shows an increase in the incidences of depression, anxiety, and suicidal behavior among children and adolescents [5,6]. This evidence supports the declaration of a national emergency in pediatric mental health. Primary care health care providers serving children and adolescents should know the risk factors, assessment strategies, and treatment modalities for pediatric mental health issues. Furthermore, pediatric health care providers should be aware of the increasing incidences of mental illness among American youth and advocate for the resources to combat this national emergency. Further research should be conducted to observe the efficacy of various mental health treatments in pediatric patients, advance the assessment tools available to screen for and diagnose mental health conditions in children and adolescents, and how the presentation and incidence of pediatric mental health issues change as the COVID-19 pandemic evolves.

CLINICS CARE POINTS

- In April 2022, a national emergency in children's mental health was declared in the United States [1].
- Due to an increase in environmental stressors, social isolations and shutdowns, many children and adolescents are experiencing increased incidences of mental health disorders during the COVID-19 pandemic.
- Emergency department visits for suicide attempts in adolescents aged 12-17 years increased by more than 50% from 2019 (pre-pandemic) to early 2021.
- Advanced practice nurses should be prepared to advocate for access to mental health services for all children and adolescents.
- Advanced practice nurses serving children and adolescents should be prepared to identify and treat emerging mental health conditions in children and adolescents, as well as provide the education and resources to help families and their children.

DISCLOSURE

The authors have nothing to disclose.

References

[1] Ray G. Pediatricians, child and adolescent psychiatrists and children's hospitals declare national emergency in children's mental health. Indiana State Nurse's Association; 2022. Available at: http://www.publications.nursingald.com/indiana-bulletin-february-2022/66246745/5. Accessed June 1, 2022.

[2] Miller R, Moran M, Shomaker LB, et al. Health effects of covid-19 for vulnerable adolescents in a randomized controlled trial. Sch Psychol 2021;36(5):293–302.

[3] Murthy VH. Protecting youth mental health. The U.S. Surgeon General's Advisory. 2021. Available at: http://www.hhs.gov/sites/default/files/surgeon-general-youth-mental-health-advisory.pdf. Accessed June 1, 2022.

[4] Centers for Disease Control and Prevention. New CDC data illuminate youth mental health threats during the covid-19 pandemic. CDC Newsroom Releases. 2022. Available at: https://www.cdc.gov/media/releases/2022/p0331-youth-mental-health-covid-19.html. Accessed June 21, 2022.

[5] Racine N, McArthur BA, Cooke JE, et al. Global prevalence of depressive and anxiety symptoms in children and adolescents during covid-19. JAMA Pediatr 2021; https://doi.org/10.1001/jamapediatrics.2021.2482.

[6] Hawes MT, Szenczy AK, Klein DN, et al. Increases in depression and anxiety symptoms in adolescents and young adults during the covid-19 pandemic. Psychol Med 2021; https://doi.org/10.1017/S0033291720005358.

[7] Gray H, Makowski A, Parrish E. From social distancing to social isolation: adolescent anxiety and the impact of covid-19. Kentucky Nurse; 2022. Available at: https://www.s3.amazonaws.com/nursing-network/production/files/109005/original/Kentucky_Nurse_March_2022.pdf?1647622250. Accessed June 1, 2022.

[8] Walter HJ, DeMaso DR. Psychosocial assessment and interviewing. In: Kliegman RM, St Geme JW, Blum NJ, et al, editors. Nelson textbook of pediatrics. Philadelphia, PA: Elsevier; 2020. p. 184–8.

[9] Zhang J, Zixiang Z, Zhang W. Intervention of research-based psychological counseling on adolescents' mental health during the covid-19 epidemic. Psychiatria Danubina 2021;33(2):209–16.

[10] Inscoe AB, Donisch K, Cheek S, et al. Trauma-informed care for youth suicide prevention: a qualitative analysis of caregivers' perspectives. Psychol Trauma Theor Res Pract Policy 2022;14(4):653–60.

[11] Garzon DL, Starr NB, Chauvin J. Neurodevelopmental, behavioral, and mental health disorders. In: Maaks DLG, Starr NB, Brady MA, et al, editors. Burns' pediatric primary care. Philadelphia, PA: Elsevier; 2020. p. 421–55.

[12] Walter HJ, DeMaso DR, Mood disorders, In: Kliegman RM, St Geme JW, Blum NJ. (Eds.), et al., Nelson textbook of pediatrics, Elsevier: Philadelphia, PA, 2020, pp. 217–224.

[13] Walter HJ, DeMaso DR. Suicide and attempted suicide. In: Kliegman RM, St Geme JW, Blum NJ, et al, editors. Nelson textbook of pediatrics. Philadelphia, PA: Elsevier; 2020. p. 225–8.

[14] Rosenberg DR, Chiriboga JA. Anxiety disorders. In: Kliegman RM, St Geme JW, Blum NJ, et al, editors. Nelson Textbook of Pediatrics. Elsevier: Philadelphia, PA; 2020. p. 211–6.

Advances in Family Practice Nursing 5 (2023) 255–266

ADVANCES IN FAMILY PRACTICE NURSING

Attention-Deficit/Hyperactivity Disorder Update 2022
New Medications Are Here!

Erin O'Connor Prange, MSN, CPNP-PC

Division of Neurology, Children's Hospital of Philadelphia, 3400 Civic Center Boulevard, 10th
Floor BGR, Philadelphia, PA 19104, USA

Keywords
- Stimulants • Methylphenidate • Amphetamine • Non-stimulants • Norepinephrine
- Dopamine

Key points
- New approved attention-deficit/hyperactivity disorder medications have the same mechanism of action but have different delivery systems.
- Extended-release options are available in liquid and capsules that can be opened to ease administration in patients who cannot swallow a tablet whole.
- With different layer coatings and time-released capsules and beads, some stimulant medications have a duration of up to 16 h.

D iagnosing and treating attention-deficit/hyperactivity disorder (ADHD) is a responsibility often shared among primary care, behavioral health, and neurology providers. Over the last 20 years, the incidence of ADHD in the pediatric population has increased from 6.1% in 1998 to 10.2% in 2016 with a steady increase across ethnic backgrounds. Non-Hispanic white children increased from 8.5 to 12.5%, non-Hispanic black children 5.5 to 9.6%, and Hispanic children 3.8 to 6.4% [1]. According to survey results published in 2018, 6.1 million children have been diagnosed with ADHD in the United States leading to a large need of providers who can provide quality care to manage this disorder [2]. Based on self-report questionnaires, approximately 57% of primary care clinicians report being responsible for diagnosis, manage, or co-manage this disorder [3]. With this increase in the prevalence of ADHD, there has also been an increase in available

---

E-mail address: prangee@chop.edu

https://doi.org/10.1016/j.yfpn.2022.11.015
2589-420X/23/© 2022 Elsevier Inc. All rights reserved.

medications approved by the US Food and Drug Administration (FDA). Over the last 10 years, 17 medications have been approved with seven of these added in the last five years alone. This explosion of newly approved ADHD medications has been welcomed by many providers; however, trying to discern what is the best medication for a specific patient can be daunting. The purpose of this article is to provide information about the new medications to help guide provider's decision-making.

MEDICATION OVERVIEW

The two broad categories of medication used to manage ADHD are stimulant and non-stimulant medications. Both categories directly impact catecholamine neurotransmitters that are active in several brain regions associated with ADHD symptoms. The two catecholamines targeted in ADHD treatment are norepinephrine and dopamine. Norepinephrine is a neurotransmitter that increases alertness and arousal, speeds up reaction time, increases the ability to concentrate, and positively affects mood. Dopamine is a neurotransmitter that directly impacts the pleasure and reward system in the brain which provides motivation and encourages repetition of desired behavior to improve attention, learning, cognitive function, and motor control.

The two classes of stimulant medications are methylphenidate products that block reuptake of norepinephrine and dopamine, and amphetamine products that promote release of dopamine and norepinephrine. Stimulant medications increase norepinephrine and dopamine in the synapse to decrease hyperactivity and impulsivity and improve inattention. There is strong evidence that stimulant medications are effective in managing elementary school-aged and adolescent patients with ADHD [4]. Non-stimulant medications selectively inhibit the reuptake of norepinephrine which secondarily increases norepinephrine in the synapse with little to no effect on other neurotransmitters. Although there is also evidence showing efficacy in treating ADHD symptoms such as hyperactivity and inattention with the non-stimulants, its effect size is less in comparison to stimulants [4].

Stimulant medications have been used for ADHD for over 60 years and some non-stimulants for over 20 years. The benefit of most newly approved medications is that they vary in terms of their delivery system and provide extended symptom control. The prolonged duration decreases the need for booster doses later in the day which can result in mood changes as shorter acting medications wear off and boosters have not yet taken effect. The variability in duration and delivery systems offers the provider more options to meet individual patient needs.

Short-acting stimulants have about 4-h duration of effectiveness, intermediate-acting stimulants have a 5 to 10 h duration of effectiveness, and the newer medications have up to 16 h of effectiveness. With early start times for middle and high school students, this author has many patients who report intermediate-acting medication wear off by the afternoon and they struggle with homework, after-school activities, sports, and after-school jobs. For that reason, many patients require a short-acting stimulant referred to as a "booster" given at lunch or after school to support these afternoon and evening activities. Unfortunately, when intermediate-acting stimulants wear off in the afternoon and booster doses have not yet taken effect, many patients report mood dysregulation. The booster stimulant can also suppress appetite around dinner exacerbating weight loss concerns in a subset of patients. Booster dosing in afternoon can make it more difficult for patients to fall asleep. Therefore, although the combination of intermediate-lasting stimulants and boosters has been used for years, this author has found that the availability of the newly approved longer acting medications decreases the need for boosters and improves tolerability while providing coverage throughout the whole day. Also, all medications have the potential of side effects so increasing the number of medications approved for use, offers the provider more choices for a patient who is not tolerating a specific medication.

Choosing stimulant versus non-stimulant medication

Open dialogue with patients and families, reviewing side effects and pharmacokinetics facilitates the decision-making process to start a stimulant versus a non-stimulant medication. Stimulant medications can suppress appetite and lead to weight loss or mild growth suppression; therefore, a non-stimulant would be the preferred first option for a child who is underweight or has a history of growth failure. Stimulant medications also can exacerbate an underlying tic disorder, so the provider needs to weigh the risks versus benefits of starting a stimulant medication in a patient with co-morbid tics or Tourette's syndrome. Although tics are not a contraindication to using a stimulant medication, if the patient is medication naïve, this author would suggest starting with a non-stimulant. If a non-stimulant medication is ineffective in managing the ADHD symptoms, then the provider could consider transitioning to a stimulant medication and educate the family to reach out if tics increase in frequency or severity and are interfering with the patient's function.

Onset of sleep can be affected by stimulant medication use. If a young child already has trouble falling asleep, this author recommends starting with a non-stimulant medication, such as clonidine which is FDA approved for the treatment of ADHD and can be helpful with sleep onset [5]. Clonidine, however, in this author's opinion may not provide adequate treatment of ADHD symptoms throughout the day, specifically for older patients so be aware that preexisting sleep issues are not a contraindication to stimulant use.

Unmanaged ADHD can lead to hyperactivity and decreased ability to settle to fall asleep, so some parents report improvement in bedtime routine and sleep onset after stimulant medication has been initiated. Therefore, sleep concerns are not a contraindication to stimulant medication, but rather another point for discussion. By discussing risks and benefits with the patient and family, an educated decision regarding medication choice can be made. In addition, the importance of observation and follow-up needs to be reviewed with the patient and family so that ADHD medication can be adjusted appropriately with a goal of maximum efficacy with tolerable side effects [4].

After discussion, if the recommendation is to start a stimulant, the provider should take a thorough cardiac history of both the patient and family before prescribing this medication. If the patient has a history of cardiac diseases such as structural abnormalities or ventricular arrhythmias or if there is a family history of sudden death, Wolff-Parkinson-White syndrome, cardiomyopathy, or prolonged QT, the provider needs to weigh the risks and benefits of stimulant medication use and strongly consider ordering an electrocardiogram (ECG or EKG) before initiation of stimulant medication [4].

Choosing methylphenidate versus amphetamines in a stimulant naïve patients

Because both classes of stimulants, methylphenidate, and amphetamines, are similar in their mechanism of action and side effect profile, the decision regarding which stimulant medication to start in a stimulant naïve patient depends on the age of patient, available dose formulation, and insurance coverage. There is no current method to determine which stimulant will be more effective for a given patient at onset of treatment [4]. A good starting point for the provider is to review which medications are FDA approved for the age of the patient to be treated, then determine which of these have formulations that the patient is able to take. This will guide the discussion with the patient and family regarding medication choices. Choosing a formulation the child is willing and able to take can increase compliance, which in turn improves their outcome. Lastly, the provider or family can check with the insurance to determine if the medication is covered and what tier it is classified. For some families, even if the insurance covers the medication, the copay for name-brand stimulant medications can be cost-prohibitive. In this case, the provider can research co-pay assistance offers from pharmaceutical companies which provide a cost-effective way to trial a medication to determine its effectiveness and tolerability. This information can inform the appeal to the insurance company for coverage of the chosen stimulant medication.

New amphetamine products

The newest amphetamine products to be released are Adzenys, Dyanavel, and Mydais. Adzenys was approved in 2016 for patients aged 6 years and older and is effective for about 13 h. It is available in suspension and oral disintegrating tablets providing options for patients who cannot/will not swallow a tablet or when greater titration control is desired. The oral disintegrating tablets should not be crushed or chewed but allowed to dissolve in the mouth [6]. Dyanavel was approved in 2015 for patients aged 6 years and older and has 13-h duration of effectiveness. It is available in a suspension and chewable tablet [7]. Mydayis was approved in 2017 for patients aged 13 years and older with duration of effectiveness up to 16 h. It is available in a capsule that can be swallowed whole or opened and contents sprinkled on food [8]. Refer to Table 1 for

Table 1
Newly approved attention deficit/hyperactivity disorder medications: quick reference

Name	Class	FDA	Min Age	Onset	Peak	Duration	Formulation	Open/ Crush
Adzenys ER	Amphetamine	2016	6 yr	1 h	5 h	13 h	Suspension	N/A
Adzenys ODT	Amphetamine	2016	6 yr	1 h	5 h	13 h	ODT	No
Dyanavel	Amphetamine	2015	6 yr	1 h	4.5 h	13 h	Suspension	N/A
Mydayis	Amphetamine	2017	13 yr	2 h	7 to 10 h	16 h	Capsule	Yes
Cotempla	Methylphenidate	2017	6 yr	1 h	4.5 h	12 h	ODT	No
Aptensio	Methylphenidate	2015	6 yr	1 h	2 h and 8 h	12 h	Capsule	Yes
Jornay	Methylphenidate	2019	6 yr	10 h	14 h	18 h	Capsule	Yes
Qelbree	Nonstimulant	2021	6 yr	2 days	5 h	16- 24 h	Capsule	No

author's quick reference guide of these medications. Refer to Table 2 for links to drug websites for full dosing and prescribing information [6–11].

New methylphenidate products
The newest methylphenidate products are Aptensio, Cotempla, and Jornay. Aptensio was FDA approved in 2015 for patients aged 6 years and older and has 12-h duration of effectiveness. Aptensio is available in capsule form that can be swallowed whole or opened and sprinkled on food [9]. Cotempla was approved in 2017 for patients aged 6 years and older with 12-h duration of effectiveness. It is available as an oral disintegrating tablet which should not be crushed or chewed. Rather the tablet should be allowed to dissolve in the mouth [10]. Jornay was FDA approved in 2019 for ages 6 years and older with 18-h duration. It is the first delayed release formulation indicated to take before bed with onset of action about 10 hours later providing early morning effectiveness. It is available in capsule form that can be swallowed whole or opened and sprinkled on food [11]. Refer to Table 1 for author's quick

Table 2
Resource links

ADHD Medication Guide	The ADHD Medication Guide
Adzenys	Adzenys XR-ODT (adzenysxrodt.com)
Aptensio	Aptensio XR: Package Insert/Prescribing Information— Drugs.com
Cotempla	Cotempla XR-ODT: Package Insert/Prescribing Information - Drugs.com
Dyanavel	Dyanavel XR: Uses, Dosage & Side Effects - Drugs.com
Jornay	JORNAY PM® (methylphenidate HCl) l Official Patient Site
Mydayis	MYDAYIS® (mixed salts of a single-entity amphetamine product)
Quelbree	https://www.qelbree.com

reference of these medications. Refer to Table 2 [6-11] for links to drug-specific websites for full dosing and prescribing information.

New non-stimulant products
A newly approved non-stimulant that does not adversely affect sleep onset is Qelbree. This is the first FDA-approved non-stimulant medication for use in the treatment of ADHD symptoms in over a decade [12]. This non-stimulant medication is approved for patients aged 6 years and older and is available in a capsule formulation that can be opened and sprinkled on food [13]. Steady state is reached within two days of consecutive use. Owing to risk of hypertensive crisis, Qelbree should not be used in patients taking monoamine oxidase inhibitors (MAOI) or within 14 days of stopping an MAOI [13].

Changing stimulant medication
When the provider needs to consider a medication change, they should think about "the why" to determine if a change in medication class is necessary versus changing to an alternative formulation within the same class. For example, if the patient is doing well on Concerta in terms of side effects and effectiveness but duration of effectiveness is not long enough, it is prudent to stay in the same methylphenidate class but choose a longer acting medication such as Cotempla. Alternatively, if the patient tried Aptensio and is experiencing mood lability but duration of effectiveness is appropriate, the provider should consider transitioning the child to an amphetamine product with similar duration of effectiveness such as Mydayis. In summary, if the child is tolerating the chosen medication well but the duration of effectiveness is not optimal, the provider should move through the formulations within that stimulant category before switching to an alternative class. If the stimulant medication does not have an adequate duration of effectiveness or side effects limit the patient or family's use of the medication, the provider should consider switching the stimulant medication to an alternative class. Having a list of all available FDA-approved ADHD medications can be very helpful when making these decisions. Reference Figs. 1 and 2 for a comprehensive overview of all the stimulant medications available as of August 2022 [14].

Managing side effects
Although there are many new stimulant medications that have been approved, they have similar side effect profiles to the stimulant medications that have been available for years. The most common side effects include decreased appetite, difficulty sleeping, and mood dysregulation. Strattera and Quelbree have a black box warning for suicidal ideation. Implementation of strategies to mitigate side effects for 4-6 weeks should be trialed to support the decision to continue or discontinue the medication.

Decrease in appetite
Stimulant medications increase dopamine that suppresses appetite. Therefore, it is highly likely that a child will have a decreased appetite during the effective duration of the medication. Managing the side effects of decreased appetite, poor weight gain, and growth suppression includes patient and family

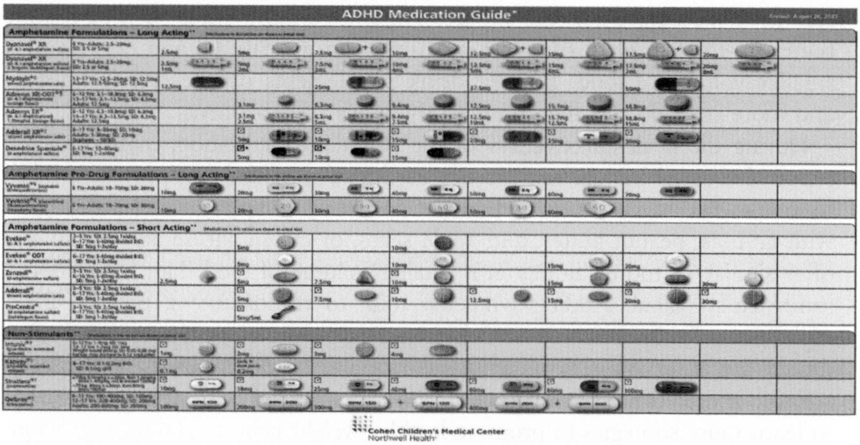

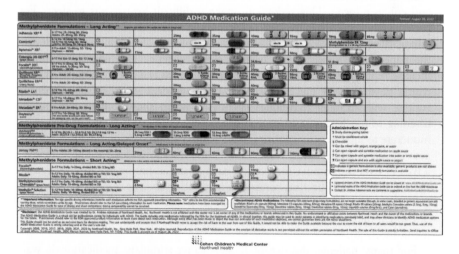

Fig. 1. ADHD amphetamine and non-stimulant medication guide. (*From Cohen Children's Medical Center. ADHD Medication Guide. August 2022 via* http://www.adhdmedicationguide.com/.)

education regarding increasing nutrient-dense foods, snack strategies, and appetite-enhancing medications.

Providing patients with a list of nutrient-dense foods such as nuts, trail mix, whole-fat yogurt, cheese, avocados, cream cheese, and supplemental shakes/ meal replacement drinks can be helpful. Advising patients to eat breakfast before they take their stimulant medication in the morning can ensure adequate

Fig. 2. ADHD methylphenidate medication guide. (*From Cohen Children's Medical Center. ADHD Medication Guide. August 2022 via* http://www.adhdmedicationguide.com/.)

caloric intake before appetite suppression is a concern. Ideas such as peanut butter on toast in place of cereal with milk can increase fat and calories in a smaller volume of food. Powder drink supplements can be calorie-building and more cost-effective than most ready-to-drink supplements.

During the peak effectiveness of the stimulant medication, many patients report decreased hunger and do not eat lunch at school but may be willing to snack. Packing a lunch with items such as cheese and crackers, yogurt with granola, peanut butter, and apple slices, or cream cheese and celery can offer similar or more calories in a smaller volume of food than a traditional sandwich or salad. Adding whole-fat milk to reconstitute a powder meal replacement for breakfast or adding ice cream to a protein shake as a treat after dinner are other ways to increase calories and support growth. Consider a referral to a dietician or nutritionist who can work with the child and family to learn more strategies to promote healthy weight gain.

If these interventions alone do not promote weight gain, in the author's experience, medications like cyproheptadine can be used concurrently to enhance appetite. Cyproheptadine is an antihistamine medication available in liquid and tablet form that can enhance appetite and support efforts to gain weight. Dosing schedules vary but starting around 0.25 mg/kg/day divided twice daily or 2 mg twice daily, whichever is lower, and increase as needed and tolerated to max of 8 to 12 mg per day can be tried [15]. Although adding a second medication to treat the side effects of the first medication is not ideal, this should be considered if the risks and benefits are discussed with the patient and family and benefits of staying on the stimulant medication are substantial.

Sleep disturbance
Stimulant medications act on the central nervous system to increase alertness and enhance focus. This action can make it difficult for patients to sleep. For patients who experience the benefits of stimulant medication but have difficulty falling asleep, the provider should assess the patient's sleep routine and educate the patient and family about healthy sleep hygiene. This education should include reminders of no electronics 2 hours before bed and removing all electronic devices from the bedroom to promote sleep. A consistent bedtime routine with calming techniques such as a warm shower, light reading, or listening to music can be helpful in promoting sleep onset. Encourage regular moderate to intense activity throughout the day to provide an outlet for hyperactivity can also be helpful. When lifestyle modifications alone are not effective, a trial of over-the-counter medication such as melatonin or magnesium can be tried. If these are ineffective, consider a medication such as clonidine. Clonidine is FDA approved for ADHD but can also help with sleep onset and decrease in tics which makes it a versatile medication to use in conjunction with stimulant medications [5].

For many patients, the use of longer acting stimulant medication is warranted to promote school success and support healthy self-esteem, so adding a medication to manage side effects may be worthwhile. Cyproheptadine has a side effect of fatigue so in the author's opinion, administering this medication at night can help with sleep onset in patients who struggle with sleep, in addition to its appetite-enhancing effect, as noted above.

Tics

The dopamine increase that occurs with stimulant medication can exacerbate tics in some patients, but this is not a contradiction for use. Patients with tics or Tourette's syndrome who experience an increase in tics after the initiation of a stimulant medication but report effectiveness in the management of their ADHD symptoms should consider *Cognitive-Behavioral Intervention for Tics* (CBIT). CBIT helps patients identify the urge before they tic and teaches the patient strategies to stop or change the tic. If this is ineffective and tics are interfering with the quality of life, this author recommends referral to neurology to consider pharmacologic management. The goal of therapy is to decrease tics to promote quality of life, but complete resolution of tics is not always realistic. Educating the patient and family regarding this goal is necessary to manage the expectation for this treatment.

Black box warning for suicidal ideation

Non-stimulant medications are not without concerns. Strattera and Quelbree have a black box warning for suicidal ideation which needs to be discussed with the patient and family before starting treatment. The provider needs to consider the patient's history in relation to depression and suicidal ideations or attempts. If risks and benefits are discussed with the patient and family, and the provider recommends starting one of the non-stimulant medications, the patient should have regular surveillance with a therapist or frequent follow-up with the prescribing provider. For example, the provider may consider asking the family to send weekly emails providing an update on effectiveness and mood as well as monthly follow-up visits with the prescribing provider if they are not under the care of a therapist. If the patient is seeing a therapist, the provider may consider requesting a phone call, email, or letter from the therapist every 2-4 weeks during initiation of the non-stimulant medication until dosing is stable and the therapist is satisfied that there are no concerns for suicidal thoughts or attempts.

Implication for advanced practice nurses. Staying up to date with new medication options is pivotal in providing cutting-edge care to patients. Recent shifts to online learning during COVID, self-directed learning, and more independent work make it more important than ever to support patients with shortened attention spans and hyperactivity. With seven new FDA-approved medications for use in pediatrics over the last five years, understanding the pharmacokinetics and side effects helps the provider offer optimal treatment options for their patients.

Choosing which medications to use should be a discussion between the provider, patient, and their family. Key questions to focus on during the history should target determining the needs and expectations of the patient and family.

What are the most problematic symptoms and what causes the most barriers in feeling successful academically, socially, and personally? Does the patient have after-school activities, work, or evening commitments that require a longer acting medication? For these patients, choosing medications that last 12+ h would be beneficial (Refer to Table 1). Does the patient have co-morbid tics, anxiety, or risk of abuse in the home where a non-stimulant medication such as Clonidine or Qelbree should be considered first? Are mornings particularly difficult resulting in tardiness to school/work or increased stress on other family members where a nighttime dosing of a delayed release stimulant such as Jornay may be beneficial? Having an open discussion with the patient and family reviewing the risks and benefits of each drug is critical in finding the best medication to increase compliance and meet the family and patient's outcome expectations.

After a medication has been initiated, the author recommends follow-up every 4 to 6 weeks while dosing is being adjusted and then every 3 to 6 months for routine surveillance to assess tolerability and effectiveness. The use of telehealth has expanded in many areas since the start of the COVID pandemic and can provide better access to connecting with patients more frequently while limiting their time missed from school. In this author's experience, patients have the option to complete telehealth visits from their car with the parent in the school parking lot which can decrease time missed from school to 20 min rather than an hour or more for a traditional office visit due to travel time. Once the patient is stable on a medication, routine surveillance in 3 months and then every 3 to 6 months over the first year is helpful so that adjustments can be made to maximize efficacy while monitoring issues such as weight, sleep, and school performance. ADHD follow-up scales such as the *Vanderbilt Follow-up Assessment*, which is a brief 18-question rating scale for parents and teachers, can provide an objective means to monitor effectiveness, ongoing need for therapy, and evidence to escalate or change therapy [16]. This author recommends these assessment forms be completed each time medication is changed or at least once yearly.

Questions to focus on during follow-up visits should include asking if the patient is experiencing trouble falling asleep at night, decrease in appetite, mood changes, or increase in tics since these are commonly reported side effects. If these are problematic, a shorter acting agent such as an intermediate release like metadate, Focalin XR, or Adderall XR (see Fig. 2) may be better tolerated than one of the new longer acting formulations because the intermediate medications typically wear off in the afternoon allowing the patient to eat dinner and fall asleep easier.

SUMMARY

In conclusion, with ADHD diagnoses on the rise, all providers are likely to be faced with the opportunity to diagnose and manage patients with this disorder. By educating providers regarding the benefits, side effects, and differences of each medication available, they can feel empowered to manage this chronic disorder to improve patient and family experience and promote school success.

Effectively differentiating between the categories of medications and delivery systems available, providers can partner with patients to individually determine which medication to use. It is vital that primary care providers stay up to date on the newest medications available as access to child psychiatrists and behavioral health specialists are becoming more difficult.

CLINICS CARE POINTS

- FDA-approved medications should be prescribed for school aged children with ADHD along with behavioral and classroom accomodations (4)
- ADHD medications should be titrated with a goal of maxium efficacy and tolerable side effects (4)

DISCLOSURES
The author has nothing to disclose.

References
[1] Children and Adults with Attention Deficit Disorder (CHADD). ADHD Data and Statistics. General Prevalence of ADHD. 2022. Available at: https://chadd.org/about-adhd/general-prevalence.
[2] Danielson ML, Bitsko RH, Ghandour RM, et al. Prevalence of Parent-Reported ADHD Diagnosis and Associated Treatment Among US Children and Adolescents, 2016. J Clin Child Adolesc Psychol 2018; https://doi.org/10.1080/15374416.2017.1417860.
[3] Stein REK, Storfer-Isser A, Kerker BD, et al. Beyond ADHD: how well are we doing? Acad Pediatr 2016;16(2):115–21.
[4] Wolraich ML, Hagan JF, Allan C, et al. Clinical Practice Guideline for the Diagnosis, Evaluation and Treatment of Attention-Deficit/Hyperactivty Disorder in Children and Adolescents. Pediatrics 2019;144(4). Available at: https://publications.aap.org/pediatrics/article/144/4/e20192528/81590/Clinical-Practice-Guideline-for-the-Diagnosis.
[5] Nguyen M, Tharani S, Rahmani M, et al. A review of the use of clonidine as a sleep aid in the child and adolescent population. Clin Pediatr 2014;53(3):211–6.
[6] Aytu BioPharma. Adzenys. 2021. Available at: https://www.drugs.com/dyanavel-xr.html.
[7] Stewart J. Dyanavel. Drugs.com. 2021. Available at: https://www.drugs.com/dyanavel-xr.html.
[8] Takeda Pharmaceuticals. Mydais. 2022. Available at: https://www.mydayis.com.
[9] Drugs.com. Aptensio. 2021. Available at: https://www.drugs.com/pro/aptensio-xr.html.
[10] Stewart J. Cotempla. Drugs.com. 2014. Available at: https://www.drugs.com/pro/cotempla-xr-odt.html.
[11] Ironshore Pharmaceuticals. Jornay. Available at: https://www.jornaypm.com.
[12] Associated Press. FDA approves 1st new ADHD drug for kids in over a decade. Today. 2021. Available at: https://www.today.com/health/what-qelbree-fda-approves-new-adhd-drug-kids.
[13] Supernus Pharmaceuticals. Qelbree. Available at: https://www.qelbree.com.

[14] Cohen Children's Medical Center. ADHD Medication Guide. 2022. Available at: http://www.adhdmedicationguide.com/.

[15] Harrison ME, Norris ML, Robinson A, et al. Use of cyproheptadine to stimulate appetite and body weight gain: A systematic review. Appetite 2019;137:62–72.

[16] Vanderbilt Scales. Available at: https://www.nichq.org/sites/default/files/resource-file/NICHQ-Vanderbilt-Assessment-Scales.pdf.

Advances in Family Practice Nursing 5 (2023) 267–281

Primary Care Management of Autonomic Dysfunction

June Bryant, DNP, APRN, CPNP-PC

Department of Nursing, University of Tampa, 400 North Ashley Drive, Suite 1900, Tampa, FL 33602, USA

Keywords

- Autonomic dysfunction • Primary care • Dysautonomia • Therapeutic management
- Long-COVID

Key points

- Autonomic dysfunction (AD) presents heterogeneously throughout the life span leaving many advanced practice nurses feeling uncomfortable with accurately diagnosing and managing those with this condition.
- Recognition of AD symptoms as they present in our patients leads to better quality of life due to early management, including pharmacologic and non-pharmacological therapies, specialists' consults, and lifestyle recommendations.
- Symptom acknowledgment is sometimes just as important as diagnosis because countless patients feel hopeless after many trips to health-care providers and specialists to have their symptoms dismissed or misdiagnosed.

INTRODUCTION

Autonomic dysfunction (AD) in the primary care setting can often be masked by other conditions or met with provider bias due to subjectivity of symptoms. Without specific diagnostic test markers, underdiagnosis or misdiagnosis is common in those conditions that fall under the umbrella of dysautonomia. Dysfunction of the autonomic nervous system (ANS) can present with symptoms starting at birth (such as development failure), extending through adolescence and adulthood (such as after viral onset) and into the geriatric years (as with neurodegenerative diseases; Table 1). Symptoms of dysautonomia depend on the location and the type of AD and can present heterogeneously, spontaneously, and develop from multiple body systems. The ability for the primary care provider to recognize these symptoms at all stages of life is imperative to

E-mail address: jbryant@ut.edu

https://doi.org/10.1016/j.yfpn.2022.11.010
2589-420X/23/© 2022 Elsevier Inc. All rights reserved.

Table 1
Types of dysautonomia and their characteristics

Dysautonomia presentations throughout the life span	
Examples of Types of Dysautonomia	Top 3 Notable Characteristics
Pediatric Onset	*Disruption in development of autonomic nervous system
	Familial dysautonomia
	• Impaired pain
	• Impaired temperature sensation
	• Blood pressure instability
	Phenylketonuria (PKU)
	• Low birth weight
	• Microcephaly
	• Behavior problems
	• Convulsions
	Menkes disease
	• Sparse kinky hair
	• Failure to thrive
	• Dry Skin
	Hereditary sensory and autonomic neuropathy (HSAN)
	• Inflamed fingers and toes
	• Numbness and tingling in hands and feet
	• Impaired temperature sensation
	Congenital central hypoventilation syndrome (CCHS)
	• Shallow breathing
	• Cardiac systoles
	• Hirschsprung disease
	Catecholaminergic polymorphic ventricular tachycardia (CPVT)
	• Lightheadness
	• Palpitations
	• Loss of consciousness
	Hirschsprung disease
	• Protruding abdomen
	• Vomiting/diarrhea
	• Delayed meconium passage
Adolescent/ adult onset	*Functional changes in the autonomic nervous system
	POTS
	• Difficulty standing still
	• Fatigue
	• Lightheadedness
	• Brain fog/mental clouding
	Autonomically mediated syncope (vasovagal syncope)
	• Seizures
	• Orthostatic
	• Hypotension
	• Decrease in heart rate and blood pressure
Geriatric onset	*Results from degeneration of the nerves
	Multiple system atrophy (MSA)
	• Loss of muscle control
	• Loss of bladder control

(continued on next page)

Table 1 (continued)		
Dysautonomia presentations throughout the life span		
PAF	• Erectile dysfunction • Orthostatic hypotension • Visual disturbances • Impotence	

*indicates the causes of the onset of AD.

decrease the burden of the diagnosis and enhance every AD patient's quality of life. Management of the condition also depends on the severity of the AD, the form and the symptoms that are present. This article will provide a broad overview of the common types of AD presenting in the primary care setting, how providers should recognize, diagnose, and manage these types of AD, as well as when and what patients should be referred out.

PATHOPHYSIOLOGY

As a broad overview, the nervous system is divided into the central nervous system (CNS) including the brain and spinal cord, and the peripheral nervous system, which comprises the motor and sensory branches, where the motor branch houses the somatic nervous system and the ANS. The ANS controls involuntary functions, such as digestion, temperature regulation, and cardiac ability. AD occurs when all or part of the ANS is not functioning properly and can be a primary dysregulation from a disruption in the ANS itself or the ANS reacting to a primary problem as commonly seen in diabetes or Parkinson disease. Failure of or an overreaction of the sympathetic and parasympathetic nervous systems leads to AD. The pathophysiology of AD is not fully understood; however, AD leads to activation of the sympathetic nervous system and excessive catecholamine (such as epinephrine and norepinephrine) release, which causes hypertension, tachycardia, tachypnea, diaphoresis, and hyperthermia [1].

HISTORY

Onset of AD can begin at birth due to the failure of the autonomic system to develop properly, as seen with familial dysautonomia; between puberty and adulthood, as seen with postural orthostatic tachycardia syndrome (POTS) or autonomically mediated syncope; and in the geriatric population that presents due to neurodegenerative disease as seen with multiple system atrophy or pure autonomic failure (PAF). Recognizing the age of onset of symptoms is one of the first steps in aiding to identify the type of AD.

The presenting chief complaint or symptom may not be as simple as a single problem. Dysautonomias are multifactorial and heterogeneous in presentation. Most patients present with symptoms that are neurologic, cardiovascular, or gastrointestinal. Understanding that many of the symptoms manifest in these

System	Symptoms
Cardiovascular	tachycardia, bradycardia, hypotension, exercise intolerance, shortness of breath
Neurological	fatigue, syncope, dizziness, anxiety, mood changes, disrupted sleep, brain fog, temperature dysregulation, migraines
Gastrointestinal	gastroesophageal reflux, dysphagia, nausea, vomiting, bloating, diarrhea, gastroparesis

Fig. 1. Common symptoms of dysautonomias.

3 body systems can help the advanced practice nurse (APN) focus their history taking to make the visit more efficient. The reader is referred to Fig. 1 for information on the common system-specific symptoms of dysautonomia. Because there are several symptoms that present more frequently than others, APNs asking questions surrounding these specific symptoms may be beneficial. For this reason, the reader is referred to Fig. 2 for the top 7 signs and symptoms of AD.

APNs have access to a variety of tools to enhance history taking for patients with suspected dysautonomia. Mayo Clinic created an 84-question self-assessment tool for identifying ANS dysfunction symptom severity called *Compass 31* [2]. This assessment tool screens patients aged as young as 8 years on 6 domains of dysfunction including orthostatic intolerance, gastrointestinal, vasomotor, secretomotor, bladder, and pupillomotor [2]. The *Dysautonomia Project*

difficulty standing still	fatigue
lightheadedness	nausea and other GI symptoms
brain fog mental clouding	palpitations/chest discomfort
shortness of breath/difficulty breathing	

Fig. 2. Top 7 signs and symptoms of autonomic dysfunction. (*Adapted from* Freeman, K, Goldstein, DS, Thompson, CR. The Dysautonomia Project: Understanding autonomic system disorders for physicians and patients. Bardolf & Company; 2015; with permission.)

Table 2
Guide for taking an autonomic history

Chief Complaint	In a few words, what is the main problem bothering you that brings you here today?
History of present illness	When was the last time you felt completely healthy?
	What was the first thing that went wrong?
	What happened next?
	Have you noticed anything that makes the problem worse or better?
	What treatments have been tried, and how did you respond?
	(Note: These questions only cover some aspects of autonomic screening.)
Autonomic Review of Systems	Who does your shopping?
	Are you able to tolerate standing, exercise, heat, a large meal?
	Do you sweat like other people?
	Do you make spit like other people?
	Have you noticed any problems with urination?
	Have you noticed any problems with bowel movements?
	Have you noticed any problems with sexual function?
Prescribed or OTC medications and supplements	(Make note of any which may affect hemodynamics and/or main chemical messengers of the ANS such as NE, EPI, and/or Ach.)
Past Hx	
Family Hx	
Personal and soical Hx	
Physical examination	Water bottle sign?
	Signs of pooling of blood in feet? Cyanosis, dependent edema?
Orthostatic vitals test	Normal/abnormal?

(From Freeman, K, Goldstein, DS, Thompson, CR. The Dysautonomia Project: Understanding autonomic system disorders for physicians and patients. Bardolf & Company; 2015; with permission)

tool provides APNs with a fillable instrument to guide them to taking a complete autonomic history [3]. This history-taking tool is appropriate for patient of any age, and the parent can complete the form to report subjective symptoms in their children [3]. The reader is referred to Table 2 for the guide to taking an autonomic history.

ASSESSMENT
Important elements of history taking
Because of the heterogenous presentation of AD, APNs should approach the history component similar to that of a typical sick visit. However, the history may be very complex and need to occur during multiple visits to help narrow the differential diagnosis. Understanding the ANS pathophysiology is important when determining the proper questions to ask a patient. For example, the ANS is responsible for regulating breathing, blood pressure, heart rate, digestion, excretions, and sexual arousal. The pertinent questions that the

APN needs to ask as part of the review of systems (ROS) include episodes of dizziness or syncope, decreases or increases in heart rate when standing up, nausea, diarrhea, constipation or gastroparesis, fatigue, shortness of breath, anxiety, brain fog, sensory sensitivity, and disruptions in sleep. Additionally, the ROS should include the patient's diet history, weight history, past medical history, surgical history, current medications, prescription and over the counter, and supplements.

History of present illness

Asking about the onset of symptoms is important with AD to determine the timeline and sequence of symptoms. Because many types of dysautonomia present in different ages, identifying the timeline when symptoms first started or when the patient last felt "healthy" is important to the final diagnosis. Aggravating factors are also important to elicit because different environmental/emotional situations may exacerbate symptoms. For example, stress exacerbates POTS symptoms by increasing catecholamine release, which then leads to a spiral of autonomic symptoms. The waxing and waning of symptoms contribute to confusion in the history making it difficult for the APN to formulate a differential diagnosis list that includes AD. [4]. Common signs and symptoms that present with AD patients usually stem from 3 body systems: cardiovascular, neurologic, and gastrointestinal. Fig. 1 includes an expanded symptom list by system. Of note, 85% of adult patients and 91% of children with familial dysautonomia have some degree of sleep-disordered breathing, which includes low pulse oximetry (SpO_2) and low end-tidal capnography ($EtCO_2$) that can lead to sudden unexpected death in sleep [5].

Past medical history

Determining the possible presence of coexisting conditions is important for an accurate diagnosis. Rather than strictly focusing on the ROS related to the chief complaint, it is beneficial for the APN to complete an extensive review of history in determining the final diagnosis because a recent viral illness or coexisting autoimmune disorders could be clues to a possible trigger of the AD symptomology. Diabetes and the associated autonomic neuropathy, autoimmune disorders, Ehlers Danlos syndrome (EDS), mast cell activation syndrome, and depression are highly correlated to the diagnosis of dysautonomia.

Trigger identification

In adolescent or adult-onset AD, the history of viral illness such as Epstein Barr virus, hepatitis C virus, human immunodeficiency virus, or coronavirus-19 (COVID-19) supports the diagnosis of AD. [6]. In these cases, patients will contract the illness and will never truly feel recovered as the APN would typically suspect. Head injuries, concussions, cardiac arrest, brain tumors, and CNS infections are also common precursor to the onset of AD. Typically, the presence of symptoms of AD occurs within the first several weeks of injury [7]. Provocative triggers that exacerbate AD symptoms include emotional or physical stressors. Some of these triggers may include emotional stress (good or bad), pain, atmospheric stress (high heat, changes in barometric pressure), or physical stress (standing over a hot stovetop in the kitchen, standing in a warm shower, long walks, or trips to theme parks).

DIAGNOSIS

There is much variability in the types of testing that can be performed to support the diagnosis of AD. Most of these tests are performed at autonomic laboratories or centers that primary care providers can refer to if the case is difficult or more severe. Autonomic laboratories are performed by autonomic medicine specialists, advanced practice providers with training specifically in AD, nurses, neurodiagnostic technologists, and physicists. Physiologic testing such as orthostatic vitals, tilt table testing, or environmental changes (changing the temperature) may aid in the diagnosis and recognition of AD. Neuropharmacological tests include giving a provocative medication that may lead to a response on a physiologic measure or biochemical measure. Neurochemical tests measure the amount of catecholamines under rest as a baseline and then in response to stressors. Reliable neuroimaging tests can be hard to pinpoint, and there are no accepted neuroimaging tests that can be used to visualize parasympathetic nerves [8]. Testing is individualized based on the patient's AD type and the ability of the center that is conducting the testing. Depending on the type and severity of dysautonomia, diagnosis and management plans may be left up to the primary APN or referred to an autonomic specialist.

To quantify autonomic severity and distribution, many providers will use the validated *Composite Autonomic Severity Score* (CASS) [9]. This tool assesses the symptoms in 3 subdomains including sudomotor (sweat test), cardiovagal (response to tilt table testing including deep breathing and Valsalva maneuver), and adrenergic (blood pressure responses to Valsalva maneuver). CASS ranges from 0 to 10, with 0 to 3 indicated mild AD and 7 to 10 with severe autonomic failure. This scale can be used across the life span from school-aged children to the elderly [9]. The Valsalva maneuver and tilt table testing are 2 hallmark assessments that provide complementary information about autonomic responses.

Valsalva maneuver

The Valsalva maneuver includes forced expiration against resistance of at least 40 mm Hg for 15 seconds while the patient is in a sitting position [10]. This indirect measurement of adrenergic activity detects changes in sympathetically medicated blood pressure. Straining, by the means of forced expiration as exampled above, "bearing down" or a cold stimulant to the patients face, increases the intrathoracic pressure therefore decreasing cardiac preload [11]. The Valsalva maneuver is especially useful as a noninvasive measurement of adrenergic stability, especially when determining cardiovascular vagal and AD.

Tilt table testing

Tilt table testing has been used for more than 50 years to evaluate the autonomic response to positional changes, as well as hemodynamic and neuroendocrine responses to heart failure, hypertension, and orthostatic hypotension [12]. Although tilt table testing is known as the gold standard for diagnosis of some AD conditions, such as POTS, the test does not necessarily provide additional information about other disease processes associated with dysautonomia. The tilt table test is reliable only for diagnosing conditions that have an orthostatic component. The tilt table test is a provocative test where the patient is safely strapped to a table, and the table will tilt at different angles to elicit a symptom response in blood pressure or heart rate. Passive tilting is better at promoting an orthostatic stimulus rather than having the patient actively stand, which can cause a greater reduction in blood pressure and larger increase in cardiac output [11]. These symptoms may include syncope, greying out, dizziness, lightheadedness, or unsteadiness [12]. This specific test is administered in the presence of health-care staff and an electrophysiologist.

Orthostatic intolerance testing

Nurses typically recall using orthostatic blood pressures for orthostatic hypotension. However, this simple, inexpensive, and noninvasive tool can be used to help determine hemodynamic stability. For example, in POTS, you will see an increase of 30 beats per minute in adults and 40 bpm in adolescents aged 12 to 19 years with symptoms of syncope or presyncope. Orthostatic intolerance alone can be diagnosed by taking the heart rate of a patient and if a pulse greater than 120 beats per minute in the first 10 minutes of an upright position, or an elevation in pulse greater than 30 beats per minute in the first 10 minutes of an upright position [13]. In Neurogenic Orthostatic Hypotension, practitioners will see a drop in systolic/diastolic blood pressure in the absence of tachycardia [12]. For patients that do not have the financial means to undergo further testing and if the AD symptoms are mild, this test could be a means to diagnose certain conditions, such as POTS. The reader is referred to Fig. 3 for an Orthostatic Vitals Test Form. The proper way to conduct an Orthostatic Vitals Test can be reviewed by viewing this YouTube video: https://youtu.be/kFG66qaxcuM.

MANAGEMENT

A multimodal approach to treatment is important in AD patients. Treatment is individualized based on the specific condition and severity of symptoms. Management is focused on environmental modifications, pharmaceutical interventions, nonpharmaceutical interventions, and referrals to appropriate specialists.

Nonpharmacological

Water hydration and sodium intake

Water and sodium are known to help regulate the sympathetic nervous system, especially with vasoconstriction. For example, in patients with POTS, increasing water intake increases peripheral vascularity, which assists with decreasing the incidence of orthostatic tachycardia and vasovagal syncope without a change in resting blood pressure. A healthy increase in both sodium and water will increase fluid volume, which helps protect patients with the

Orthostatic Vitals Test Form

Before the Test	Explanation of Procedure:
	• Use of blood pressure cuff and heart rate measurement
	• Important not to speak unless answering a question
	• Goal, first 5-10 minutes: to be as relaxed as possible (no phone, reading, etc.)
	• Explain why we do the test

1. **RESTING PHASE =** 5-10 Minutes	Ensure proper position with feet extended.	
Notes:	Resting Supine HR:	Supine BP:
	Reported Symptoms:	
	Transition (Explain before sitting):	
	• Sit upright as much as possible at the edge, feet on floor	
	• Avoid leaning, moving their body and, if possible, without supporting weight with hands	

2. **SITTING PHASE =** 2 Minutes	Ensure proper position.	
Notes:	Sitting HR:	Sitting BP:
	Reported Symptoms:	
	Transition (Explain before standing):	
	• Stand for up to five minutes	
	• If at any time they begin to feel faint, sit down immediately	
	• Do not ask to sit because their safety is most important	
	• It is not a problem if they do not finish the entire test	
	• It is important to stand as still as possible, avoid leaning	

3. **STANDING PHASE =** 5 Minutes	Ensure proper position.	
Notes:	1 Minute Standing HR:	1 Minute Standing BP:
	Reported Symptoms:	
	3 Minute Standing HR:	3 Minute Standing BP:
	Reported Symptoms:	
	5 Minute Standing HR:	5 Minute Standing BP:
	Reported Symptoms:	

Explain that the test is done. They can either sit or lie down during the next few minutes to rest.

Summary:

Resting HR: _____	Resting BP: _____
Sitting HR: _____	Sitting BP: _____
Standing HR 1: _____	Standing BP 1: _____
Standing HR 3: _____	Standing BP 3: _____
Standing HR 5: _____	Standing BP 5: _____

Orthostatic HR Increase: _____ bpm *(difference between resting & highest standing)*

Fig. 3. Orthostatic vitals test form. (*From* Freeman, K, Goldstein, DS, Thompson, CR. The Dysautonomia Project: Understanding autonomic system disorders for physicians and patients. Bardolf & Company; 2015; with permission.)

diagnosis of PAF from hypotension. Contraindications for increasing fluid and sodium intake include hypertensive or heart failure patients. Standard of care for adolescent and adult patients would be more than a gallon of water a day (132 oz) and a target amount of added sodium (preferably sea salt and non-iodized) of 10 g/d [14]. Salt tablets are recommended if there is not enough sodium intake from diet alone but patients should be educated that this can cause abdominal discomfort. Increasing salt in the adolescent population by adding up to 1 to 2 teaspoons of salt per day will aid with fluid retention [15]. In children, consuming 500 mL of water orally can increase systolic blood pressure by 30 mm Hg within 5 minutes due to a hyperosmolar reflex and can last for up to an hour to provide relief with an upright posture [4]. For young children with other conditions that are not orthostatic, collaborating with a dietitian is recommended for dietary restrictions and additions.

Movement
Patients with AD are at high risk for deconditioning of the muscles due to chronic fatigue, pain, or other extrinsic/intrinsic factors depending on the type of dysautonomia. Any type of tolerable movement, exercise, or activity will help decrease muscle wasting, improve cardiac flow, increase overall vascular tone and enhance circulation. As the primary care provider, stressing the importance of overall low-impact movements, even in recumbent positions, will lead to positive outcomes and a better quality of life for patients with any type of autonomic disorder. Avoiding high-intensity exercise is important because this can increase peripheral vasodilation [15]. Referral to a physical therapist can be helpful for patients with AD because they can help with exercises to strengthen the legs to help with venous return in those with POTS, EDS, and any AD disorder that could use conditioning of the muscles [4].

Compression wear
To prevent blood pooling and counteract peripheral vasodilation, compression wear at about 30 to 40 mm Hg in strength should be considered [16,17]. Leggings/hose are helpful to prevent pooling in the legs, and arm sleeves would help promote circulation in the arms and hands. Coupling thigh high compression wear and abdominal binders are helpful when combatting orthostatic hypotension and intolerance, as most pooling occurs in the splanchnic-mesenteric bed [15]. Readers are referred to Fig. 4 for an example of a prescription for compression wear.

Dietary recommendations
Small, frequent meals are typically recommended for AD patients. Larger meals lead to blood shunting to the stomach and intestines for digestion and can trigger postprandial syncopal episodes due to hypotension. Meals that are low in fiber, sugar, and carbohydrates are better tolerated. Many patients with AD have gastroparesis (delayed gastric emptying), which causes moderate nausea, making it difficult to adhere to a well-rounded diet. In some cases, chopped or pureed food is better to aid in digestion. Antiemetics such as

Patient Name:
Date:
Diagnosis: Autonomic Dysfunction/POTS
Compression Class: 30–40mmHG
Style: Waist stocking   # of pairs: 3

APN Name (Print):
APN name (Signature):

Fig. 4. Compression stocking prescription sample.

ondansetron and diphenhydramine can be used for the management of nausea. Skipping of meals and caffeine intake is not recommended due to the possibility of hypoglycemia and diuresis [4]. The APN should be prepared for frequent follow-ups with patients that have gastroparesis to monitor their weight. For those with severe gastroparesis related to AD, biweekly weight checks would be warranted. Referral to an age-appropriate dietitian should also be considered.

Education

Patient and family education is the single most important treatment/management plan the APN can provide. There are reputable sources the APN can refer patients to for further information that can empower the patient to manage their symptoms. The reader is referred to Fig. 5 for these resources. The first level of intervention involves talking with patients and their families about the patient's ability to return to activities of daily living such as school or work after being homebound [4]. This provides hope and empowerment to the patient and family. Providing patients with information about support groups or directing them to local nonprofit organizations that help educate and provide resources to support patients that are still undergoing testing can combat feelings of loneliness or hopelessness. This is especially important because these feelings can exacerbate symptoms of AD [18].

Pharmacologic

The purpose of pharmacologic treatment focuses on catecholamines and increasing, decreasing, or blocking their uptake depending on the type of AD and the individual patient's symptoms. Because AD patients are typically heterogeneous in their presentation for symptoms, what may work for one patient may not work for another. The literature supports using *fludrocortisone* off label to help retain salt in exchange for potassium and is used mostly in those patients with hypotensive episodes [19]. This medication expands plasma volume and increases cardiac afterload therefore aids with fluid retention. Checking serum potassium routinely is important because hypokalemia can present in patients on this medication, and recommendation include checking

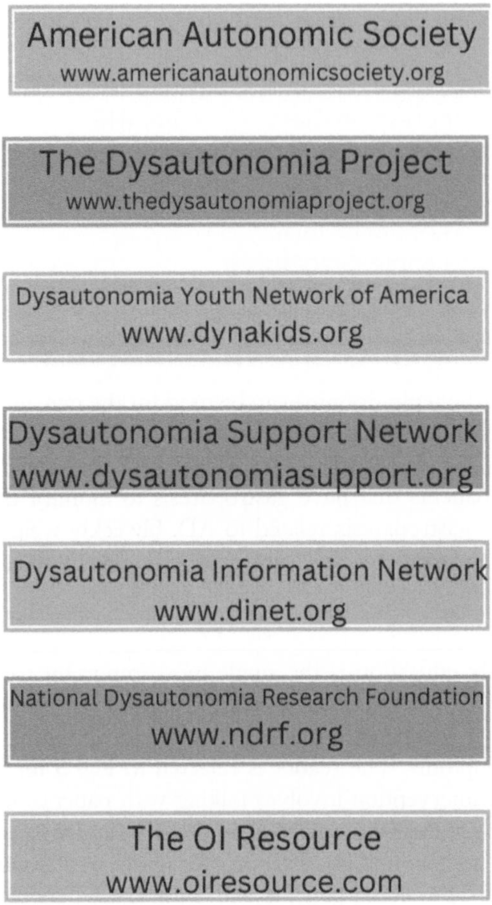

American Autonomic Society
www.americanautonomicsociety.org

The Dysautonomia Project
www.thedysautonomiaproject.org

Dysautonomia Youth Network of America
www.dynakids.org

Dysautonomia Support Network
www.dysautonomiasupport.org

Dysautonomia Information Network
www.dinet.org

National Dysautonomia Research Foundation
www.ndrf.org

The OI Resource
www.oiresource.com

Fig. 5. Dysautonomia reference sites.

potassium at baseline, before initiation of the medication, and then 1 week after initiation, and every 3 months or if symptomatic [19]. *Midodrine* is a vasoconstrictor and is approved for use in those with orthostatic hypotension and tachycardia and helps with increasing venous return to the heart [19]. Intravenous therapy (up to 2L for acute clinical decompensation) with saline can also be considered for those that are not able to consume the recommended amount of water, especially in patients with gastroparesis [20]. Constipation and diarrhea can occur quite frequently in these patients due to decreased mobility. Conservative management in these patients includes adequate movement and increased hydration. However, if these interventions are unsuccessful, the APN should consider the use of stool softeners [5]. *Stimulants* are recommended for the treatment of brain fog, fatigue, and the decreased ability to concentrate [1]. The literature supports the use of *Melatonin* for patients with disrupted sleep hygiene as this over-the-counter medication typically has less side effects than prescription insomnia medications [4].

REFERRAL

For complicated patients with an autonomic disorder, a referral to an autonomic laboratory/autonomic medicine specialist should be the standard of care. Complicated patients include those that are not responding to nonpharmacological and/or pharmacologic treatments, those whose symptoms have a significant impact on their activities of daily living, those that have comorbidities, and any patient the APN feels would benefit with additional resources.

SPECIAL POPULATION CONSIDERATIONS

Long-COVID

As the SARS-COV-2 pandemic continues, more research is presented about the complications of COVID-19 including long-COVID. Long-COVID syndrome is defined as signs and symptoms that develop for 4 weeks or more after the onset of COVID-19, and are unexplained by alternative diagnoses [13]. There are multiple explanations for the mechanisms surrounding this occurrence, including interaction of SARS-COV-2 with the angiotensin-converting enzyme leading to dysregulation of the feedback loop, the cytokine storm leading to cardiovascular system dysfunction, neurotropism through the olfactory bulb and impairment of the ANS by means of brain impairment [21]. The number of patients reporting long-lasting symptoms post-COVID is increasing, even after mild cases. Lightheadedness, dizziness, cognitive dysfunction, tachycardia, and nausea have all been reported in patients with long-COVID [21]. Most CASS scores for those with long-COVID are mild AD and many symptoms resolve by 6 months [21]. As the pandemic progresses and multiple strains of COVID-19 circulate and evolve, more research will be conducted on the correlation between AD and COVID-19 infection, especially in the pediatric population.

Pediatrics

The most common type of dysautonomia that is seen in pediatrics is POTS, and usually presents in the pubescent adolescent population. Those patients that are typically higher risk for symptoms of AD include those that have higher stress levels, such as those considered "high achievers" in academics, athletics, or both. Lack of sleep is also an exacerbating factor for those patients with AD. Sleep habits should be monitored by the parents and special attention to educating the patient and family on sleep habits should be given by the APN. Use of pharmacologic interventions in children should only be considered in collaboration with an autonomic specialist because certain medications can cause decreased growth velocity or osteoporosis (such as seen with *fludrocortisone*) [18].

SUMMARY

AD is not a rare condition; it is just rarely diagnosed due to complex heterogenous symptomatology and lack of APN knowledge surrounding the dysfunction. AD can be recognized by taking a thorough patient history and be preliminarily diagnosed with orthostatic vitals in the primary care office. AD can be managed with nonpharmacological and pharmacologic treatment measures. Acknowledging and affirming the patients' symptoms is an essential element of the APN's role when evaluating a patient with a potential AD diagnosis to prevent mental anguish and feelings of hopelessness in patients with this multisystem disorder. APNs should take initiative to educate themselves on the most common AD disorders to be able to acknowledge, identify, and manage these patients to achieve the best possible outcomes. The reader is referred to Fig. 3 for resources.

CLINICS CARE POINTS

- AD can present throughout the life span. APNs should be able to recognize the multisystem symptoms that may present in any case (see Table 1).
- Orthostatic vitals taken in the office can offer a preliminary diagnosis of AD or rule out AD in the presence of symptomatic tachycardia [18]. AD should not be considered a diagnosis of exclusion.
- Referrals to specialists that are not familiar with AD may yield disappointment, misdiagnosis, and hopelessness in the patient and family. APNs should be aware of outside providers/specialists that are familiar with AD when deciding to refer.

DISCLOSURE

The author has nothing to disclose.

References

[1] Burton JM, Morozova OM. Calming the storm: dysautonomia for the pediatrician. Curr Probl Pediatr Adolesc Health Care 2017;47(7):145–50.

[2] Sletten DM, Suarez GA, Low PA, et al. COMPASS 31: a refined and abbreviated Composite Autonomic Symptom Score. Mayo Clin Proc 2012;87(12):1196–201.

[3] Freeman K, Goldstein DS, Thompson CR. The Dysautonomia Project: Understanding autonomic system disorders for physicians and patients. Sarasota, FL: Bardolf & Company; 2015.

[4] Do T, Diamond S, Green C, et al. Nutritional implications of patients with dysautonomia and hypermobility syndromes. Curr Nutr Rep 2021;10(4):324–33.

[5] Singh K, Palma JA, Kaufmann H, et al. Prevalence and characteristics of sleep-disordered breathing in familial dysautonomia. Sleep Med 2018;45:33–8.

[6] Barizien N, Le Guen M, Russel S, et al. Clinical characterization of dysautonomia in long COVID-19 patients. Sci Rep 2021;11(1):14042.

[7] Kirk KA, Shoykhet M, Jeong JH, et al. Dysautonomia after pediatric brain injury. Dev Med Child Neurol 2012;54(8):759–64.

[8] Goldstein DS. Principles of autonomic medicine. 2020. Available at: https://ninds-large-s3-hosted-files.s3.amazonaws.com/intramural%2F2022-07%2F1657650342_PrinciplesofAutonomicMedicinev40_508C.zip. Accessed September 15, 2022.

[9] Armstrong KR, De Souza AM, Sneddon PL, et al. Exercise and the multidisciplinary holistic approach to adolescent dysautonomia. Acta Paediatr 2017;106(4):612–8.

[10] Rasmussen TK, Hansen J, Low PA, et al. Autonomic function testing: Compliance and consequences. Auton Neurosci Basic Clin 2017;208:150–5.

[11] Cheshire WP, Freeman R, Gibbons CH, et al. Electrodiagnostic assessment of the autonomic nervous system: A consensus statement endorsed by the American Autonomic Society, American Academy of Neurology, and the International Federation of Clinical Neurophysiology. Clin Neurophysiol 2021;132(2):666–82 [published correction appears in Clin Neurophysiol. 2021 May;132(5):1194].

[12] Sutton R, Fedorowski A, Olshansky B, et al. Tilt testing remains a valuable asset. Eur Heart J 2021;42(17):1654–60.

[13] Eldokla AM, Ali ST. Autonomic function testing in long-COVID syndrome patients with orthostatic intolerance. Auton Neurosci : Basic Clin 2022;241:102997.

[14] Fu Q, Levine BD. Exercise and non-pharmacological treatment of POTS. Auton Neurosci 2018;215:20–7.

[15] Armstrong KR, De Souza AM, Sneddon PL, et al. Exercise and the multidisciplinary holistic approach to adolescent dysautonomia. Acta Paediatr 2017;106(4):612–8.

[16] Bourne KM, Sheldon RS, Hall J, et al. Compression garment reduces orthostatic tachycardia and symptoms in patients with postural orthostatic tachycardia syndrome. J Am Coll Cardiol 2021;77(3):285–96.

[17] Boris JR, Huang J, Bernadzikowski T. Orthostatic heart rate does not predict symptomatic burden in pediatric patients with chronic orthostatic intolerance. Clin Auton Res 2020;30(1):19–28.

[18] Boris JR. The role of the cardiologist in the evaluation of dysautonomia. Cardiol Young 2010;20(Suppl 3):135–9.

[19] Dani M, Dirksen A, Taraborrelli P, et al. Autonomic dysfunction in 'long COVID': rationale, physiology and management strategies. Clin Med (Lond) 2021;21(1):e63–7.

[20] Zadourian A, Doherty TA, Swiatkiewicz I, et al. Postural orthostatic tachycardia syndrome: prevalence, pathophysiology, and management. Drugs 2018;78(10):983–94.

[21] Barizien N, Le Guen M, Russel S, et al. Clinical characterization of dysautonomia in long COVID-19 patients. Sci Rep 2021;11(1):14042, Published 2021 Jul 7.

Advances in Family Practice Nursing 5 (2023) 283–297

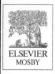

When It Is Not Just Attention-Deficit Hyperactivity Disorder
Coexisting Depression and Anxiety in Pediatric Primary Care

Valerie C. Martinez, DNP, APRN, CPNP-PC, PMHS

Department of Nursing Practice, College of Nursing, University of Central Florida, 12201 Research Parkway, Suite 300, Orlando, FL 32826, USA

Keywords
- ADHD • Anxiety • Depression • Pediatric • Primary care • Diagnosis
- Management

Key points
- Attention-deficit hyperactivity disorder (ADHD) is a common neurodevelopmental disorder that is often accompanied by coexisting conditions, including depression and anxiety.
- Primary care providers must possess a comprehensive understanding of ADHD and coexisting depression and/or anxiety to effectively diagnose and treat their patient's symptoms.
- Behavioral and pharmacologic treatment options have the potential to be effective to treat ADHD and its coexisting conditions if a comprehensive evaluation is conducted.
- A referral to mental health subspecialists should be made if the coexisting conditions lead to moderate to severe functional impairments or if the primary care provider is not confident in diagnosing and treating ADHD with coexisting conditions.

INTRODUCTION

Attention-deficit hyperactivity disorder (ADHD) is one of the most common neurodevelopmental disorders of childhood and may negatively affect a child or adolescent's academic performance, social interactions, and quality of life [1–3]. ADHD includes persistent and impairing symptoms of inattention,

E-mail address: Valerie.Martinez@ucf.edu

https://doi.org/10.1016/j.yfpn.2023.01.007

disorganization, hyperactivity, and/or impulsivity that occur across multiple settings [4]. ADHD often exists along with other psychiatric disorders, including depression and anxiety [1,2,4,5], but these conditions may be misdiagnosed or undertreated due to often overlapping symptomatology [6]. Although pediatric primary care providers (PCPs) regularly manage mild-to-moderate ADHD, depression, and anxiety as standalone conditions [2], the care of youth with ADHD who have coexisting psychiatric conditions is often challenging, complicated, and can prevent optimal ADHD management [7]. Although interprofessional care is recommended for children and adolescents with ADHD and coexisting conditions [1], there are significant systemic and structural barriers to accessing specialized mental health care [8]. Therefore, pediatric PCPs must possess a comprehensive understanding of ADHD and coexisting depression and/or anxiety to effectively diagnose and treat their patient's symptoms when subspecialty care is not accessible. Untreated symptoms of ADHD, depression, and/or anxiety may increase the risk of substance abuse, poor academic and social functioning, and suicidal behavior in youth [1]. The purpose of this article is to review the prevalence of ADHD with coexisting depression and anxiety in youth and outline assessment, diagnostic, and management considerations for PCPs when it is not just ADHD that requires clinical decision-making.

PREVALENCE

ADHD has a worldwide prevalence of 7.2% among children and adolescents [9]. In the United States, 9.4% of children and adolescents in 2016 had ever received a diagnosis of ADHD, and more than 5 million children currently had ADHD (8.4%) [10]. Of those children and adolescents currently affected by ADHD, approximately 17% also had depression and one-third of children with ADHD reported coexisting anxiety [10]. Among youth with ADHD and a coexisting condition, only 41% had received both pharmacologic and behavioral treatment, whereas 16.7% had not received either pharmacologic or behavioral treatment [10]. Further, children living in rural areas were 30% more likely to have ever received an ADHD diagnosis [10]. These disparities make it essential to ensure that youth who have limited access to specialized mental health services receive appropriate care from their PCP [10], especially in cases of coexisting psychiatric conditions.

CLINICAL PRACTICE GUIDELINES

To aid primary and subspecialty care providers, the American Academy of Pediatrics (AAP) [2] and the Society for Developmental and Behavioral Pediatrics (SDBP) [1] released clinical practice guidelines aimed at caring for children with ADHD and coexisting conditions. The 2019 update to the AAP guideline focuses on all children ages 4 to 17 years presenting to primary care with academic or behavioral problems and symptoms of inattention, hyperactivity, or impulsivity [2]. The 2020 SDBP guideline complements the AAP guideline and guides all professionals managing care of children and adolescents with "complex ADHD," including those with coexisting conditions, such as depression and anxiety, to improve long-term functional outcomes [1]. In addition to these clinical practice guidelines, the AAP also developed a resource toolkit for PCPs to facilitate effective diagnosis and management of ADHD and coexisting conditions [7].

ASSESSMENT

The diagnostic process of evaluating a child or adolescent for ADHD and/or coexisting conditions begins with a comprehensive, developmentally appropriate, and culturally sensitive assessment. Without a thorough assessment, coexisting depression and/or anxiety may be undetected or inadequately treated because symptoms often overlap [6]. An important aspect of a comprehensive assessment is collaboration among the PCP, child, family, and school personnel. Collaborative care and communication provide the greatest potential for accurate diagnosis and effective treatment [7].

History

An adequate assessment of youth with ADHD and potential coexisting depression or anxiety requires a detailed history focused on functional difficulties across settings. Caregiver and child interviews should be conducted to obtain a thorough history, which includes the present concerns, past medical history, behavioral history, review of systems, medication use, social history, and family mental health and medical history. Obtaining this comprehensive history is necessary to assess and differentiate symptom significance among the coexisting conditions. It helps determine the most important functional impairments for targeted intervention and treatment or if an immediate referral or crisis management is necessary.

Screening and diagnostic assessment tools

In addition to caregiver and child interviews, several broadband and condition-specific standardized screening and diagnostic assessment tools can aid PCPs in the identification of symptoms and level of functional impairment (Table 1). These tools may also be used during follow-up to monitor treatment response. Broadband assessment tools focus on a variety of behavioral symptoms, whereas targeted assessment tools focus on core symptoms of a specific condition, such as ADHD.

Broadband screening tools are helpful to evaluate the overall behavioral and social-emotional functioning of a child. They allow a PCP to screen for multiple issues, including ADHD, depression, and anxiety, without targeting any specific diagnosis. Three common, valid, and reliable broadband screening tools include the Pediatric Symptom Checklist (PSC), the Child Behavior Checklist (CBCL), and the Strengths and Difficulties Questionnaire (SDQ). The PSC consists of questions assessing internalizing (ie, depression, anxiety) and externalizing (ie, hyperactivity, impulsivity) symptoms as well as attention difficulties in children [11]. Likewise, the CBCL consists of questions assessing internalizing and externalizing symptoms in children [12]. The SDQ screens

Table 1
Selected parent-report screening and assessment tools

Broadband	ADHD	Depression	Anxiety
Pediatric Symptom Checklist (PSC) • 17 or 35 items • 4–16 y	ADHD Rating Scale-5 (ADHD-RS-V) • 18 items • 5–17 y	Patient Health Questionnaire Modified for Adolescents (PHQ-A) • 9 items • 11–17 y	Screen for Child Anxiety and Related Emotional Disorders (SCARED) • Ranges from 38 to 71 items • ≥8 y
Child Behavior Checklist (CBCL) • 113 items • 6–18 y	Vanderbilt Assessment Scales • 55 items (parent scale); 43 items (teacher scale) • 6–12 y	Center For Epidemiological Studies Depression Scale for Children (CES-DC) • 20 items • 6–17 y	Spence Children's Anxiety Scale (SCAS) • 44 items • 21/2–12 y
Strengths and Difficulties Questionnaire (SDQ) • 25 items • 2–17 y	Conners 3rd Edition Short-Form Assessment Scales • 62 items (parent scale);69 items (teacher scale) • 6–18 y	Short Mood and Feelings Questionnaire (SMFQ) • 13 items • 8–16 y	Generalized Anxiety Disorder-7 (GAD-7) • 7 items • 11–17 y

for issues with attention, internalizing symptoms, conduct, peer relationships, and prosocial behaviors [12].

To diagnose ADHD in primary care, AAP guidelines recommend that PCPs obtain information using a rating scale based on the *Diagnostic and Statistical Manual (DSM)* [2]. Because there were minimal changes to the specific behaviors of ADHD from the *DSM-IV* to the *DSM-5-TR* criteria, the AAP endorses the use of any *DSM*-based rating scale to obtain the necessary information. Three frequently used valid and reliable ADHD-specific rating scales are the ADHD Rating Scale–5 (ADHD-RS-V), the Vanderbilt Assessment Scales, and the Connors' Assessment Scale. Each of these scales include both parent and teacher rating scales and have been updated using *DSM-5* criteria for ADHD [7,13,14]. The ADHD-RS-V consists of items specific to the core symptoms of ADHD and functional impairments in children and adolescents [13]. The Vanderbilt consists of items that focus on core symptoms of ADHD, functional impairments, and symptoms of externalizing and internalizing disorders in children [7]. The short-form Conners scale includes items regarding executive functioning, aggression, peer relations, learning problems, hyperactivity/impulsivity, and inattention subscales in children and adolescents [14].

Some of the same tools used to screen for ADHD may also be used to identify depression and anxiety in children, such as the Vanderbilt subscale questions on internalizing symptoms and the PSC broadband screener [7]. In addition, valid and reliable depression-specific screening tools may be used to identify core symptoms of depression. The Patient Health Questionnaire–9 (PHQ-9), a screening tool for persons older than 18 years, has been modified for Adolescents (PHQ-A) [15]. Another screening tool that may be useful to PCPs is the Center for Epidemiologic Studies Depression Scale for Children (CES-DC), which targets depressive symptoms and emotional turmoil in children and adolescents [16]. Another brief screening tool for depression is the Short Mood and Feelings Questionnaire (SMFQ), which was adapted from the longer Mood and Feelings Questionnaire (MFQ) [17].

Common targeted screening tools for anxiety include the Screen for Child Anxiety and Related Emotional Disorders (SCARED), the Spence Children's Anxiety Scale (SCAS), and the Generalized Anxiety Disorder–7 (GAD-7). The SCARED tool screens for generalized anxiety disorder (GAD), along with separation anxiety disorder (SAD), panic/somatic disorder, social anxiety disorder, and school avoidance, with revised versions expanding to also screen for obsessive-compulsive disorder (OCD) and posttraumatic stress disorder [18]. The SCAS assesses the severity of symptoms in the most common childhood anxiety disorders, including GAD, panic attacks, agoraphobia, SAD, OCD, social phobia, and physical injury fears [19]. Finally, the GAD-7 screens for symptoms consistent with GAD and is best used in adolescents [7].

Physical examination

In addition to a comprehensive history and use of standardized diagnostic tools, it is essential to conduct a complete physical examination with particular attention to neurologic, cardiac, endocrine, or genetic issues [7]. Although no specific diagnostic laboratory test is required to make a diagnosis of ADHD, depression, or anxiety, it may be helpful to obtain laboratory tests to rule out medical conditions, such as anemia, lead exposure, thyroid disorders, and vitamin deficiency, which may present similarly to depression or anxiety. A nonexhaustive list of laboratory tests that may aid the PCP in assessment and clinical decision-making include a complete blood cell count, vitamin B12 and folate, lead level, thyroid function tests, and chemistry panel [7,20].

DIAGNOSIS
In order to make a diagnosis of ADHD, anxiety, and/or depression, the PCP should ensure that *DSM-5-TR* criteria has been met for any condition diagnosed [2]. *DSM-5-TR* criteria for ADHD, major depressive disorder, and GAD are outlined in Boxes 1–3, respectively [4]. Although differentiating symptom presentation between ADHD and depression can be difficult, it may be more apparent if a comprehensive history was obtained. For example, markedly diminished interest in activities is part of the diagnostic criteria for depression, and with ADHD it is common to enjoy an activity intensely and then lose interest and move on to something new and more stimulating. However, with depression, a patient may not find any enjoyment with any activity; this would be discernible with a thorough history. Likewise, anxiety makes it difficult to sleep, but often children or adolescents who are taking stimulant medication also report difficulty sleeping [21]. Without a complete history it may be challenging to determine if symptoms such as these are related to ADHD or anxiety, especially because many symptoms of ADHD mimic anxiety symptoms [20,21].

MANAGEMENT
On making a diagnosis, it is important to collaboratively communicate the diagnosis to the family and empower them in shared decision-making for treatment approaches [1]. The PCP can help the child and caregivers identify and prioritize their goals for treatment [7]. If ADHD was already previously diagnosed, but a coexisting depression and/or anxiety was identified, the child or adolescent's ADHD treatment may need to be altered [2]. Youth with ADHD and either coexisting depression or anxiety may have a decreased response to their medications [22] and require evaluation of their treatment plan. However, if ADHD is the primary condition, once it is appropriately treated with stimulant medication, coexisting anxiety and/or depression symptoms may also improve [23]. At times, even with a comprehensive assessment, it is difficult to determine if ADHD or one of its coexisting conditions is the primary issue; in this case it is appropriate to address the symptoms that cause the greatest impairment first [7].

Psychoeducation
The first step in every treatment plan should be developmentally and culturally appropriate psychoeducation about ADHD and its coexisting depression or

Box 1: Attention-deficit hyperactivity disorder DSM-5-TR criteria

A. A persistent pattern of inattention and/or hyperactivity-impulsivity that interferes with functioning or development as characterized by (1) and/or (2)

1. *Inattention*: 6 (or more) of the following symptoms have persisted for at least 6 months to a degree that is inconsistent with developmental level and that negatively affects directly on social and academic/occupational activities:

   Note: the symptoms are not solely a manifestation of oppositional behavior, hostility, or failure to understand tasks or instructions. For older adolescents and adults (17 years and older), at least 5 symptoms are required.

   a. Often fails to give close attention to details or makes careless mistakes in schoolwork, at work, or during other activities (eg, overlooks or misses details, work is inaccurate).

   b. Often has difficulty sustaining attention in tasks or play activities (eg, has difficulty remaining focused during lectures, conversations, or lengthy reading).

   c. Often does not seem to listen when spoken to directly (eg, mind seems elsewhere, even in the absence of any obvious distraction).

   d. Often does not follow through on instructions and fails to finish schoolwork, chores, or duties in the workplace (eg, starts tasks but quickly loses focus and is easily sidetracked).

   e. Often has difficulty organizing tasks and activities (eg, difficulty managing sequential tasks; difficulty keeping materials and belongings in order; messy, disorganized work; has poor time management; fails to meet deadliness).

   f. Often avoids, dislikes, or reluctant to engage in tasks that require sustained mental effort (eg, schoolwork or homework; for older adolescents and adults, preparing reports, completing forms, reviewing lengthy papers).

   g. Often loses things necessary for tasks or activities (eg, school materials, pencils, books, tools, wallets, keys, paperwork, eyeglasses, mobile telephones).

   h. Is often easily distracted by extraneous stimuli (for older adolescents and adults, may include unrelated thoughts).

   i. Is often forgetful in daily activities (eg, doing chores, running errands; for older adolescents and adults, returning calls, paying bills, keeping appointments).

2. *Hyperactivity and impulsivity*: 6 (or more) of the following symptoms have persisted for at least 6 months to a degree that is inconsistent with developmental level and that negatively affects directly on social and academic/occupational activities:

   Note: the symptoms are not solely a manifestation of oppositional behavior, defiance, hostility, or a failure to understand tasks or instructions. For older adolescents and adults (age 17 years and older), at least 5 symptoms are required.

   a. Often fidgets with or taps hands or feet or squirms in seat.

   b. Often leaves seat in situations when remaining seated is expected (eg, leaves his or her place in the classroom, in the office or other workplace, or in other situations that require remaining in place).

   c. Often runs about or climbs in situations where it is inappropriate. (Note: in adolescents or adults, may be limited to feeling restless).

   d. Often unable to play or engage in leisure activities quietly.

   e. Is often "on the go," acting as if "driven by a motor" (eg, is unable to be or uncomfortable being still for extended time, as in restaurants, meeting; may be experienced by others as being restless or difficult to keep up with).

   f. Often talks excessively.

   g. Often blurts our answer before a question has been completed (eg, completes people's sentences; cannot wait for turn in conversation).

   h. Often has difficulty waiting his or her turn (eg, while waiting in line).

   i. Often interrupts or intrudes on others (eg, butts into conversations, games, or activities; may start using other people's things without asking or receiving permission; for adolescents and adults, may intrude into or take over what others are doing).

B. Several inattentive or hyperactive-impulsive symptoms were present before age 12 years.

C. Several inattentive or hyperactive-impulsive symptoms are present in 2 or more settings (eg, home, school, or work; with friends or relatives; in other activities).

D. There is clear evidence that the symptoms interfere with, or reduce the quality of, social, academic, or occupational functioning.

From American Psychiatric Association. Diagnostic and Statistical Manual of Mental Disorders, Fifth Edition, Text Revision (DSM-5-TR™). American Psychiatric Association Publishing; 2022; with permission.

anxiety. Psychoeducation is a systematic and structured educational approach to promote understanding of a patient's condition, treatment options, and personal management skills [24]. Psychoeducation should be provided to the child or adolescent and their family and include evidence-based behavioral and psychosocial intervention approaches as well as potential pharmacologic treatment approaches [1]. Psychoeducation should be updated at every patient encounter with considerations of the youth's developmental level. Although parents of young children are often the recipient of psychoeducation, it is important for PCPs to increasingly direct psychoeducation toward the patient as the child progresses toward adolescence [1].

Nonpharmacologic treatment approaches

Evidence-based behavioral, educational, and psychosocial interventions targeted at impairments can improve functioning in children and adolescents with ADHD and coexisting depression or anxiety [1]. Behavioral parent training, behavioral classroom management, behavioral peer interventions,

Box 2: Major depressive disorder DSM-5-TR criteria

A. Five (or more) of the following symptoms have been present during the same 2-week period and represent a change from previous functioning; at least one of the symptoms is either (1) depressed mood or (2) loss of interest or pleasure.

Note: do not include symptoms that are clearly attributable to another medical condition.

1. Depressed mood most of the day, nearly every day, as indicated by either subjective report (eg, feels sad, empty, or hopeless) or observation made by others (eg, seems tearful). (Note: children and adolescents can be in irritable mood.)

2. Markedly diminished interest or pleasure in all, or almost all, activities most of the day, nearly every day (as indicated by either subjective account or observation).

3. Significant weight loss when not dieting or weight gain (eg, a change of more than 5% of body weight in a month) or decrease or increase in appetite nearly every day. (Note: in children, consider failure to make expected weight gain.)

4. Insomnia or hypersomnia nearly every day.

5. Psychomotor agitation or retardation nearly every day (observable by others, not merely subjective feelings of restlessness or being slowed down).

6. Fatigue or loss of energy nearly every day.

7. Feelings of worthlessness or excessive or inappropriate guilt (which may be delusional) nearly every day (either by subjective account or as observed by others).

8. Diminished ability to think or concentrate, or indecisiveness, nearly every day (either by subjective account or as observed by others).

9. Recurrent thoughts of death (not just fear of dying), recurrent suicidal ideation without a specific plan, or a suicide attempt or a specific plan for committing suicide.

B. The symptoms cause clinically significant distress or impairment in social, occupational, or other important areas of functioning.

C. The episode is not attributable to the physiologic effects of a substance or another medical condition.

Note: criteria A–C represent a major depressive episode.

Note: responses to a significant loss (eg, bereavement, financial ruin, loss from a natural disaster, a serious medical illness, or disability) may include the feelings of intense sadness, rumination about the loss, insomnia, poor appetite, and weight loss noted in criterion A, which may resemble a depressive episode. Although such symptoms may be understandable or considered appropriate to the loss, the presence of a major depressive episode in addition to the normal response to a significant loss should also be carefully considered. This decision inevitably requires the exercise of clinical judgment based on the individual's history and the cultural norms for the expression of distress in the context of loss.

D. At least one major depressive episode is not better explained by schizoaffective disorder and is not superimposed on schizophrenia, schizophreniform disorder, or other specified and unspecified schizophrenia spectrum and other psychotic disorders.

E. There has never been a manic episode or a hypomanic episode.

Note: this exclusion does not apply if all of the maniclike or hypomaniclike episodes are substances induced or are attributable to the physiologic effects of another medical condition.

From American Psychiatric Association. Diagnostic and Statistical Manual of Mental Disorders, Fifth Edition, Text Revision (DSM-5-TR™). American Psychiatric Association Publishing; 2022; with permission.

Box 3: Generalized anxiety disorder DSM-5-TR criteria

A. Excessive anxiety and worry (apprehensive expectation), occurring more days than not for at least 6 months, about several events or activities (such as work or school performance).

B. The individual finds it difficult to control the worry.

C. The anxiety and worry are associated with 3 (or more) of the following 6 symptoms (with symptoms having been present for more days than not for the past 6 months):

   Note: only one item is required in children.

   1. Restlessness or feeling keyed up or in edge

   2. Being easily fatigue

   3. Difficulty concentrating or mind going blank

   4. Irritability

   5. Muscle tension

   6. Sleep disturbance (difficulty falling or staying asleep or restless, unsatisfying sleep)

D. The anxiety, worry, or physical symptoms cause clinically significant distress or impairment in social, occupational, or other important areas of functioning.

E. The disturbance is not attributable to the physiologic effects of a substance (eg, a drug of abuse, a medication) or another medical condition (eg, hyperthyroidism).

F. The disturbance is not better explained by another mental disorder (eg, anxiety or worry about having panic attacks in panic disorder, negative evaluation in social anxiety disorder, contamination or other obsessions in obsessive-compulsive disorder, reminders of traumatic complaints in somatic symptom disorder, perceived appearance flaws in body dysmorphic disorder, having a serious illness in illness anxiety disorder, or the content of delusional beliefs in schizophrenia or delusional disorder).

From American Psychiatric Association. Diagnostic and Statistical Manual of Mental Disorders, Fifth Edition, Text Revision (DSM-5-TR™). American Psychiatric Association Publishing; 2022; with permission.

and organizational skills training are well-supported nonpharmacologic treatment options to decrease undesirable behaviors in youth with ADHD and can also reduce symptoms of coexisting depression and/or anxiety [1]. These interventions require collaborative communication from the PCP and significant engagement from caregivers and teachers. In addition, cognitive behavioral therapy (CBT) is a first-line nonpharmacologic option for both coexisting depression and/or anxiety [25].

Pharmacologic treatment approaches

If nonpharmacologic treatment options do not sufficiently improve functioning, a comprehensive treatment plan for individuals with ADHD and coexisting depression and anxiety should include a psychopharmacologic approach. Psychopharmacologic interventions used in the primary care setting for ADHD and coexisting depression and anxiety include stimulants, alpha-2 adrenergic agonists, selective serotonin reuptake inhibitors (SSRIs), and selective norepinephrine reuptake inhibitors (SNRIs).

Food and Drug Administration (FDA)-approved stimulant medications for children 6 years of age and older, which include methylphenidate and amphetamine, are considered first-line pharmacologic treatment of ADHD symptoms because they have demonstrated a greater degree of improvement in ADHD symptoms than other medications. Use of stimulant treatment of ADHD typically does not exacerbate symptoms of depression or anxiety and may have a beneficial effect on these symptoms [1,26]. FDA-approved alpha-2 adrenergic agonists, which include guanfacine and clonidine, are also approved medications for ADHD in children 6 years of age and older. However, guanfacine has a more favorable side-effect profile than clonidine [27]. Likewise, atomoxetine, an SNRI, is FDA-approved for the treatment of ADHD in children at least 6 years old, but has a much longer effect onset than other approved medications, ranging from 1 to 2 weeks for initial effect and 4 to 6 weeks for full effect [27].

SSRIs are considered first-line pharmacologic treatment of depression in youth and can be combined with CBT [27]. Fluoxetine is the SSRI with the most evidence to support its use in pediatric populations [28] and is FDA-approved for children 8 years of age and older. Escitalopram is another FDA-approved SSRI to treat depression in children at least 12 years old. The American Academy of Child and Adolescent Psychiatry (AACAP) also recommend SSRIs and CBT for the treatment of anxiety in children and adolescents [29]. However, no specific SSRIs have been approved by the FDA for anxiety. Further, an important consideration for PCPs is that all SSRIs have a boxed warning for suicidal thinking and behavior even though they are typically well tolerated by youth [29], so close monitoring for suicidality in patients taking SSRIs is essential. SNRIs are also recommended for pediatric anxiety, of which duloxetine is the only SNRI to be approved for the treatment of GAD in children greater than 7 years of age [29]. Despite the medication chosen for psychopharmacologic treatment, therapy should be initiated at a low dose and slowly titrated [27]. Once an optimal dose has been reached, continued monitoring every 1 to 3 months is recommended [27]. Specific dosing and monitoring of psychopharmacologic treatments should follow FDA or AAP/AACAP guidelines [2,28,29]. Although many medications are effective for ADHD, depression, and anxiety in youth, it is essential that prescribing PCPs have a comprehensive understanding of medication side effects and safety profiles to effectively prescribe and monitor use of these medications [7,16].

Suicide risk

Although effective treatment options for ADHD and coexisting depression and anxiety exist, ensuring appropriate suicide risk assessment has been completed is vital to the safety of the child or adolescent. There is a well-established link between ADHD and risk for suicidal behavior, which is even more elevated in the presence of comorbid psychiatric disorders [30,31]. Conducting a brief suicide safety assessment using an evidence-based tool, such as the Ask Suicide-Screening Questionnaire (ASQ) [32], can help PCPs determine if it is safe to send the patient home or whether the patient is at imminent risk of suicide and immediate safety interventions are necessary.

Referral to mental health specialists

Assessing and managing ADHD with coexisting psychiatric conditions may require more time than a busy primary care setting allows. When PCPs cannot assess for or adequately manage coexisting conditions, they should refer children to appropriate subspecialists for further evaluation [1,2,33]. Specifically, guidelines include recommendations to refer patients with ADHD who present diagnostic challenges, have failed to respond to treatment, or have coexisting disorders or other complicating factors [1,2]. However, some youth with ADHD and coexisting depression or anxiety who respond well to treatment by their PCP and maintain good function may not require a referral [1]. Despite guideline recommendations for referral to subspecialists when ADHD coexists with another psychiatric disorder, many are never referred. In fact, in a study evaluating ADHD care practices among PCPs, less than one-third of children diagnosed with ADHD who screened positive for a comorbid mental health condition were referred for additional assessment and treatment [33].

Follow-up monitoring

Youth with ADHD and coexisting depression or anxiety may require more intensive follow-up monitoring than if only one condition was present. Regular follow-up visits should include monitoring of progress toward treatment goals, effectiveness of treatment on target symptoms, and side effects of medications [7]. In addition, standardized rating scales should be obtained at least 2 to 4 times per year [1].

IMPLICATIONS FOR CLINICAL PRACTICE

When initiating the diagnostic process of evaluating a child or adolescent for ADHD, it is important to recognize that ADHD often coexists with depression and anxiety. Therefore, it is critical that PCPs conduct a comprehensive assessment of these patients to identify any coexisting psychiatric disorders. Further, it would be prudent to comprehensively assess all patients with ADHD for coexisting conditions at regular intervals. A comprehensive assessment and treatment plan with parental engagement for ADHD and coexisting depression and/or anxiety has the potential to greatly improve functioning for these children [1]. With an increased risk for suicide among those with ADHD and coexisting psychiatric disorders, it is imperative that PCPs closely monitor these children and adolescents in order to implement prevention efforts [31]. Finally, PCPs should understand their knowledge and comfort limitations to determine when a referral to a subspecialist is warranted.

SUMMARY

Care for a child or adolescent with ADHD who also has coexisting depression or anxiety is complicated and requires the PCP to be aware of the presentation of these conditions and treatment options. It is important to take a comprehensive approach when a child or adolescent with ADHD presents with new concerns that may be related to anxiety or depression. A comprehensive assessment should be completed so that treatment strategies can be discussed, and family shared decision-making can proceed. With proper assessment and diagnosis, treatment of both coexisting conditions is feasible in primary care, especially in the case of patients with milder functional impairments.

CLINICS CARE POINTS

- Clinical practice guidelines exist to aid primary care nurse practitioners in the care of children with ADHD and coexisting conditions.
- The diagnostic process begings with a comprehensive, developmentally appropriate, and culturally sensitive assessment.
- The PCP should ensure that DSM-5-TR criteria has been met for any condition diagnosed.
- If it is difficult to determine if ADHD or one of its coexisiting conditions is the primary issue, it is appropriate to address the symptoms that cause the greatest impairment first.
- Management includes psychoeducation, nonpharmacologic treatment approaches, and potentially pharmacologic treatment approaches.
- Refer to subspecialists when children with ADHD present diagnostic challenges, fail to respond to treatment, or have complicating factors.

DISCLOSURE
The author has nothing to disclose.

References

[1] Barbaresi WJ, Campbell L, Diekroger EA, et al. Society for Developmental and Behavioral Pediatrics clinical practice guideline for the assessment and treatment of children and adolescents with complex attention-deficit/hyperactivity disorder. J Dev Behav Pediatr 2020;41(Suppl 2S):S35–57.

[2] Wolraich ML, Hagan JF, Allan C, et al. Clinical practice guideline for the diagnosis, evaluation, and treatment of attention-deficit/hyperactivity disorder in children and adolescents. Pediatrics 2019;144(4):e20192528.

[3] Velő S, Keresztény Á, Ferenczi-Dallos G, et al. Long-term effects of multimodal treatment on psychopathology and health-related quality of life of children with attention deficit hyperactivity disorder. Front Psychol 2019;10:2037.

[4] American Psychiatric Association. Diagnostic and Statistical Manual of Mental Disorders. 5th edition. Washington, DC: Text revision (DSM-5-TRTM), American Psychiatric Association Publishing; 2022.

[5] D'Agati E, Curatolo P, Mazzone L. Comorbidity between ADHD and anxiety disorders across the lifespan. Int J Psychiatry Clin Pract 2019;23(4):238–44.

[6] Gnanavel S, Sharma P, Kaushal P, et al. Attention deficit hyperactivity disorder and comorbidity: A review of literature. World J Clin Cases 2019;7(17):2420–6.

[7] Zurhellen W, Lessin HR, Chan E, et al. ADHD – caring for children with ADHD: a practical resource toolkit for clinicians. 3rd edition. Itasca, IL: American Academy of Pediatrics; 2019.

[8] Radez J, Reardon T, Creswell C, et al. Why do children and adolescents (not) seek and access professional help for their mental health problems? A systematic review of quantitative and qualitative studies. Eur Child Adolesc Psychiatry 2021;30(2):183–211.

[9] Sayal K, Prasad V, Daley D, et al. ADHD in children and young people: Prevalence, care pathways, and service provision. Lancet Psychiatr 2018;5(2):175–86.

[10] Danielson ML, Bitsko RH, Ghandour RM, et al. Prevalence of parent-reported ADHD diagnosis and associated treatment among U.S. children and adolescents, 2016. J Clin Child Adolesc Psychol 2018;47(2):199–212.

[11] Murphy JM, Bergmann P, Chiang C, et al. The PSC-17: Subscale scores, reliability, and factor structure in a new national sample. Pediatrics 2016;138(3):e20160038–2016.

[12] Warnick EM, Bracken MB, Kasl S. Screening efficiency of the Child Behavior Checklist and Strengths and Difficulties Questionnaire: A systematic review. Child Adolesc Ment Health 2008;13(3):140–7.

[13] DuPaul GJ, Power TJ, Anastopoulos AD, et al. ADHD rating scale-5 for children and adolescents revised edition: checklists, norms, and clinical interpretation. New York, NY: Guilford Press; 2016.

[14] Conners CK. Conners 3rd Edition™ (Conners 3™): DSM-5 update, Multi-Health Systems. Cheektowaga, NY: Inc; 2014.

[15] Johnson JG, Harris ES, Spitzer RL, et al. The Patient Health Questionnaire for Adolescents: Validation of an instrument for the assessment of mental disorders among adolescent primary care patients. J Adolesc Health 2002;30(3):196–204.

[16] Earls MF, Foy JM, Green CM. Addressing mental health concerns in pediatrics: a practical resource toolkit for clinicians. 2nd edition. Itasca, IL: American Academy of Pediatrics; 2021.

[17] Rhew IC, Simpson K, Tracy M, et al. Criterion validity of the Short Mood and Feelings Questionnaire and one- and two-item depression screens in young adolescents. Child Adolesc Psychiatry Ment Health 2010;4(1):8.

[18] Runyon K, Chesnut SR, Burley H. Screening for childhood anxiety: A meta-analysis of the screen for child anxiety related emotional disorders. J Affect Disord 2018;240:220–9.

[19] Orgilés M, Fernández-Martínez I, Guillén-Riquelme A, et al. A systematic review of the factor structure and reliability of the Spence Children's Anxiety Scale. J Affect Disord 2016;190:333–40.

[20] Ilipilla G, Pranckun ZD, Wernick H, et al. Attention Deficit Hyperactivity Disorder and Anxiety. In: Driver D, Thomas SS, editors. Complex disorders in pediatric Psychiatry: a clinician's guide. Elsevier; 2018. p. 23–35.

[21] Wajszilber D, Santisteban JA, Gruber R. Sleep disorders in patients with ADHD: Impact and management challenges. Nat Sci Sleep 2018;10:453–80.

[22] Chen M-H, Pan T-L, Hsu J-W, et al. Attention-deficit hyperactivity disorder comorbidity and antidepressant resistance among patients with major depression: A nationwide longitudinal study. Eur Neuropsychopharmacol 2016;26(11):1760–7.

[23] Golubchik P, Weizman A. Management of anxiety disorders in children with attention-deficit hyperactivity disorder: A narrative review. Int Clin Psychopharmacol 2021;36(1): 1–11.

[24] Powell LA, Parker J, Weighall A, et al. Psychoeducation Intervention Effectiveness to Improve Social Skills in Young People with ADHD: A Meta-Analysis. J Atten Disord 2022;26(3): 340–57.

[25] Friesen K, Markowsky A. The diagnosis and management of anxiety in adolescents with comorbid ADHD. J Nurse Pract 2021;17(1):65–9.

[26] Soul O, Gross R, Basel D, et al. Stimulant treatment effect on anxiety domains in children with attention-deficit/hyperactivity disorder with and without anxiety disorders: A 12-week open-label prospective study. J Child Adolesc Psychopharmacol 2021;31(9): 639–44.

[27] Riddle MA. Pediatric psychopharmacology for primary care. 2nd edition. Itasca, IL: American Academy of Pediatrics; 2018.

[28] Cheung AH, Zuckerbrot RA, Jensen PS, et al. Guidelines for adolescent depression in primary care (GLAD-PC): Part II. Treatment and ongoing management. Pediatrics 2018;141(3):e20174082.

[29] Walter HJ, Bukstein OG, Abright AR, et al. Clinical practice guideline for the assessment and treatment of children and adolescents with anxiety disorders. J Am Acad Child Adolesc Psychiatry 2020;59(10):1107–24.

[30] Fitzgerald C, Dalsgaard S, Nordentoft M, et al. Suicidal behaviour among persons with attention-deficit hyperactivity disorder. Br J Psychiatry 2019;215(4):615–20.

[31] Sun S, Kuja-Halkola R, Faraone SV, et al. Association of psychiatric comorbidity with the risk of premature death among children and adults with attention-deficit/hyperactivity disorder. JAMA Psychiatr 2019;76(11):1141–9.

[32] Aguinaldo LD, Sullivant S, Lanzillo EC, et al. Validation of the Ask Suicide-Screening Questions (ASQ) with youth in outpatient specialty and primary care clinics. Gen Hosp Psychiatry 2021;68:52–8.

[33] Al Ghriwati N, Langberg JM, Gardner W, et al. Impact of mental health comorbidities on the community-based pediatric treatment and outcomes of children with attention deficit hyperactivity disorder. J Dev Behav Pediatr 2017;38(1):20–8.

Moving?

Make sure your subscription moves with you!

To notify us of your new address, find your **Clinics Account Number** (located on your mailing label above your name), and contact customer service at:

Email: journalscustomerservice-usa@elsevier.com

800-654-2452 (subscribers in the U.S. & Canada)
314-447-8871 (subscribers outside of the U.S. & Canada)

Fax number: 314-447-8029

Elsevier Health Sciences Division
Subscription Customer Service
3251 Riverport Lane
Maryland Heights, MO 63043

*To ensure uninterrupted delivery of your subscription, please notify us at least 4 weeks in advance of move.

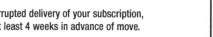

Printed and bound by CPI Group (UK) Ltd, Croydon, CR0 4YY

03/10/2024

01040477-0006